Veterinary Science: Animal Pathology and Clinical Aspects

Veterinary Science: Animal Pathology and Clinical Aspects

Editor: Gerardo Bailey

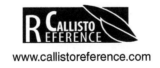

www.callistoreference.com

Callisto Reference,
118-35 Queens Blvd., Suite 400,
Forest Hills, NY 11375, USA

Visit us on the World Wide Web at:
www.callistoreference.com

© Callisto Reference, 2017

ISBN: 978-1-63239-880-2 (Hardback)

Cataloging-in-Publication Data

Veterinary science : animal pathology and clinical aspects / edited by Gerardo Bailey.
    p. cm.
Includes bibliographical references and index.
ISBN 978-1-63239-880-2
1. Veterinary medicine. 2. Veterinary pathology. 3. Animals--Diseases.
4. Veterinary clinical pathology. I. Bailey, Gerardo.
SF615 .V48 2017
636--dc23

Table of Contents

Permissions

List of Contributors

Index

Preface

Every book is a source of knowledge and this one is no exception. The idea that led to the conceptualization of this book was the fact that the world is advancing rapidly; which makes it crucial to document the progress in every field. I am aware that a lot of data is already available, yet, there is a lot more to learn. Hence, I accepted the responsibility of editing this book and contributing my knowledge to the community.

This book attempts to understand the multiple branches that fall under the discipline of veterinary science and how such concepts have practical applications. It delves into the anatomy and clinical pathology of animals. This field incorporates the study and treatment revolving around domesticated as well as wild animals. The topics included in this book on veterinary science are of utmost significance and bound to provide incredible insights to readers. The various advancements in this field are glanced at and their applications as well as ramifications are looked at in detail. This book, with its detailed analyses and data, will prove immensely beneficial to professionals and students involved in this area at various levels.

While editing this book, I had multiple visions for it. Then I finally narrowed down to make every chapter a sole standing text explaining a particular topic, so that they can be used independently. However, the umbrella subject sinews them into a common theme. This makes the book a unique platform of knowledge.

I would like to give the major credit of this book to the experts from every corner of the world, who took the time to share their expertise with us. Also, I owe the completion of this book to the never-ending support of my family, who supported me throughout the project.

Editor

VALIDATION OF SCREENING METHOD FOR DETERMINATION OF METHYLTESTOSTERONE IN FISH

Uzunov Risto[1], Hajrulai-Musliu Zehra[1], Stojanovska-Dimzoska Biljana[1],
Dimitrieska-Stojkovic Elizabeta[1], Todorovic Aleksandra[1], Stojkovski Velimir[2]

[1]*Food Institute, Faculty of Veterinary Medicine, Skopje, Republic of Macedonia*
[2]*Institute for Reproduction and Biomedicine, Faculty of Veterinary Medicine-Skopje,
Republic of Macedonia*

ABSTRACT

Anabolic androgenic steroids are synthetic derivatives of testosterone, which is the primary male sex hormone. These anabolic agents are used to increase the weight gain, to improve the food efficiency, storing proteins and to decrease fatness. However, depending on the use of anabolic agent in animal feed, anabolic residues that may occur in meat and meat products present risks to human health. The aim of this study was the validation of screening ELISA method for determination of methyltesterone anabolic steroid in fish. The validation process was carried out according to Commission Decision 2002/657/EC criteria. The detection limit for methyltestosterone was 140.95 ng/kg and the detection capability was 564.43 ng/kg. The overall recoveries and the coefficients of variation (CV) were in the range of 82.4%-97.4% and 1.5%-6.9%, respectively, a working range between 50 to 4050 ng/kg, and the regression equation of the final inhibition curve was: y= -0,1741x + 1,5082, R^2= 0.9927. Because of the good recovery and precision, and satisfactory detection capability, this method is applicable in official control laboratories as a rapid screening method for determination of methyltestosterone in fish.

Key words: methyltestosterone, fish, ELISA, anabolic steroids, validation.

INTRODUCTION

Methyltestosterone is a synthetically produced anabolic and androgenic steroid hormone (1, 2). Anabolic steroids are potentially useful compounds in aquaculture due to their ability to increase weight gains and muscle deposition of treated fish. Methyltestosterone promotes both muscle growth and the development of male sexual characters (1, 2). The increased growth rate in fishes, through the administration of androgenic hormone has been reported from many authors (3). The enhanced growth rate, obtained in *Cyprinus carpio* using 17α-Methyltestosterone revealed that this hormone would induce faster growth by acting probably in three different ways and they are activation on secretion of other androgenic anabolic hormones, increased food conversion and direct effect of 17α-Methyltestosterone on the gene expression in the muscle cells (3, 4). The increase in body weight gain may attribute to that androgenic steroids enhance the release of growth hormone from the pituitary somatotrops of the fish and/or induce the feed digestion and absorption rate causing increase in body weight (5). Moreover the higher level (60 mg/kg of feed) of 17-alpha methyltestosterone produced some testicular degeneration (1). After they are used in fish, a portion is discharged into the water environment by excretion and the rest remain in the animal's body. These compounds may be transfered into water, foods and food products if not well controlled and much evidence has been documented indicating that exposure to synthetic chemicals at low levels may lead to potential risk to human and wildlife health. For this reason the European Economic Community (EEC)

Corresponding author: Uzunov Risto, DVM

e-mail address: risteuzunov@gmail.com
Present address: Food institute, Faculty of Veterinary medicine-Skopje,
"Ss. Cyril and Methodius" University,
Lazar Pop- Trajkov 5-7, 1000 Skopje, R. Macedonia

prohibited the use of anabolic compounds as growth accelerators in the food animals. The Minimum required performance limit for methyltestosterone in muscle is 1 μg/kg (6). In Republic of Macedonia, the use of anabolic hormones as growth promoters has been made illegal also. The aim of this study was to validate of the screening ELISA method for determination of methyltestosterone in fish muscle.

MATERIAL AND METHODS

For validation of this screening ELISA method for determination of methyltestosterone anabolic steroid in fish we used blank fish muscle from untreated fish (*Species Carp, Cyprinus Carpio*).

Reagents. Most of the reagents that were used are contained in the RIDASCREEN Methyltestosterone test kit (Art. No. R3603) from R-Biopharm AG, Darmstadt, Germany. Kit contents was: Microtiter plate with 96 wells (12 strips with 8 removable wells each) coated with capture antibodies, 6 standard solutions: (0 ng/kg, 50 ng/kg, 150 ng/kg, 450 ng/kg, 1350 ng/kg, 4050 ng/kg methyltestosterone in 40% methanol ready to use), conjugate (peroxidase conjugated methyltestosterone, concentrate), anti-methyltestosterone antibody (concentrate), substrate/chromogen solution who contains tetramethyl-benzidine, stop solution which contained 1 N sulfuric acid, conjugate and antibody dilution buffer. Methanol (code I649035230) and tertiary butyl methyl ether (code K38520849) were of analytical grade and purchased from Merck. 20mM Phosphate buffer (PBS), pH 7.2, was prepared by mixing 0.55 g Sodium dihydrogen phosphate hydrate (NaH_2PO_4 x H_2O (code A689146545, Merck)) with 2.85 g Disodium hydrogen phosphate dihydrate (Na_2HPO_4 x 2 H_2O (code FI639486105, Merck)) and 9 g Sodium chloride (NaCl (code K36586304638, Merck)) and was filled up to 1000 ml distilled water. 67 mM PBS buffer, pH 7.2, was prepared by mixing 1.8 g Sodium dihydrogen phosphate hydrate (NaH_2PO_4 x H_2O) with 9.61 g Disodium hydrogen phosphate dihydrate (Na_2HPO_4 x 2 H_2O) and 9 g Sodium chloride (NaCl) and was filled up to 1000 ml with distilled water (7).

For fortified samples and calculation of recovery for this method we used external standard methyltestosterone from Fluka (code: 46444). From this standard we prepared standard solutions of methyltestosterone in methanol with concentration of 20 μg/kg and with this concentration of standard we fortified the blank sample on three levels: 1000, 1500 and 2000 ng/kg.

Extraction procedure. Fat was removed from muscle and the muscle was grinded. Ten grams from grounded muscle was homogenized with 10 ml of 67 mM PBS buffer by mixer (Typ T25 B, serial number 895944, IKA® Werke GmbH & Co.KG, Staufen, Germany) 5 min. Two gram from homogenized sample was mixed with 5 ml Tertiary butyl methyl ether in a centrifugal screw vial and shaken carefully for 30 - 60 min and then samples were centrifuged for 10 min at 3000 rpm on 10 - 15°C. The supernatant (ether layer) was transferred to another centrifugal vial and extraction procedure was repeated with 5 ml Tertiary butyl methyl ether. Then the samples were evaporated to dryness and dissolved in 1 ml methanol/water (80:20; v:v). The methanolic solution was diluted with 2 ml of 20mM PBS buffer and applied to a RIDA C_{18} column in the following manner: column was rinsed by flowing of 3 ml methanol (100%); then the column was equilibrated by injection of 2 ml of 20 mM PBS buffer; a sample (3 ml) was applied on column; column was rinsed by injection of 2 ml methanol/water (40:60; v:v); column was dried by pressing N_2 trough it for 3 min; the sample was diluted slowly by injection of 1 ml methanol/water (80:20; v:v) (flow rate: 15 drops/min) and then sample was diluted with distilled water 1:2. In the test 50 μl of the samples per well was used (7).

Validation procedure. The limit of detection (LOD) of the assay was defined as the concentration corresponding to the mean signal of 20 blank fish muscle samples plus 3 times of standard deviation of the mean. Blank fish muscle samples were obtained from untreated fish. The accuracy was evaluated by determining the recovery of spiked fish muscle samples on three concentrations of methyltestosterone external standards (1000, 1500 and 2000 ng/kg). Precision was expressed as the CV (Coefficient of variation) (%) of the calculated standards and sample concentrations. Detection capabilities (CCβ) were required to be at or lower than the MRPL (8). CCβ were evaluated by analyzing of 20 spiked fish muscle samples at 0.5 times MRPL (1000 ng/kg for methyltestosterone in muscle) for methyltestosterone and calculated in accordance with European Commission Decision 2002/657/EC (7).

Test procedure. RIDASCREEN® Methyltes-tosterone ELISA kits (R-Biopharm AG, Darmstad, Germany) were used for validation of Methyltestosterone in fish muscle. All reagents in the kit had to be brought to room temperature (20 - 25 °C) before use. Standards used for methyltestosterone were containing 0 ng/kg, 50 ng/kg, 150 ng/kg, 450 ng/kg, 1350 ng/kg, 4050 ng/kg methyltestosterone in 40% methanol.

50 µl of each standard solution or prepared sample were added and after that 50 µl of the diluted enzyme conjugate and 50 µl of anti-methyltestosterone antibody solution to each well were added. The solution in the microplate was carefully mixed by shaking of the plate manually. The plate was then incubated at 4 °C for 16 hours. The liquid was poured out of the wells and after the complete removal of liquid, all wells were filled with distilled water. After rinsing, the water was also discarded; the washing was repeated two more times. Then, 50 µl of substrate and 50 µl of chromogen were added, and after mixing thoroughly and incubating for 30 min at room temperature in the dark, 100 µl of stop solution (1 N sulphuric acid) was added. After mixing, the absorbance was read at 450 nm by using of the spectrophotometer (BIO RAD model 680) (7).

RESULTS

In this study a commercial ELISA kit was used for validation of methyltestosterone in fish muscle. The ELISA technique showed very high correlation between methyltestosterone concentration (ng/kg) and maximum absorbance (%).

The correlation between the absorbance ratio and methyltestosterone concentration was evaluated over the range from 50 to 4050 ng/kg. Linear regression analysis showed good correlation, with R^2 values 0.9927, (y= -0,1741x + 1,5082), where y was relative absorbance (%) and x was methyltestosterone concentration in ng/kg (Fig. 1).

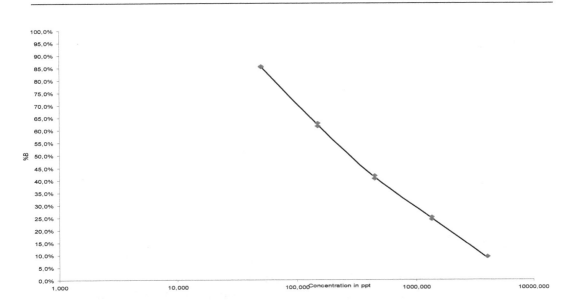

Figure 1. Linearity of the screening ELISA method for determination of methyltestosterone in fish muscle

Results for the precision of the method are presented in Table 1. The precision (Coefficient of variation (CV) %) in methyltestosterone standards ranged from 0.2% to 11.5%. The precision (CV %) in spiked fish muscle sample ranged from 2.5% to 6.8%.

Table 1. Precision of the screening ELISA method for determination of methyltestosterone in fish muscle

	Concentration (ng/kg)	CV (%)
methyltestosterone standards	0	2.5
	50	0.2
	150	1.4
	450	2.1
	1350	2.8
	4050	11.5
CV % for spiked sample	1000	6.8
	1500	2.5
	2000	3.1

The accuracy was expressed as the recovery (%) of the estimated concentration. For the three target concentration (1000, 1500 and 2000 ng/kg) the recoveries in fish muscle sample were 97.4%, 82.4% and 85.1% respectively and they are presented in Table3. From Table 2 we can see that value of recovery is highest in the first case when the level of fortified sample is lowest.

Table 2. Accuracy of the screening ELISA method for determination of methyltestosterone in fish muscle (recovery %)

Fish muscle samples n (number of replicates)	Methyltestosterone		Recovery %
	Added (ng/kg)	Found (ng/kg)	
n = 8	1000	974	97.4
n = 8	1500	1236	82.4
n = 8	2000	1702	85.1

Detection limit for methyltestosterone was found to be 140.95 ng/kg. The detection capability (CCβ) for methyltestosterone was 564.43 ng/kg, less than MRPL level of 1000 ng/kg (6).

DISCUSSION

Raw fish and fish products, which play an important role in human nutrition, should be safe and should not contain any factors or substances harmful for human health. However, the anabolic agents used for various purposes in animal husbandry tend to leave residues and this causes some problems in consumer health (9, 10). Androgen excess leads to the development of insulin resistance during both hyperglycemic and euglycemic hyperinsulinemia and these findings provide direct evidence for a relationship between hyperandrogenemia and insulin resistance, and its associated risk factors for cardiovascular disease (11). Moreover, after administration high dose of methyltestosteron in humans causes negative mood as irritability, mood swings, violent feelings, and hostility, then cognitive impairment as distractibility, forgetfulness, and confusion (12). Other negative effects on the humans are increased risk of injury, increased blood pressure, gastrointestinal complications, benign and malignant liver tumours, Peliosis hepatis (blood-filled cysts), virilisation, clitoral hypertrophy, deepened voice, painful breast lumps in women, gynaecomastia and testicular atrophy in men, abnormalities of sperm count, motility and morphology, sterility, benign prostatic hypertrophy cutaneous striae (13). Because of negative effects the European Economic Community (EEC) prohibited the use of anabolic compounds as growth accelerators in food animals and fishes (14). In the presented study, the ELISA method was used to achieve the unambiguous identification of methyltestosterone in fish muscle. This method was validated in accordance to the criteria of Commission Decision 2002/657/EC. Due to the simplicity, rapidness, and cost-effectiveness of the method and its good recovery and precision it is applicable in the official control laboratories as a screening method. But in the case when the target analyte is clearly identified above CCβ the sample is considered as non compliant and the results must be confirmed with confirmation method on GC/MS, LC/MS or with another confirmatory method (14, 15).

REFERENCES

1. Khalil, W. K. B., Hasheesh, W. S., Marie, M. A. S.,Abbas H. H.,Zahran E.A.(2005).Assessment the impact of 17α-methyltestosterone hormone on growth, hormone concentration, molecular and histopathological changes in muscles and testis of Nile tilapia; Oreochromis niloticus. Life Sci J, 8: 329-343.

2. Schanzer, W. (1996). Metabolism of anabolic androgenic steroids. Clin Chem, 42: 1001-1020.

3. K. P. Lone, A. J. Matty. (1981). The effect of feeding androgenic hormones on the proteolytic activity of the alimentary canal of carp *Cyprinus carpio* L. J Fish Biol, 18 (3): 353–358.

4. Felix, S. (1989). Effect of 17 a methyltsetosterone on the growth ornamental fish, Xiphophorus maculates. Indian J. Fish, 36 (3): 263-265.

5. Yamazaki, F. (1976). Application of hormones in fish culture. J. Fish. Res, 33: 948-958.

6. CRL Guidance paper. (2007). CRLs view on state of the art analytical methods for National residue control plans, 3-7.

7. R-Biopharm AG, Darmstadt, Germany: RIDASCREEN® 17 methyltestosterone, Enzyme immunoassay for the quantitative analysis of 17 methyltestosterone, R3601.

8. Commission of the European Communities: European Commission Decision of 12 August 2002 Implementing Council Directive 96/23/EC Concerning the Performance of Analytical Methods and the Interpretation of Results (2002/657/EC), Off J Eur Comm, L 221: 8-36.

9. Hoffman, B. (1996). Problems of residue and health risks of anabolic agents with hormone like activities. Proceedings of the Scientific Conference on Growth Promotion in Meat Production, European Comm. Dir. Gen. VI. Agric., Official Pub. European Comm., Brussels; 271-296.

10. Nazli, B., Colak, H., Aydin A, Hampikyan, H. (2005). The Presence of Some Anabolic Residues in Meat and Meat Products Sold in Istanbul. Turk J Vet Anim Sci, 29: 691-699.

11. Diamond, P., M., Grainger, D., Diamond, C.,M., Sherwin, S., R., DeFronzo, A., R. (1998). Effects of Methyltestosterone on Insulin Secretion and Sensitivity In Women. JCEM, 83 (12): 4420.

12. Su, T., P., Pagliaro, M., Schmidt, P., J., Pickar, D., Wolkowitz, O., Rubinow, D., R. (1993). Neuropsychiatric effects of anabolic steroids in male normal volunteers. JAMA, 269 (21): 2760-2764.

13. Rashid, H., Ormerod, S., Day, E. (2007). Anabolic androgenic steroids: what the psychiatrist needs to know. Adv. Phys, 13: 203-211.

14. Commission of the European Communities: European Commission Decision of 12 August 2002 Implementing Council Directive 96/23/EC Concerning the Performance of Analytical Methods and the Interpretation of Results (2002/657/EC), Off J Eur Comm, L 221: 8-36.

15. Commission of the European Communities: European Commission Decision of 29 April 1996 on measures to monitor certain substances and residues thereof in live animals and animalproducts and repealing Directives 85/358/EEC and 86/469/EEC and Decisions 89/187/EEC and 91/664/EEC (2002/657/EC), Off J Eur Comm, L 125: 1-28.

2

PUDENDAL NERVE BLOCK IN MALE GOATS: COMPARISON OF ISCHIORECTAL FOSSA AND ISCHIAL ARCH APPROACHES USING LOW VOLUME 1% LIGNOCAINE HYDROCHLORIDE

Mujeebur Rehman Fazili[1], Nida Handoo[2], Mohd Younus Mir[2], Beenish Qureshi[2]

[1]*Veterinary Clinical Complex, Faculty of Veterinary Sciences & Animal Husbandry, Shere Kashmir Universityof Agricultural Sciences & Technology of Kashmir, Shuhama, Srinagar, Kashmir, India*
[2]*Division of Veterinary Surgery & Radiology, Faculty of Veterinary Sciences & Animal Husbandry, Shere Kashmir University of Agricultural Sciences & Technology of Kashmir, Shuhama, Srinagar, Kashmir, India*

ABSTRACT

Thirty (30) adult male goats were injected xylazine (0.05 mg/kg, IM) and randomly divided into three equal groups. Internal pudendal nerve block was tried using 3.5 ml (on each side) of 1% lignocaine hydrochloride byischiorectal fossa or ischial arch approaches in goats from Group 1 and Group 2 respectively, 15 minutes after giving xylazine. Inadvertent puncture of the rectal wall and prick to the finger placed in the rectum was experienced once in Group 1 animal. None of the animals showed protrusion of the penis without manual manipulation. Prolapse of the prepucial ring was noticed in three animals from Group 1 and two each from Group 2 and 3. The application of mild manual push percutaneously resulted in the exposure of the penis in eight and six animals belonging to Group 1 and Group 2 respectively, 15 minutes after injection of the local anaesthetic. Statistically significant (P>0.05) difference between Group 1 and 2 values was detected only once at 90 minutes following injection of the local anaesthetic. The block lasted longer in animals of Group 1. The exposed organ was flaccid and insensitive. The organ retracted into the prepucial cover within five minutes of its release in all the animals. The penile exposure could not be achieved by similar manipulation in any of the Group 3 animals. From this study it was concluded that the ischiorectal fossa approach is cumbersome and may lead to inadvertent punctures, but the block develops in more number of animals for a longer period than with the ischial arch approach.The outcome of the two techniques did not show statistically significant (P>0.05) difference for most of the assessment period. Reducing the concentration of lignocaine hydrochloride may reduce the chances of continued relaxation of the penis beyond the required period and also the drug toxicity. However, studies using larger volume of 1% lignocaine hydrochloride may be undertaken for short term exposure of the penis without manual manipulation.

Key words: pudendal nerve block, goat**,** penis, prepuce, ischiorectal, ischial arch

INTRODUCTION

Bilateral pudendal nerve block is used in the male ruminants for penile analgesia along with its relaxation. Examination and excision of the urethral process or management of penile and prepucial pathology like infections, tumours, trauma and

Corresponding author: Dr. Mujeebur Rehman Fazili, PhD
E-mail address: fazili_mr@yahoo.co.in
Present address: Veterinary Clinical Complex, Faculty of Veterinary Sciences & Animal Husbandry, Shere Kashmir University of Agricultural Sciences & Technology of Kashmir, Shuhama, Srinagar, Kashmir, India
Pin code: 91-190006

pizzle rot are some of the common indications of the block in small ruminants (1). The pudendal nerve arises from the ventral branches of the second to fourth sacral nerves and provides motor supply to the retractor penis muscle and, via the dorsal nerve of penis, sensory innervation of the penis (2). The internal pudendal nerve block using an ischiorectal fossa approach was described for the first time by Larson (3) in bulls. An alternate lateral approach for rams was developed by McFarlane (4). El-Kammar and Alsafy (5) described the ischial arch approach in goats. In addition to the maintenance of the tail tone, the most important advantage of the internal pudendal nerve desensitization over lumbosacral epidural analgesia is the maintenance of the motor power of the hind limbs (6). The undue delay in the retraction of the protruded penis beyond the period required for clinical examination or surgery and the consequent risk of trauma to this organ (7) is a serious concern precluding the frequent use of this procedure in clinical practice. Perusal of the available literature indicates very few reports of the use of pudendal nerve block in goats. This study was therefore planned to compare two techniques of this block in male goats. Use of low volume of the 1% lignocaine hydrochloride was hypothesized to reduce the duration of penile protrusion and the risk of drug toxicity.

MATERIAL AND METHODS

Thirty clinically healthy adult male goats of different breeds (Bakerwal, Pashmina and their cross) were randomly divided into three equal groups. The goats were maintained under standard welfare guidelines at Mountain Research Centre for Sheep and Goats of the University. The study was undertaken after the Institutional Animal Ethics Committee (IAEC) approved the design of the work. All animals were administered xylazine (0.05 mg/kg, IM). They were let loose in the paddock for 15 minutes and then restrained in a standing posture. Two assistants were required, one holding the head of the goat and the other the hind quarters and the tail.

Following the routine aseptic measures, the goats of Group 1 were subjected to the pudendal nerve block using 3.5 ml (on each side) of 1% lignocaine hydrochloride (2% preparation diluted with equal volume of normal saline) following the ischiorectal fossa technique (Fig. 1) described by Larson (3). The finger of the gloved hand was introduced into the rectum of these goats and directed laterally to detect the slit-like lesser sacrosciatic foramen, 4.0 to 5.0 cm inside the anal opening. Hypodermic (18-G)

needle was introduced percutaneously in the deepest depression of the ishiorectal fossa and guided by the finger inside the rectum of the animal to the sacrosciatic foramen for deposition of the local anaesthetic. The procedure was similarly repeated on the contralateral side of the goat. In Group 2 goats the ischial arch approach (5) was followed for deposition of 3.5 ml lignocaine hydrochloride (1%) on each side (Fig. 2). The needle (18-G) was inserted 2.0 cm dorsomedial to the ischial arch and 2.0 cm lateral to the anus. It was advanced in the medioventral direction till it stroked the ischial arch and the local anaesthetic deposited. The Group 3 goats were not injected a local anaesthetic.

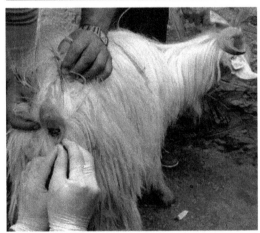

Figure 2. Ischial arch approach for pudendal nerve block in a goat: G-18 hypodermic needle inserted dorsomedial to the right ischial arch and lateral to the anus

The animals were let loose in the open paddock and observed continuously for protrusion of the prepuce and penis up to 2 hours. All of them were restrained 15 minutes after xylazine administration in a standing posture. While sitting on the right side of the animal, the penis was held percutaneously with the left hand and pushed cranially with mild manual force. The right hand was simultaneously used to push the prepucial sheath in the opposite direction so that the penis could be exposed. The goats belonging to Group 1 and Group 2, but not the Group 3 goats, were injected local anaesthetic for blocking their pudendal nerves. All the animals were repeatedly restrained in a standing posture 15 minutes, 30 minutes, 60 minutes, 90 minutes and 120 minutes after injection of the local anaesthetic (Group 1 and Group 2) or xylazine (Group 3) for exposure of the penis following the above mentioned procedure.

The body weight values of the goats belonging to the various groups are presented as mean with

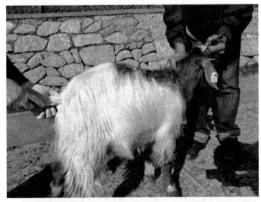

Figure 1. Ischiorectal fossa approach for pudendal nerve block in a goat: Left hand first finger in the rectum guiding the hypodermic needle (inserted via right ischiorectal fossa) to the sacrosciatic foramen

standard deviation (mean±SD) after application of the one-way ANOVA. The outcome of the approaches for inducing pudendal nerve block was analysed by the Fisher's Exact Test. Statistically significant differences were accepted at P<0.05.

RESULTS

The outcome of the pudendal nerve block in male goats has been presented in Table 1.

The mean ±S.D body weight of the goats included in Group 1 was 29.80±6.03 kg, Group 2,31.50±7.26 kg and Group 3,30.10±5.74 kg. The mean values between the groups did not differ significantly (P>0.05).

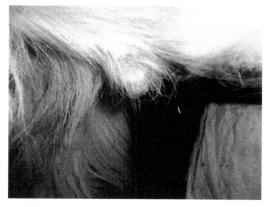

Figure 3. Relaxed prepucial ring of a goat after xylazine administration

Table1. Outcome of the pudendal nerve block using 1% lignocaine hydrochloride (3.5 ml/side) in male goats

Male Goats			Time interval (minutes)					
Groups	Body weight (kg) (mean±S.D)	N	0	15	30	60	90	120
I	29.80±6.03[a]	10	nil[x]	8[y]	8[y]	9[y]	9[y]	6[y]
II	31.50±7.26[a]	10	nil[x]	6[y]	7[y]	6[y]	3[z]	3[y]
III	30.10±5.74[a]	10	nil[x]	nil[x]	nil[x]	nil[x]	nil[x]	nil[x]

Values with different superscripts vary significantly (P>0.05) between the groups.

Xylazine induced sedation was mild so that it could allow injection of the local anaesthetic without frequent movement of the animals. Most of them remained standing throughout the observation period however, eight showed tendency to lie down after the first 15 minutes of administration of xylazine. Five urinated and three showed dribbling of saliva for a variable period.

The passage of the lubricated gloved finger into the rectum of the animals belonging to Group 1 was resisted by the animals in the beginning of the procedure. Inadvertent puncture of the rectal wall and prick to the finger placed in the rectum was experienced once. Accidental puncture of a blood vessel (indicated by backflow of blood drops through the needle hub) also occurred once while guiding the tip of the percutaneously inserted needle.

None of the animals of any group showed prolapse of the penis without manipulation throughout the observation period. However, three animals from Group 1 showed prolapse of the prepucial ring from 60 minutes to 90 minutes post injection. In Group 2 and Group 3 goats, two animals developed prepucial prolapse at 15 minutes/30 minutes that continued up to 60 minutes (Fig. 3).

In none of the animals included in the study, the penis could be exposed manually immediately before xylazine administration and also 15 minutes later. In Group 3 goats, the organ could not be exposed even beyond that period.

In eight of the ten goats belonging to Group 1, the glans penis could be exposed manually from 15 minutes to 90 minutes after injection of the local anaesthetic (Fig. 4). One more goat from this group also responded at 60 minutes and 90 minutes. At 120 minutes post-injection, the exposure of the penis was possible in six animals only.

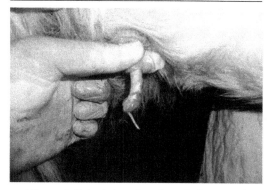

Figure 4. Extruded penis and urethral process in a standing goat after pudendal nerve block

In Group 2 goats, the penis could be exposed in six animals at 15 minutes and 60 minutes, seven at 30 minutes and three animals only during last two examinations.

The outcome of the goats belonging to Group 1 and Group 2 differed significantly with that of Group 3 animals at all assessment intervals. However, the outcome between the first two groups showed no significant difference (P>0.05) except at 90 minutes following injection of the local anaesthetic. At this interval, the Group 1 outcome was significantly better than that of Group 2 animals.

In all the animals of both groups, wherein the penis could be exposed, the manual holding and mild traction of the urethral process or glans penis did not result in local or general reaction indicative of pain or discomfort to the animal. The penis retracted into the prepucial cover within five minutes of its release in all of these animals.

DISCUSSION

Relaxation and analgesia of the penis in male animals is certain following epidural injection of the local anaesthetic. However in practice, the prolonged recumbency as a serious objection to this technique cannot be ignored (8).

The temperament of the goat to resist physical restrain often demands use of a sedative. Xylazine is used as an effective calming agent in ruminants. It is accompanied by some muscle relaxant effect, but unlike phenothiazine derivatives, it has not been found to cause relaxation of the penis in male animals. The low dose (0.05 mg/kg, IM) of the agent used in the present study provided standing sedation in majority of the goats. The ones that showed tendency of lying down got up when approached for examination at repeated intervals. Major effects of the xylazine develop within 10 to 15 minutes after IM injection (6). The goats included in Group 1 and Group 2 were therefore injected local anaesthetic 15 minutes after xylazine administration.

They were injected low volume (3.5 ml/side) dilute (1%) lignocaine hydrochloride. Different techniques for desensitization of internal pudendal nerves in small ruminants, using 3.0 ml to 10.0 ml of 2% lignocaine hydrochloride (with or without 1:100000 adrenaline) on either side have been described (3, 5, 6). McFarlane (4) used 7.0 ml of a 2% or 5.0 ml of a 5% procaine hydrochloride solution in ovine. It has been found that increasing the dose prolongs the duration of the block (5).

In this study, 2% lignocaine hydrochloride preparation was diluted with equal volume of normal saline immediately before its use to reduce the total dose of the injected drug. Systematic toxicity is a potential complication in small ruminants, so the limited dosage and diluted solutions of xylocaine hydrochloride 2% in nerve blocking has been advocated (9, 10). Restricting the initial administration dose of lignocaine hydrochloride to 6.0 mg/kg is considered safe in these species (8).

The rectal wall puncture in a goat and injury to the finger of the anaesthetist occurred once during an ischiorectal fossa approach. The danger of puncturing the finger is obvious in such procedures, as the needle is directed by per rectal palpation to locate the appropriate landmarks (11). This places surgeons at high risk for accidentally puncturing their fingers with the needle particularly when the animal moves during the procedure. The ischial approach does not require rectal palpation, it is therefore safer on this account.

Desired results were obtained in eight of the animals in Group 1 and six of those included in Group 2, when examined at 15 minutes following injection of the local anaesthetic. One more goat from each group responded later. The exposed penis was flaccid and insensitive when held manually and pulled lightly. Better outcome in the Group 1 animals (indicated by more number responding positively for longer period) was possible due to the exact identification of the pelvic landmarks by rectal palpation of the injection site. In cattle, 38 of the 40 cattle subjected to this block by the lateral approach obtained relaxation and anaesthesia (4).

None of the animals included in our study showed protrusion of the penis without manipulation. In the animals where the organ was exposed manually, it returned into the prepucial cover within 5 minutes after its release, thus avoiding the risk of injury to it. Using a 2% preparation of the local anaesthetic, the penis continues to hang outside from one and half to four hours (3, 5). In order to avoid trauma of the protruded penis, this delay necessitates manual retraction of penis into the prepuce and application of a tape or purse string suture around the prepucial orifice (7).

CONCLUSION

From the study it is concluded that the ischiorectal fossa approach is cumbersome and may lead to 3, 5, 6 inadvertent punctures. However, the block develops in a higher number of male goats for a longer period than with the ischial arch approach. Reducing the concentration of the lignocaine hydrochloride may avoid the major disadvantage of protracted relaxation of the penis and also the chances of drug toxicity. However, studies using larger volume than used in this study of 1% lignocaine hydrochloride may be undertaken for obtaining short-term exposure of the penis without manual manipulation.

ACKNOWLEDGEMENT

The authors express their gratitude to Dr. Z.A Pampori, Senior Scientist, Mountain Research Centre for Sheep and Goats, Prof. R.A Shah, Head Division of Animal Biotechnology and Prof. B.A. Moulvi Head, Division of Veterinary Surgery & Radiology, Faculty of Veterinary Sciences & AH, SKUAST-K for providing animals and the facilities required to undertake the study.

REFERENCES

1. Galatos, A.D. (2011). Anesthesia and analgesia in sheep and goats. Vet. Clin. Food Anim. Pract. 27, 47-59.
   http://dx.doi.org/10.1016/j.cvfa.2010.10.007
   PMid:21215889

2. Gilbert, R.O., Fubini, S.L. (2004). Surgery of the bovine reproductive system and urinary tract. In: Fubini, S.L & Ducharme, N.G. (Ed.), Farm animal surgery (pp. 353-354). First edition, Elsevier (USA), St. Louis

3. Larson, L.L. (1953). The internal pudendal (pudic) nerve block for anaesthesia of the penis and relaxation of the retractor penis muscle. J. Am. Vet. Med. Assos. 123, 18-27.
   PMid:13061360

4. McFarlane, I.S. (1963). The lateral approach to pudendal nerve block in the bovine and ovine. J. S. African Vet. Med. Ass. 34, 73-76.

5. El-Kammar, M.H., Alsafy, M.A. (2006). Pudendal nerve blockage: Surgical and topographical anatomical study in goat. Kafr El-Sheikh Vet. Med. J. 4, 1011-1030.

6. Tranquilli, W.J., Thurmon, J.C., Grimm, K.A. (2007). Lumb and Jone's veterinary anesthesia and analgesia (pp. 662-663). Fourth edition. Iowa: Blackwell Publishing, USA

7. Elmore, R.G. (1981). Food-animal regional anesthesia. Edwardsville, KS, Veterinary Medicine Publishing

8. Clarke, K.W., Trim, C.M., Hall, L.W. (2014). Veterinary Anaesthesia. (pp.319, 325-326, 347). Eleventh edition. London: Saunders Elsevier, England

9. Gray, P.R., McDonnell, W. (1986). Anaesthesia in sheep and goat. Part1. Local analgesia. Compend. Contin.Educ. 8, S3.

10. Turner, S.A., Mellwaraith, W.C. (1989). Techniques in large animal surgery. Lea & Febiger (Ed). Third edition, Philladelphia, London

11. Abdi, S., Shenouda, P., Patel, N., Saini, B., Bharat, Y., Calvillo, O. (2004). A novel technique for pudendal nerve block. Pain Physician. 7, 319-322.
    PMid:16858468

3

PRELIMINARY INVESTIGATION OF THE POSSIBILITY FOR IMPLEMENTATION OF MODIFIED PHARMACOPOEIAL HPLC METHODS FOR QUALITY CONTROL OF METRONIDAZOLE AND CIPROFLOXACIN IN MEDICINAL PRODUCTS USED IN VETERINARY MEDICINE

Marjan Piponski, Tanja Bakovska, Marina Naumoska, Tatjana Rusevska, Gordana Trendovska Serafimovska, Hristina Andonoska

Pharmaceutical Company Replek Farm Ltd., Quality Control Department st. Kozle 188, 1000 Skopje

ABSTRACT

Quality control of veterinary medicine products containing two different frequently used antibiotics metronidazole and ciprofloxacin hydrochloride, was considered and performed, using modified pharmacopoeial HPLC methods. Three different HPLC systems were used: Varian ProStar, Perkin Elmer Series and UPLC Shimadzu Prominence XR. The chromatographic columns used were LiChropher RP Select B 75 mm x 4 mm with 5 µm particles and Discovery C18 100 mm x 4,6 mm with 5 µm particles. Chromatographic methods used for both analytes were compendial, with minor modifications made for experimental purposes. Minor modifications of the pharmacopoeia prescribed chromatographic conditions, in both cases, led to better chromatographic parameters, good resolution and shorter analysis times. Optimized methods can be used for: determination of metronidazole in gel formulation, for its simultaneous quantification with preservatives present in the formulation and even for identification and quantification of its specified impurity, 2-methyl-5-nitroimidazole; determination of ciprofloxacin hydrochloride in film coated tablets and eye drops and identification and quantification of its specified impurities. These slightly modified and optimized pharmacopoeial methods for quality control of metronidazole and ciprofloxacin dosage forms used in veterinary medicine can be successfully applied in laboratories for quality control of veterinary medicines.

Key words: metronidazole, ciprofloxacin hydrochloride, veterinary medicines, pharmacopoeia, quality control

INTRODUCTION

We considered and performed quality control of two different antibiotics used in human and veterinary medicine, metronidazole and ciprofloxacin hydrochloride, which are frequently used worldwide. Metronidazole (Fig. 1a) is a nitroimidazole antibiotic used for prevention and treatment of bacterial and parasitic infections in animals and is usually administered as tablet, capsule, oral liquid or injectable or is topically applied as gel, cream or ointment. It is not intended for use in food producing animals, i.e. according to EU Regulation 37/2010 it is a prohibited substance (1).

Corresponding author: Marjan Piponski, PhD
E-mail address: piponski@yahoo.com
Present address: Replek Farm Ltd., Quality Control Department
st. Kozle 188, Skopje, Republic of Macedonia

Ciprofloxacin hydrochloride (Fig. 1b) is a second-generation fluoroquinolone antibiotic used for treatment of bacterial infections in animals and is administered as injectable, oral liquid, tablet, capsule and eye or ear medication (2, 3). Both antibiotics are also used in human medicine.

Quality control of veterinary medicines is regulated by various directives (such as Directive 2001/82/EC and 2004/28/EC of the European Parliament and of the Council) (4, 5, 6) and guidelines (such as European Medicine Agency - EMEA guidelines for specific veterinary dosage forms) (6, 7). Methods used for quality control of veterinary medicines can be found in specific medicine monographs listed in Veterinary pharmacopoeias (which usually are companion volumes to pharmacopoeias), such as British Pharmacopoeia (Veterinary) (8), China Veterinary Pharmacopoeia (9), Indian Pharmacopoeia – Veterinary (10) etc. If there is not an official monograph in veterinary pharmacopoeias for some drug product used in veterinary medicine, its quality can be controlled according to the monographs

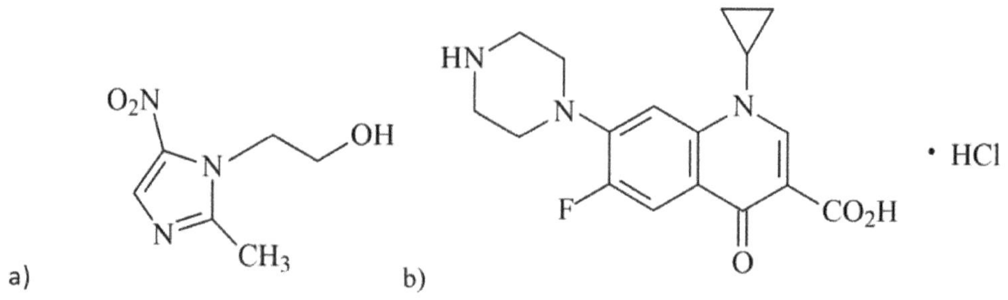

Figure 1. Structural formulas of: a) metronidazole and b) ciprofloxacin hydrochloride

given in European Pharmacopoeia (11), British Pharmacopoeia (12), United States Pharmacopoeia (13), Japanese Pharmacopoeia (14), International Pharmacopoeia (15) etc., or with some other new, completely validated analytical methods developed especially for this purpose.

Metronidazole is included in the British Pharmacopoeia (Veterinary) 2012 with a full monograph, which includes sample preparation, method for quality control and propositions for quality interpretation. Ciprofloxacin hydrochloride is not covered by the British Pharmacopoeia (Veterinary) 2012, but has a monograph in the main part of the British Pharmacopoeia 2012. In our investigation we used the method for assay determination of ciprofloxacin hydrochloride given in the BP monograph, with slight methodological modifications.

The aim of this work was to investigate the quality of some veterinary medicinal preparations containing metronidazole and ciprofloxacin hydrochloride, which can be purchased in Macedonia and to check the compliance of the obtained results with the compendial requirements of the respective drug monographs.

Also, our general aim was to investigate the possibility for implementation of improved, more rapid and more reliable procedures for quality control of the above mentioned veterinary medicinal products.

MATERIAL AND METHODS

In this research three different HPLC system were used:
- Varian ProStar with ternary high pressure mixing pump, autosampler 410 with column oven and Photo Diode Array detector 330, controlled by software Varian-Star Version 6.31;
- Perkin Elmer Series 200 with autosampler, Photo Diode Array detector, column oven and quaternary pump controlled by TotalChrom software;
- UPLC Shimadzu Prominence XR with quaternary pump, autosampler, Photo Diode Array detector, column oven and controller, controlled by Lab Solutions software.

The chromatographic columns used on these HPLC systems were: LiChropher RP Select B 75 mm x 4 mm with 5 μm particles (Merck Darmstadt, Germany) and Discovery C18 100 mm x 4,6 mm with 5 μm particles (Supelco Bellefonte, USA).

All used chemicals were of Ph.Eur. grade: methanol, acetonitrile, trifluoroacetic acid, 85 % o-phosphoric acid, ammonium dihydrogen phosphate and triethylamine, all purchased from Merck Darmstadt, Germany. The demineralized water was an in-house product with conductivity of less than 2 μS/cm. Working standards for active substances (metronidazole working standard with potency 99,6 % and ciprofloxacin hydrochloride working standard with potency 99,8 %, both standardized using referent standards purchased from European Pharmacopoeia), Metronidazole gel 0,75 % and Ciprofloxacin film coated tablets 500 mg were purchased from the pharmaceutical company Replek Farm Ltd. Skopje, Macedonia and Ciprofloxacin hydrochloride eye drops 3 mg/ml were purchased from a local pharmacy.

All the test solutions prepared from the active substances and pharmaceutical products used for examination were prepared in the respective mobile phase used for the chromatographic system.

Chromatographic methods used for both analytes in their pharmaceutical formulations were compendial, given in the monographs contained in British Pharmacopoeia BP 2012 (for ciprofloxacin hydrochloride) and British Pharmacopoeia (Veterinary) 2012 (for metronidazole), with slight modifications for experimental purposes. The modifications made are described in the following parts for each active substance, respectively.

RESULTS

Metronidazole Analysis

Method used for examination of Metronidazole gel 0,75 % was according to the Metronidazole monograph published in British Pharmacopoeia (Veterinary) 2012. It prescribes the use of: Spherisorb ODS 200 mm × 4,6 mm column with 5 μm particle size, column temperature 30°C, mobile phase consisted of 30 % methanol and 70 % 10 mM ammonium dihydrogen phosphate buffer, mobile phase flow rate 1,0 ml/min, wavelength for UV detection 315 nm and injection volume of 10 μl. The chromatogram given in Figure 2 is obtained using the pharmacopoeial prepositions using Waters Spherisorb ODS2 150 mm x 4,6 mm and 5μm particle size column, which is slightly shorter than the prescribed one, but within the permitted limits. The main peak with RT = 3.857 min is from metronidazole and the other two smaller peaks are from its impurities.

Minor modifications in these prescribed chromatographic conditions were made in order to obtain better chromatographic parameters, better resolution and shorter run times. All the modifications made are within the allowed *"Adjustments of chromatographic conditions"* described in the European Pharmacopoeia, current edition (11).

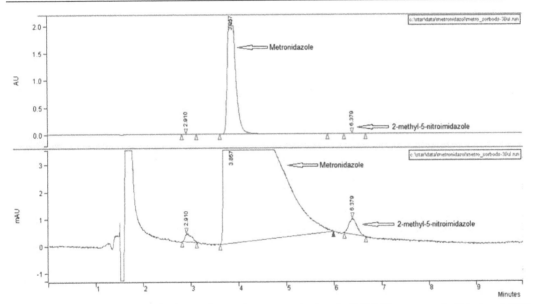

Figure 2. Chromatogram obtained according to the monograph given in British Pharmacopoeia (Veterinary) 2012 for quality control of active substance metronidazole. The lower chromatogram is extended X and Y-axis chromatogram from the upper full peak size chromatogram

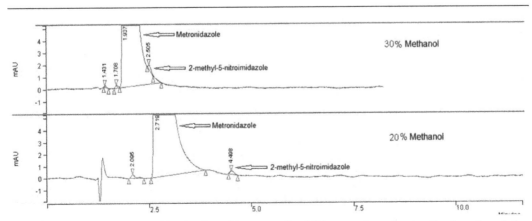

Figure 3. Mobile phase modification for achievement of satisfying retention of metronidazole and resolution between metronidazole and its specified impurity, 2-methyl-5-nitroimidazole

Furthermore, with these slight changes in various parameters the system suitability criteria can still be satisfied without fundamentally modifying the pharmacopoeia prescribed method. For this purpose, a shorter chromatographic column was used, i.e. Discovery C18 100 mm × 4,6 mm column with 5 μm particle size. Also, slight changes were made in the composition of the mobile phase. The concentration of methanol in the mobile phase was decreased from 30 % (v/v) as prescribed in the monograph to 20 % (v/v). All other chromatographic conditions are the

are present in Metronidazole gel formulation, and should be also quantified during quality control of this pharmaceutical product. It can easily be noticed that parabens cannot be quantified at 315 nm because they do not show any absorbance at this wavelength, whereas metronidazole absorbance decreases significantly at a wavelength of 254 nm, which can be clearly noticed from 3-D contour diagram analysis in the middle part of Figure 4. This is due to their different spectral characteristics, which are shown in the bottom part of Figure 4.

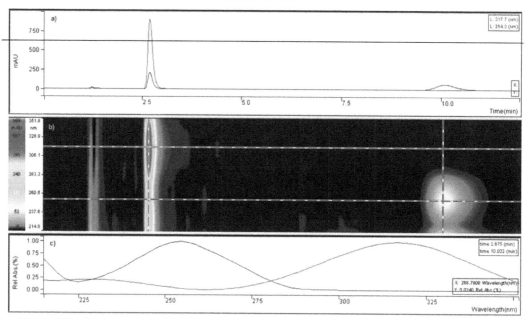

Figure 4. Simultaneous presentation of chromatogram at two wavelengths, 315 nm - red colored chromatogram and 254 nm - blue colored chromatogram (a); 3-D contour diagram of chromatogram from Metronidazol gel (b) and UV spectrums of metronidazole – red colored spectrum and Nipagin – blue colored spectrum (c)

same as the above cited pharmacopoeial conditions. Presented chromatograms are from 0,5 mg/ml metronidazole working standard solution in mobile phase.

A test solution made of Metronidazole gel 0,75 % dissolved in mobile phase, with the same concentration of metronidazole as in the standard solution (0,5 mg/ml), was examined at the same above described chromatographic conditions. One chromatogram, presented at 2 different wavelengths, is given in Figure 4. Both monitoring wavelengths are extracted from a PDA detector, and compare peak signals monitored at 315 nm, wavelength prescribed for quantification of metronidazole, with the signals monitored at 254 nm, wavelength prescribed for quantification of methyl-p-hydroxybenzoate (Nipagin) and propyl-p-hydroxybenzoate (Nipasol). These two preservatives

On the following two figures (Fig. 5 and Fig. 6), a real case of quality investigation is presented, where it can be seen that this modified pharmacopoeial method also successfully separates metronidazole and its specified impurity, 2-methyl-5-nitroimidazole, in the pure active substance and also in the gel formulation. The UV spectral analysis (Fig. 6) illustrates the spectral characteristics of chromatogram peaks labeled with their retention times, and in this way contributes to qualitative analysis, i.e. for their identification and peak purity determination.

Additional changes were made to the chromatographic method for complete chemical assay determination of Metronidazole gel, including the active pharmaceutical ingredient (metronidazole) and formulation participants with preserving functions (Nipagin and Nipasol), in order to obtain shorter analysis times, and thus obtaining higher sample throughput in industrial quality control laboratories. The following changes were made: even shorter chromatographic column, RP Select B 75 mm × 4 mm column with 5 μm particle size was used, the composition of the used mobile phase was 55 % (v/v) methanol and 45 % (v/v) water and viewing wavelength 240 nm. The test solution was prepared by dissolving 1 g of gel into 50 ml mobile phase in mixture of methanol and water in ratio 1:5.

Since there is a significant decrease in the absorbance of metronidazole at 254 nm, and of parabens at 315 nm, the wavelength of 240 nm is chosen as a compromise for quantitative determination of both, the active substance and the preservatives within the formulation. This enables use even of older types of HPLC systems with single channel UV detectors, because the signal monitoring of all three components of interest is performed at one wavelength, 240 nm, instead at two, 315 nm for metronidazole and 254 nm for preservatives.

All other chromatographic conditions are the same as the pharmacopoeial conditions cited at the beginning of this part. This method was tested also with 0.05 % TFA at pH value of 2.15 as part of the mobile phase, instead of pure water, but a peak splitting of metronidazole was observed (Fig. 7). Test solution of Metronidazole gel was prepared with dissolving ~ 1,0 g gel in 50 ml mobile phase.

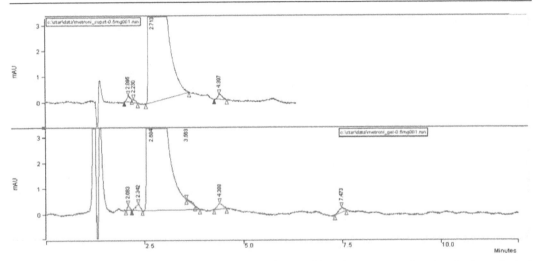

Figure 5. Comparison of chromatograms of active substance (blue chromatogram above) and gel-sample (red chromatogram below), monitored at 315 nm. The peak with RT ~4,4 min present on both hromatograms is the specified impurity 2-methyl-5-nitroimidazole

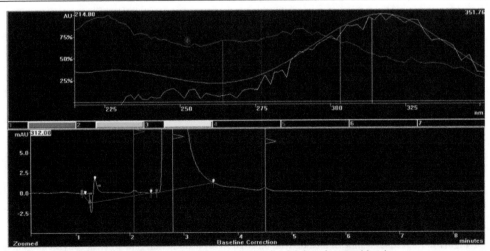

Figure 6. Spectral characteristics of impurities eluting in vicinity of metronidazole

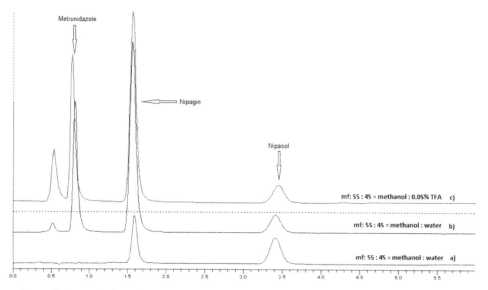

Figure 7. Determination of metronidazole, Nipagin and Nipasol using RP Select B 75 mm × 4 mm with 5 μm particle size HPLC column, at absorbance of 240 nm, with different mobile phase composition as indicated in the figure; a) Paraben mixture; b) and c) Metronidazol gel

The chromatogram a) on Figure 7 shows separation times of standards of preservatives Nipagin and Nipasol without presence of the active substance, metronidazole. The next chromatogram above this one, chromatogram b) is from a sample of Metronidazol gel, containing both parabens and active pharmaceutical substance, obtained with mobile phase composed of water and methanol.

The last chromatogram c), at the top, illustrates separation problem occurred during use of 0.05 % trifluoroacteic acid with pH=2.15 instead of water, which yields metronidazole peak splitting probably induced by acidity of mobile phase which is in vicinity of the pKa value of metronidazole, which equals 2.6 (16). It can be clearly seen that the peak of metronidazole in this chromatogram is wider

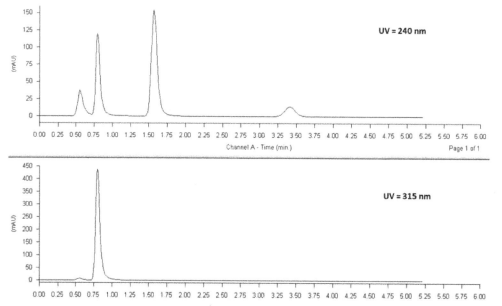

Figure 8. Ruggednes testing of method with other HPLC system, Perkin Elmer Series 200. Monitoring at 240 nm and at 315 nm

than the same peak in the chromatogram below this one in the same figure, which means that at this pH value metronidazole starts to ionize. But there is also something from the gel formulation that elutes at the same time as the split peak. This can also be seen from the comparison of the chromatograms b) and c): first peak in the chromatogram b) obtained with water is much smaller than the first peak in the chromatogram c), obtained with 0.05 % trifluoroacteic acid with pH=2.15. The first small peak in the chromatogram b) originates from the gel formulation, whereas the first peak in the chromatogram c) is a combination of gel formulation ingredients and the active substance,

which is also confirmed by spectral analysis. The performed spectral analysis showed that it contains several spectral lines and the peak is not pure. That is why we excluded this type of mobile phase from our investigation.

This method was also tested for ruggedness by performing it on another, different type of HPLC instrument, Perkin Elmer Series 200 with quaternary low-pressure mixing pump and dual beam PDA detector, compared with previous analysis which were performed on Varian ProStar with ternary high-pressure mixing pump and single beam PDA detector. Obtained chromatographic separations with both systems were satisfactory,

Table 1. Summary of method validation study

Analytical technique	HPLC		
Apparatus	Varian ProStar HPLC with PDA detector		
Validation parameters	**Acceptance criteria (17)**	**Results**		
		Metronidazole	Nipagin	Nipasol
RANGE:	min. accepted conc. 80 – 120 %	0,105 – 0.195 Metronidazole / mL (70 – 130 %)	0,035 – 0.065 Nipagin / mL (70 – 130 %)	0,007 – 0.013 Nipasol / mL (70 – 130 %)
LINEARITY: Correlation coefficient R^2:	$\geq 0,9900$	$R^2 = 0,9999$	$R^2 = 0,9999$	$R^2 = 0,9997$
ACCURACY: Recovery:	$98,0 – 102,0\%$	Recovery = 99.28 %	Recovery = 100.15 %	Recovery = 98,71 %
PRECISION: System repeatability	$RSD \leq 2,0\%$	RSD = 0.0003 %	RSD = 0.002 %	RSD = 0.0991 %
Method repeatability	$RSD \leq 2,0\%$	RSD = 1,85 %	RSD = 1,52 %	RSD = 1,64 %

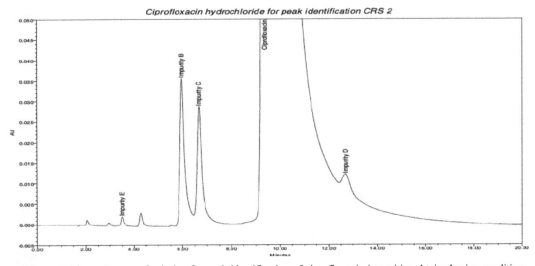

Figure 9. Chromatogram of solution for peak identification of ciprofloxacin impurities obtained using conditions prescribed in British Pharmacopoeia monograph, originating originally from the pharmacopoeia itself

and the chromatogram obtained from the analysis performed on Perkin Elmer series 200 is presented on Figure 8.

Summary of the method validation for simultaneous quantitative determination of metronidazole and both parabens, present in the gel formulation is presented in Table 1.

Ciprofloxacin Analysis

The method used for examination of Ciprofloxacin film coated tablets 500 mg and Ciprofloxacin eye drops 3 mg/ml was according to Ciprofloxacin hydrochloride monograph given in British Pharmacopoeia 2012. It prescribes the use of: Nucleosil C18 250 mm × 4,6 mm column with 5 μm particle size, column temperature 40 ℃, mobile phase consisted of 13 volumes of acetonitrile and 87 % 2,45 g/l phosphoric acid R, previously adjusted to pH 3,0 with triethylamine, mobile phase flow rate 1,5 ml/min, wavelength for UV detection 278 nm and injection volume of 10 μl. The chromatogram obtained using this pharmacopoeia prescribed conditions is presented in Figure 9.

Some minor modifications in this prescribed chromatographic conditions were made: a shorter chromatographic column was used, Discovery C18 100 mm × 4,6 mm column with 5 μm particle size and thus the mobile phase flow rate was also decreased to 1,2 ml/min. Temperature was decreased to 30 ℃. All modif cations made are within the allowed "*Adjustments of chromatographic conditions*" described in the European Pharmacopoeia, current edition. Ph. Eur./BP, current editions, under General Notices Part III, General Notices of the European Pharmacopoeia, 1.1. General Statements, under "Validation of Pharmacopoeial Methods" states:

"The test methods given in monographs and general chapters have been validated in accordance with accepted scientific practice and current recommendations on analytical validation. Unless otherwise stated in the monograph or general chapter, validation of the test methods by the analyst is not required." (8, 11).

Furthermore, with these slight changes in various parameters the system suitability criteria can still be satisfied without fundamentally modifying the pharmacopoeia prescribed method.

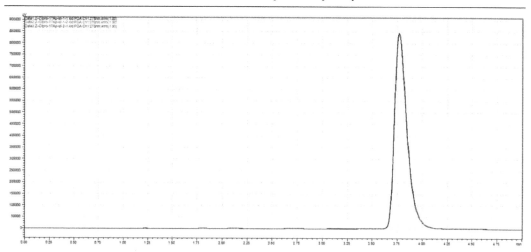

Figure 10. Overlaid chromatograms of three consecutive injections of ciprofloxacin hydrochloride working standard solution with concentration of 0,5 mg/ml

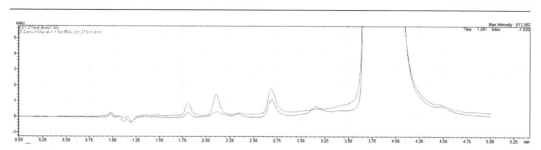

Figure 11. Demonstrative chromatograms with satisfying separation and resolution between active substance, ciprofloxacin hydrochloride and its impurities in chromatograms of standard solution for peak identification (red coloured chromatogram) and Ciprofloxacin film coated tablets test solution (green coloured chromatogram)

In Figure 10, the full size and shape of ciprofloxacin peak in 3 consecutive standard solution injections can be seen. Figure 11 illustrates expanded views of chromatograms of sample, film coated tablets solution and peak identity solution, in PDA overlay mode. Thus, an optimal retention of the active substance ciprofloxacin hydrochloride and good resolution between the active substance and its impurities, were achieved. The repeatability of this chromatographic method is excellent which can be seen from the three consecutive, overlaid injections presented on Figure 10. Presented chromatograms are from 0.5 mg/ml ciprofloxacin hydrochloride working standard solution and Ciprofloxacin film coated tablets test solution, in mobile phase.

Ciprofloxacin eye drops 5 mg/ml were prepared in the same way, with the same concentration of the active ingredient in the test solution and were tested under the same above described chromatographic conditions. The obtained complete PDA record is presented in Figure 12. It can be seen that the main peak of the active substance is well separated from the other peaks present in the chromatogram, originating from all related substances or formulation excipients. The left top part is a contour or 3-D chromatogram, below is the extracted chromatogram at 278 nm with peak report on the bottom left side. The right upper diagram is UV spectrum of ciprofloxacin and below is a peak purity graphic and presentation with calculation.

In the following figure, (Fig. 13), an expanded overlay comparison of two chromatograms is presented, one is of the solution for peak identification of specified impurities of

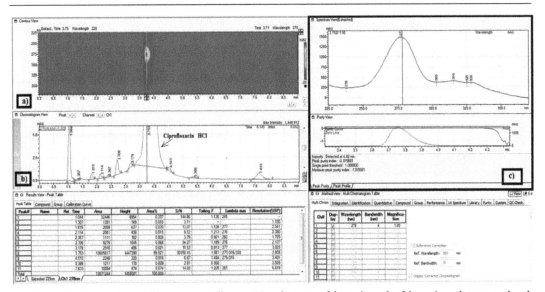

Figure 12. Presentation of: 3D or contour diagram (a) and spectra of the main peak of the active substance and peak purity of the same (c) from chromatogram of test solution prepared from Ciprofloxacin eye drops (b) with the obtained results presented in the table given below the chromatogram

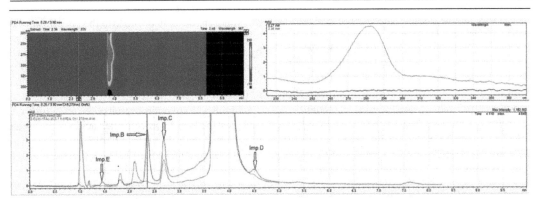

Figure 13. Comparison of chromatograms of solution for peak identification of specified impurities of ciprofloxacin (red colored chromatogram) and from Ciprofloxacin eye drops test solution (green colored chromatogram)

ciprofloxacin, for determination and quantification of its impurities (red colored chromatogram) and the other is from the test solution prepared from Ciprofloxacin eye drops (green colored chromatogram).

DISCUSSION

Metronidazole Analysis

Optimization of the pharmacopoeia prescribed method for quality control of metronidazole active substance led to achievement of better chromatographic parameters, better resolution and shorter run times, when compared to the results obtained using the original unmodified pharmacopoeial method, which can be clearly seen from Figure 2 and Figure 3.

Using a shorter chromatographic column we succeeded to achieve satisfying, optimal retention of metronidazole during shorter run times. The main reason for lowering methanol percentage in the mobile phase composition was obtaining better separation and better resolution, using this shorter column, between metronidazole (main peak in the chromatograms given on Figure 3) and its specified impurity, 2-methyl-5-nitroimidazole (peak with RT ~ 2,5 on the first and RT ~ 4,5 on the second chromatogram on the figure), which is presented on Figure 3. Thus, it is proved that this specified impurity will not interfere during assay determination of active component, and the quantity of the same, if present, can also be determined.

This modified pharmacopoeial method can also be used for quality control of Metronidazole gel, because as it is shown on Figure 4, a good separation and resolution between Metronidazole and two parabens in the composition of the gel formulation is obtained and therefore it can be used for their simultaneous determination using 240 nm as monitoring wavelength or dual wavelength monitoring at 315 nm for Metronidazole and 254 nm for Nipagin and Nipasol.

Further, Figure 5 and Figure 6 show that not only this method can be used for quantification of the constituents present in Metronidazole gel formulation, it can also serve for identification and quantification of metronidazole impurities, if present. Their determination can be performed directly in test solution prepared from the Metronidazole gel formulation, without any interference from the excipients present in the gel formulation.

The other, newly developed method for assay determination of Metronidazole gel, is even better for routine analysis of numerous samples in quality control laboratories within pharmaceutical industries. Use of an even shorter column (75 mm instead of 100 mm) with different properties from the previous one (C8 instead of C18) and different, more simple mobile phase (composed only of methanol and water instead of buffer), emphasizes the numerous benefits that this method has, when compared to the pharmacopoeial one and other methods developed for this purpose. For comparison: Tashtoush B. M., Jacobson E. L. and Jacobson M. K. developed a method for HPLC determination of Metronidazole in dermatological formulations, using 0,01 % trifluoroacetic acid and acetonitrile as mobile phase constituents, but the separation was accomplished during longer run times, ~ 10 minutes (18). When a 0.15 % TFA was used as a constituent of the mobile phase, instead of water, a peak splitting of metronidazole was observed, probably because of the close values of pH of the mobile phase (pH = 2.15 of the inorganic part) and pKa value of metronidazole which equals 2.6. Other authors (Melikyan et al.) with regards to the development of a method for determination of metronidazole benzoate and related impurities in bulk and in pharmaceutical formulations, prescribe the use of CN-RP column and mobile phase composed of acetonitrile and 0.1 % octansulfonic acid sodim salt; this method also needs longer run times, ~ 15 minutes (19).

All the changes we made during the development of our method proved to be beneficial and the goals were achieved: separation of the three main components of Metronidazole gel is successful with satisfying resolution between them and all of this can be achieved within run time of only 4,5 minutes, as can be seen from Figure 7 and Figure 8. Results obtained from the performed validation of the developed method are presented in Table 1 and are in accordance with the ICH requirements for the tested validation parameters.

Ciprofloxacin Analysis

Minor modifications made to the pharmacopeial method for quality control of ciprofloxacin hydrochloride, i.e. usage of shorter C18 chromatographic column (100 mm) instead of the prescribed one (250 mm), with slight optimization of the mobile phase flow rate (1.2 ml/min instead of 1.5 ml/min), led to optimization of the retention time of ciprofloxacin hydrochloride, achieving shorter run times (even ~ 4 times shorter when compared to the pharmacopoeial method), but still preserving the good resolution between ciprofloxacin hydrochloride and its impurities. This method was also proven to be useful in assay determination and identification and quantification of ciprofloxacin impurities for quality control of two pharmaceutical dosage forms containing ciprofloxacin: Ciprofloxacin eye drops and Ciprofloxacin film coated tablets. Excipients present in these formulations do not interfere with the active substance nor with its impurities.

CONCLUSION

As it can be clearly seen from the above presented results from the conducted research, some modifications of the pharmacopoeial methods for quality control of active substances metronidazole and ciprofloxacin led to creation of simple, fast, and reliable methods for analysis of veterinary pharmaceutical preparations containing these two active substances.

The above described, slightly modified and optimized pharmacopoeial methods for quality control of Metronidazole gel and Ciprofloxacin film coated tablets and eye drops can be successfully applied in laboratories for quality control of veterinary medicines, for assay determination and identification and quantification of specified impurities.

The new method developed for simultaneous assay determination of the active substance and the both preservatives in Metronidazole gel is simple, faster and more ecological (less methanol and time consumption) and less expensive than the compendial analytical method.

With this work we aim to prompt the establishment of laboratories for quality control of veterinary medicines sold in veterinary pharmacies and ambulances in our country and the implementation of the existing regulations for testing veterinary medicines.

REFERENCES

1. Official Journal of European Union. Commission Regulation (EU) No 37/2010 of 22 December 2009 on pharmacologically active substances and their classification regarding maximum residue limits of foodstuffs of animal origin. Pub. L. No. 15/72 (January 20, 2010).

2. WedgewoodPetRx.com [Internet]. New Jersey (USA): Wedgewood Pharmacy; c2004-13 [cited 2014 May 04]. Available from: http://www.wedgewoodpetrx.com/

3. PetMD [Internet]. Pennsylvania (USA): Pet360, Inc.; c1999-2014 [cited 2014 May 04]. Available from: http://www.petmd.com/

4. Official Journal of European Communities. Directive 2001/82/EC of the European Parliament and of the Council of 6 November 2001 on the Community code relating to veterinary medicinal products. Pub. L. No. 311/1-66 (November 28, 2001).

5. Official Journal of European Communities. Directive 2004/28/EC of the European Parliament and of the Council of 31 March 2004 on the Community code relating to veterinary medicinal products. Pub. L. No. 136/58-84 (April 30, 2004).

6. Veterinary EU Legislation: Medicines [Internet]. Brussels (EU): Federation of Veterinarians of Europe (FVE); c2014 [cited 2014 May 07]. Available from: http://www.fve.org/veterinary/medicines.php#1

7. Veterinary medicines: regulatory information [Internet]. London (UK): European Medicines Agency; c1995-2014 [cited 2014 May 07]. Available from: http://www.ema.europa.eu/ema/index.jsp?curl= pages/regulation/landing/veterinary_medicines_ regulatory.jsp&mid=

8. British Pharmacopoeia Commission. British Pharmacopoeia (Veterinary) 2012. Norwich: The Stationery Office; 2011.

9. China Veterinary Pharmacopoeia Commission. Veterinary Pharmacopoeia of the People's Republic of China. 2010 ed. Beijing: China Agriculture Press; 2010.

10. Indian Pharmacopoeia 2014: Veterinary monographs. 7th ed. Raj Nagar, Ghaziabad: Indian Pharmacopoeia Commission; 2014.

11. European Pharmacopoeia. 7th ed. Strasbourg: European Directorate for the Quality of Medicines – Council of Europe; 2010-2012.

12. British Pharmacopoeia Commission. British Pharmacopoeia 2012. Norwich: The Stationery Office; 2011.

13. United States Pharmacopeia and National Formulary (USP 33-NF 28). Rockville: United States Pharmacopeia Convention; 2009.

14. Society of Japanese Pharmacopoeia. Japanese Pharmacopoeia. 16th ed. Tokyo: Maruzen Company, Ltd.; 2012.

15. The International Pharmacopoeia. 4th ed. Geneva: World Health Organization; 2006.

16. Product Monograph. Flagyl® (Metronidazole) 10% w/w Cream, 500 mg Capsules. Quebec: Sanofi-Aventis Canada Inc.; 2013.

17. International Conference on Harmonization of Technical Requirements for Registration of Pharmaceuticals for Human Use; ICH Harmonised Tripartite Guideline. Validation of Analytical Procedures: Text and Methodology Q2(R1), Current *Step 4* version, Parent Guideline dated 27 October 1994 [cited 2014 Oct 07]. Available from: http://www.ich.org/fileadmin/Public_Web_Site/ICH_ Products/Guidelines/Quality/Q2_R1/Step4/Q2_R1__ Guideline.pdf

18. Tashtoush, BM., Jacobson, EL., Jacobson, MK. (2008). Validation of a simple and rapid HPLC method for determination of metronidazole in dermatological formulations. Drug Dev Ind Pharm. 34(8): 840-844. http://dx.doi.org/10.1080/03639040801928598 PMid:18618307

19. Melikyan, AL., Martirosyan, SS., Grigoryan, SR., Topchyan, VH., Davtyan, KT. (2013). Development and validation of HPLC method for the determination of metronidazole benzoate and related impurities in bulk and pharmaceutical formulations. IJPSR. 4(7): 2594-2599.

4

PRESENCE OF TRYPANOSOME SPECIES AND ANEMIC STATUS OF DOGS IN ZURU, NIGERIA

Rafi Rabecca Tono[1], Olufemi Oladayo Faleke[2], Abdullahi Alhaji Magaji[2],
Musbaudeen Olayinka Alayande[3], Akinyemi Olaposi Fajinmi[4],
Emmanuel Busayo Ibitoye[5]

[1]*Zonal Veterinary Clinic, Zuru Kebbi State, Nigeria*
[2]*Department of Veterinary Public Health and Preventive Medicine,
Faculty of Veterinary Medicine, Usmanu Danfodiyo University Sokoto, Nigeria*
[3]*Department of Veterinary Entomology and Parasitology, Faculty of Veterinary Medicine,
Usmanu Danfodiyo University Sokoto, Nigeria*
[4]*Nigeria Institute of Trypanosomosis and Onchocerciasis Research, Kaduna, Nigeria*
[5]*Department of Theriogenology and Animal Production, Faculty of Veterinary Medicine,
Usmanu Danfodiyo University Sokoto, Nigeria*

ABSTRACT

The aim of this research is to study the presence and prevalence of trypanosome species in local dogs between January and July, 2010 in the Zuru area of Kebbi State, Nigeria. Standard trypanosome detection methods comprising of wet blood films, thin films and microhaematocrit centrifugation technique were used to detect trypanosomes; while the degree of anemia was determined through the use of FAMACHA® eye colour chart and packed cell volume values. A total of 567 dogs were enumerated in fourteen locations within the study area out of which 192 (33.7%) were randomly examined and 4 (2.08%) were positive for the presence of trypanosomes. All positive samples morphologically belong to the *Trypanosoma brucei* group. The obtained PCV values showed that 50 (26.04%) dogs were anemic, while the FAMACHA® detected anemia status of varying degrees in 104 (77%) sampled dogs. These findings are significant as this is the first time that the trypanosome infection will be reported in dogs from the study area. This study establishes the presence of *Trypanosoma brucei* group in the study area, which is of zoonotic and economic importance.

Key words: anemia, dogs, Nigeria, trypanosomes, Zuru

INTRODUCTION

Trypanosomiasis is an important insect-borne protozoan disease and a serious constraint to livestock production and economic development in many parts of sub-Saharan Africa (1). It is widely distributed in tropical and subtropical regions and its epidemiology is determined by the ecology of its insect vector, the tsetse fly (*Glossina* spp). Canine trypanosomiasis is a devastating disease (2) characterized by anemia, severe weight loss, muscular weakness, abortion, corneal opacity, blepharitis, conjunctivitis, keratitis and death if untreated in affected dogs (3). Trypanosomiasis of dogs was first described in 1908 (4) and it is caused mainly by *Trypanosoma brucei brucei* (5), *Trypanosoma congolense* (6), *Trypanosoma cruzi* (7), *Trypanosoma evansi* (8) and *Trypanosoma caninum* (9). In Nigeria, trypanosomiasis in dogs due to *T. brucei* and *T. congolense* occurs more frequently (10). It has been established that different domestic animals including dogs are potential links for trypanosome exchange between livestock and humans i.e. *Trypanosome brucei gambiense* and *Trypanosome brucei rhodesiense*,

Corresponding author: Dr. E.B. Ibitoye, DVM, MSc
E-mail address: emmavet2001@yahoo.com
Present address: Department of Theriogenology
and Animal Production, Faculty of Veterinary Medicine
Usmanu Danfodiyo University Sokoto, Nigeria

causing a condition known as HAT, also referred to as 'sleeping sickness (11, 12, 13), while *T. brucei brucei* causes severe to fatal infections in horses, camels, dogs and cats (14).

There has been increased interest in keeping dogs in Nigeria, mainly as security or pets, and in some parts of the country for food. Similarly, the proceeds from the sales of dogs serve as additional income for the owners (15). Though dogs are known to pose minimal risk for human infection (HAT), they are important as a sentinel for infection (13). Canine trypanosomiasis has been reported as constituting a major health threat to canine population in the south-eastern part of Nigeria (10, 11, 16).

The study area is an interface between the hitherto declared 'tsetse-free' zone of the northwest and tsetse endemic areas southward in the middle belt of Nigeria. The people in the study area are predominantly crop farmers whose activities are restricted to the short period of rainfall. The long dry season is used mainly for hunting in which the expeditions takes them south, where tsetse flies abound (17). The study therefore investigated possible incursion of trypanosomes to the study area through dogs.

MATERIAL AND METHODS

Study Area

The study was undertaken in the Zuru Local Government Area, south-eastern part of Kebbi State, northwest, Nigeria. It lies within latitudes $11^0 15$' to $11^0 55$'N and longitudes $4^0 35$' to $5^0 47$ E and falls within the Sudan Savannah type of vegetation, with a mean annual rainfall of 1022 mm and a mean minimum and maximum temperatures of 24.6^0C and 28^0C respectively. The dominant group is the Lelna people whose economic activities center on crop and livestock production, with some engaging in hunting expeditions southward towards Niger and Kwara States of Nigeria. A preliminary census of household dog population was conducted in 14 selected locations using a purposive sampling method, while the dogs were sampled by a convenience sampling technique. Within the study area a representative sample size was determined using the formula: $n = Z^2PQ/L^2$. Where n = number of individuals; Z = the Z score for a given confidence interval (95%); for this study, since there was no known prevalence for canine trypanosomiasis in the study area, P was estimated at 20%; Q = 1 – P and L = is the allowable error of estimation (5%) (18). Using this formula, 167 dogs are to be sampled but

this was increased to 192 so as to increase precision. Dogs from a dog market within the study area were also sampled. Structured questionnaire comprising of information on dog usage and maintenance was designed and administered to owners in the sampled households only in relation to the veterinary health care delivery system.

About 3ml of blood was collected from the cephalic vein from each of the dogs that were sampled, using 5ml sterile syringe and needle and transferred into clean EDTA bottles. The blood in each bottle was gently mixed, placed in a cool box containing ice packs and transported in about 2hrs to the Veterinary Public Health and Preventative Medicine laboratory of Usmanu Danfodiyo University Sokoto, Nigeria for immediate analysis. The blood samples were then examined using the standard trypanosome diagnostic methods (STDM) comprising of wet blood films, thin films and microhaematocrit centrifugation technique (19, 20). Morphological identification of trypanosomes was carried out using Giemsa stained films. Packed cell volume (PCV) was determined to detect level of anemia [normal PCV range 36 – 55%] (21), while FAMACHA®, an eye colour chart with five colourscores [scores: 1=optimal, no anemia; 2=acceptable, no anemia; 3=borderline, moderate; 4=dangerous, anemic and 5=fatal, anemic] (22) were used to diagnose different levels of anemia.

Ethical approval

Ethical clearance as approved by the Research Ethical Committee of the Faculty of Veterinary Medicine, Usmanu Danfodiyo University Sokoto, Nigeria was obtained prior to this study.

Statistical Analysis

Descriptive statics was used to analyze data (23).

RESULTS

Preliminary census enumerated a total number of 510 Nigerian local breed of dogs from households in 14 locations namely: Bayan Tasha, Filin Jirgi, Gomawa, Jarkasa, Low cost, Mangorori, Rikoto, Roadblock, Sabuwar Kasuwar, Sha da Wanka, Tudun Wadata, Unguwar Zuru, Zango, Zuru Center and a dog market. As shown in Table 1, Rikoto had the highest number of dogs (n=77), while Mangorori had the lowest (n=11). A total of 192 Nigerian dogs were selected comprising of 135 dogs from the households and 57 dogs from the dog market.

Table 1. Dog population structure with the number of sampled and positive cases in households and dog market in Zuru area, Kebbi State

Location	Enumerated	Sampled No.	Percentage sampled (%)	Positive samples
Bayan Tasha	18	5	27.8	-
Dog market	57	57	100.0	1
Filin Jirgi	42	11	26.2	1
Gomawa	27	6	22.2	-
Jarkasa	46	13	28.3	-
Low Cost	27	6	22.2	-
Mangorori	11	3	27.3	-
Rikoto	76	22	28.9	1
Roadblock	39	10	25.6	-
Sabuwar Kasuwa	41	11	26.8	-
Sha da wanka	42	11	26.2	-
Tudun Wadata	39	10	25.6	-
Unguwar Zuru	49	14	28.6	1
Zango	20	5	25.0	-
Zuru Centre	33	8	24.2	-
Total	**567**	**192**	**33.7**	**4(2.08%)**

Out of 192 blood samples analyzed by STDM, 4 (2.08%) were positive for trypanosomes. Out of these wet blood film detected all the 4 positive cases, microhaematocrit detected 3, while Giemsa stain (thin blood) technique detected 2 (Table 2).

The PCV values ranges and FAMACHA scores of all sampled animals were not consistent with their anemic statuses. According to PCV values, of the 192 dogs examined 50 (26.04%) dogs were anemic (21), with 3 (1.56%) being positive for trypanosomes

Table 2. Distribution of positive samples and anemic indicator values

Areas	PCV (%)	WBC	RBC (%)	Hb	FAMACHA Score	Wet blood	Haematocrit	Thin blood
Dog market	34	12.40	3.10	10.3	NC	+	+	+
Filin Jirgi	32	10.02	3.23	10.7	4	+	+	
Rikoto	36	4.88	5.43	12.0	4	+	+	+
Unguwar Zuru	24	3.25	4.73	8.0	4	+	-	-

Key: NC = Not conducted

Morphologically, all the positive samples were identified to be in the *Trypanosoma brucei* group (Fig. 1).

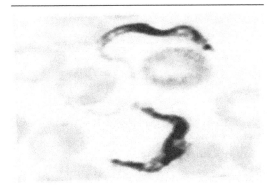

Figure 1. Giemsa stained *Trypanosomabrucei*on thin film smear

and 47 (24.47%) negative for trypanosome infection, while out of 142 (73.95%) non-anemic dogs, 1 (0.52%) was positive for trypanosomes and 141 (73.43%) were negative (Table 3). Of the 135 household-dogs sampled, FAMACHA® gave a total of 104 (77%) dogs with anemia. FAMACHA® testing was not done for dogs from the dog market (Table 4).

All the 135 respondents claimed that their dogs were kept mainly for security purposes and it was observed that dogs were mostly unleashed and found roaming about in the study area. As shown on Table 5, 21 (15.6%) of the respondents feed their dogs occasionally, 74 (54.8%) did not vaccinate their dogs against any disease, only 5 (3.7%) have their dogs receive regular veterinary health care services, while 53 (39.3%) have dogs infested with ticks and 86 (63.7%) having to dispose their dogs

Table 3. Anemic status of examined dogs at different locations in Zuru using PCV

Locations	Trypanosomal negative		Trypanosomal positive		Total
	Anemic	Non- anemic	Anemic	Non- anemic	
Bayan Tasha	2	3	-	-	5
Dog market	2	36	1	-	57
Filin Jirgin	2	8	1	-	11
Gomawa	2	4	-	-	6
Jarkasa	1	12	-	-	13
Low Cost	0	6	-	-	6
Mangorori	2	1	-	-	3
Rikoto	6	15	-	1	22
Roadblock	1	9	-	-	10
SabuwarKasuwa	2	9	-	-	11
Sha da wanka	3	8	-	-	11
Tudun Wadata	0	10	-	-	10
Unguwar Zuru	1	12	1	-	14
Zango	2	3	-	-	5
Zuru Centre	3	5	-	-	8
Total	47(24.47%)	141(73.43%)	3(1.56%)	1(0.52%)	192

Table 4. Anemic status of examined dogs at different locations in Zuru using FAMACHA®

Locations	Trypanosomal negative		Trypanosomal positive		Total
	Anemic	Non- Anemic	Anemic	Non- anemic	
Bayan Tasha	5	0	-	-	5
Dog market	NC	NC	NC	NC	NC
Filin Jirgin	5	5	1	-	11
Gomawa	6	0	-	-	6
Jarkasa	7	6	-	-	13
Low Cost	4	2	-	-	6
Mangorori	3	0	-	-	3
Rikoto	13	8	1	0	22
Roadblock	9	1	-	-	10
SabuwarKasuwa	11	0	-	-	11
Sha da wanka	11	0	-	-	11
Tudun Wadata	7	3	-	-	10
Unguwar Zuru	11	2	1	-	14
Zango	3	2	-	-	5
Zuru Centre	6	2	-	-	8
Total	101(74.81%)	31(22.96%)	3(2.22%)	0(0.0%)	135

NC = Not Conducted.

Table 5. Responses to the questionnaire survey on dog management within Zuru

Sampled questions	No. of Responses		
Purpose for keeping dog	Security 135(100%)	Commercial (Nil)	Hobby/Pet (Nil)
Duration of keeping dog sampled	1 month-1 year 12(9.8%)	2-5 years 31(23.0%)	6 year and above 93(68.9%)
Mode of feeding	More than once 92(68.2%)	Once daily 22 (16.3%)	Some times 21(15.6%)
Anti-rabies vaccination	Regularly 5(3.7%)	Sometimes 56 (41.5%)	Not at all 74(54.8%)
Acquaintance with veterinary services	Regularly 5(3.7%)	Sometimes 64 (47.4%)	Not at all 66(48.9%)
Preference to sex during purchase	Yes 6(4.4%)		No 129(95.6%)
Owing other breeds	Yes 3(2.2%)		No 132(97.8%)
Reasons leading to dog disposal	Harassment 23(17.0%)	Illness 86 (63.7%)	Accidents 26(19.3%)
Presence of ectoparasites	Yes, (ticks) 53(39.3%)		No 82(60.7%)

due to illness. Virtually all adult dogs were involved in hunting expedition during the dry season period. The hunting for game animals goes beyond the boundary of Zuru Emirate, it extends southwards into Niger and some parts of Kwara States, Nigeria.

DISCUSSION

There is little information on canine trypanosomiasis in Nigeria and its epidemiology is poorly understood. In the study area and its environs, there are no previous prevalence studies making this study a preliminary study. When compared with prevalence obtained in endemic parts of Nigeria, the obtained prevalence of 2.08% in this study could be considered higher and calls for concern as the study area is previously known to be free of trypanosomes. According to other studies, the prevalence of trypanosomiasis in dogs was 3% in Jos Plateau (24), 8.8% in two veterinary clinics in Anambra State (10) and 10% in Nsukka area of Enugu State (11). The detection of *Trypanosoma brucei* trypanosomes in the current study is in agreement with Anene et al. (11); Abenga et al. (12); Omamegbe et al. (10) and Anene et al. (16), who reported that *Trypanosoma brucei* is the predominant species involved in canine trypanosomiasis in Nigeria. The presence of trypanosomes in the study area can be attributed to factors such as the unrestricted movement of dogs through commercial purposes, hunting expeditions into endemic areas and existence of *Glossina palpalis palpalis* both in the wet and dry seasons in areas where hunting expeditions normally take place (17).

Anemia is one of the pathogenic consequences of trypanosomiasis (22). However, the high percentage of the animals showing various levels of anemia may be due to extraneous factors such as the state of nutrition, the presence of other inter-current infections such as helminthes, which is a common problem of developing countries and ubiquitous in livestock and other domestic animals (25) and stress caused by long trekking and distant transportation. From PCV values and FAMACHA® scores, all dogs infected with trypanosomes were anemic except in one dog, with PCV of 36% but a FAMACHA® score of 4. This inconsistency may be as a result of haemoconcentration in the animal (26), or could also indicate recent infection. The leucopenia observed in two of the positive samples (Rikkoto and Unguwar Zuru) could be an indication of early infection (27), but the normal leucocyte counts from the other two positive samples from the Dog market and Filin Jirgi could not be explained.

CONCLUSION

Findings of this study establish the presence of *Trypanosoma brucei* group in dogs which were found in a free-HAT zone and they pose a risk for human and livestock health. Morphologically, *Trypanosoma brucei brucei* and *Trypanosoma brucei gambiense* are indistinguishable. Therefore molecular testing is suggested in further studies in order to confirm if *Trypanosoma brucei gambiense* is present in the population. Also, appropriate measures which include public health awareness and improvement on veterinary health care delivery services be made more readily available in the study area.

ACKNOWLEDGEMENT

The authors are thankful to the authorities of the Department of Veterinary Public Health and Preventive Medicine, Faculty of Veterinary Medicine, Usmanu Danfodiyo University Sokoto, Nigeria, for the permission to use the departmental laboratory and equipment to carry out this investigation. All authors contributed financially.

REFERENCES

1. Ilemobade, A.A. (2009). Tsetse and trypanosomosis in Africa: the challenges, the opportunities. Onderstepoort J Vet Res, 76, 35-40. http://dx.doi.org/10.4102/ojvr.v76i1.59 PMid:19967926

2. Abenga, J.N., Ezebuiro, C.O., David, K., Fajinmi, A.O., Samdi, S. (2005a). Studies on anemia in Nigerian local puppies infected with *Trypanosoma congolense*. Veterinarski Arhiv, 75, 165-174.

3. Stephen, E.L. (1986). Trypanosomiasis; a veterinary perspective. In Wheaton & Co. Ltd. Exter. (Ed). (pp. 235-314).

4. Bevan, E.W. (1913). Preliminary notes on a trypanosome causing disease in man and animal in the Sebungwe district of southern Rhodesia. J. Trop. Med. Hyg., 16, 113–117.

5. Simo, G., Njitchouang, G.R., Njiokou, F., Cuny, G., Asonganyi, T. (2012). Genetic characterization of *Trypanosoma brucei* circulating in domestic animals of the Fontem sleeping sickness of Cameroon. Microbes and Infection / Institut Pasteur, 14, 651-658. http://dx.doi.org/10.1016/j.micinf.2012.02.003 PMid:22387499

6. Desquesnes, M., Ravel, S., Deschamps, J.Y., Polack, B., Roux, F. (2012). A typical hyperpachymorph *Trypanosoma (Nannomonas) congolense* forest-type in a dog returning from Senegal. Parasite, 19, 239-247. http://dx.doi.org/10.1051/parasite/2012193239 PMid:22910666 PMCid:PMC3671449

7. Quijano-Hernandez, I.A., Castro-Barcena, A., Barbabosa-Pliego, A., Ochoa-Garcia, L., Angel-Caraza, J.D., Vázquez-Chagoyán, J.C. (2012). Seroprevalance survey of American Trypanosomiasis in Central Valley of Toluca. Scientific World Journal, 450, 619. http://dx.doi.org/10.1100/2012/450619 PMid:22649293 PMCid:PMC3353279

8. Defontis, M., Richard, J., Engelmann, N., Bauer, C., Schwierk, V.M., Buscher, P., Moritz, A. (2012). Canine *Trypanosoma evansi* infection introduced into Germany. Vet. Clin. Path., 41, 369-374. http://dx.doi.org/10.1111/j.1939-165X.2012.00454.x PMid:22954298

9. Rodrigo, C.M., Fabiano, B.F., Annabel, G.W., Maria, F.M., Raquel, V.C.O., Tânia, M.P.S., Matti, K., Ingeborg, M.L. (2013). Sensitivity and specificity of in situ hybridization for diagnosis of cutaneous infection by *Leishmania infantum* in dogs. J.Clin. Microbiol., 51, 206-211. http://dx.doi.org/10.1128/JCM.02123-12 PMid:23135932 PMCid:PMC3536224

10. Omamegbe, J.O., Orajaka, L.J.E., Omehelu, C.O. (1984). The incidence and clinical forms of naturally occurring canine trypanosomosis in two vet clinics in an Anambra State of Nigeria. Bull Animal Hlth Prod Africa, 32, 23-29.

11. Anene, B.M., Obetta, S.S., Agu, W.E. (1997). Prevalence of canine trypanosomosis with regards to dog and owners characteristics in Nsukka area of Enugu State, Nigeria. Nig. Vet. J., 18, 306-310.

12. Abenga, J.N., David, K., Ezebuiro, C.O.G., Lawani, F.A.G. (2005). Observation on the prevalence of young dogs (puppies) to infection with *Trypanosoma congolense*. African Journal of Clinical Experimental Microbiology, 6, 28-33.

13. Museux, K., Boulouha, L., Majani, S., Journaux, H. (2011). African Trypanosoma infection in dog in France. Veterinary Records, 168: 590b. http://dx.doi.org/10.1136/vr.d888 PMid:21622597

14. African Trypanosomiasis http://www.vet.uga.edu/vpp/gray_book/Handheld/aat.htm

15. Oboegbulem, I.S. (1994). Rabies in man and animals. Fidelity publishers and printer Co. Ltd. Enugu. Pp. 41-42.

16. Anene, B.M., Ezeokonkwo, R.C., Mmesirionye, T.I., Tettey, J.N.A., Brock, J.M., Barret, M.P., De Koning, H.P. (2005). A diaminazine resistant strain of *Trypanosoma brucei* isolated from a dog is cross resistant to pentamidine in experimentally infected albino rats. Parasitology, 132, 127-133. http://dx.doi.org/10.1017/S0031182005008760 PMid:16393361

17. Ahmed, A.B. (2004). A peridomestic population of the tsetse flies Glossina palpalis palpalis. Robinneau-Desvoidy, 1830 (Diptera: Glossinidae) at Kotongora town, Niger State, Nigeria. Entomología Vectores, 11, 599-610. http://dx.doi.org/10.1590/S0328-03812004000400004

18. Martin, S.W., Meek, A.H., Willeberg, P. (1987). Veterinary epidemiology, principle and methods. Iowa State University Press, pg. 343.

19. Woo, P.K.T. (1969). The haematocrit centrifugation for the detection of trypanosomes in blood. Can. J. Zoolog., 47, 921–923. http://dx.doi.org/10.1139/z69-150

20. World Organization of Animal Health (2004). Manual of diagnosis tests and vaccines for terrestrial animals, 5th edition, part 2, section 2, 3 and 15.

21. Hassan, A.Z., Hassan, F.B. (2003). Basic Clinic Services. In: An Introduction to Veterinary Practice. 1st Ed. p. 57.

22. Grace, D., Himstedt, H., Sidibe, I., Randolph, T.H., Clausen, P. (2007). Comparing FAMACHA® eye colour chart and Haemoglobin colour scale tests for detecting anemia and improving treatment of bovine trypanosomosis in West Africa. Acta Trop. Aug; 111(2):137-43. http://dx.doi.org/10.1016/j.actatropica.2009.03.009. PMID: 19524082

23. Anthony, E.O. (2005). Biostatistics: A practical approach to research and data handling. Mindex Press, Ugbowo, Benin City, Nigeria

24. Fajinmi, O.A. (2008). Epidemiology of animal trypanosomosis in Sokoto State, Nigeria. A MVPH Dissertation Report, Faculty of Veterinary Medicine, Usmanu Danfodiyo University, Sokoto, p. 139.

25. Kerboeuf, D., Blackhall, W., Kaminsky, R., Samson-Himmelst Jerna, G.V. (2003). P-glycoprotein in helminthes. Function and perspectives for anthelminthic treatment and reversal of resistance. Int. J. Parasitol., 22, 332-346.

26. Evans, S.F., Hinds, C.J., Varley, J.G. (1984). A new canine model of endotoxin shock. Brit J Pharmacol., 83 (2):433-442. http://dx.doi.org/10.1111/j.1476-5381.1984.tb16504.x PMid:6435710; PMCid:PMC1987104

27. Mackenzie, P.K.I., Boyt, W.P., Nesham, V.M., Pirie, E. (1983). The aetiology and significance of the phagocytosis of erythrocytes and leucocytes in sheep infected with *Trypanosoma congolense* (Broden, 1904). Research in Veterinary Science, 24, 4-7.

5

HIGH YIELDING DAIRY COWS: TO PRODUCE OR TO REPRODUCE AND WHAT PRACTITIONERS SHOULD KNOW ABOUT THIS TO HELP THEIR CLIENTS

Opsomer Geert

Department of Reproduction, Obstetrics and Herd Health,
Faculty of Veterinary Medicine,
Ghent University, Belgium

ABSTRACT

The present article aims to 'translate' the current – mostly theoretical – knowledge on fertility disorders in modern high yielding dairy cows, towards the actual situation in the stable with a main emphasis on the resumption of the ovarian activity after calving. While some detailed research has recently been done at our department to elucidate the association between a high level of milk production and the reproductive performance of the current dairy cow, the next challenge is to 'translate' this knowledge into practice and to offer possibilities and strategies to minimize the effects of the decrease in fertility. As the negative energy balance and general health status after calving are known to be paramount factors hampering fertility, it is apparent that avoiding both is among the most important preventive measures to be taken. Improvement of the energy status by achieving a high dry matter intake and the provision of optimal and well balanced nutrition during the transition period as well as during early lactation are key goals in this effort. To achieve these goals, we should not only calculate the rations on paper, but should also check in the stable to determine whether the calculated amount is really being consumed by the cows. Furthermore, veterinarians should use their 'clinical eyes' as well as other diagnostic tools to assess the general health status of the cows and to assess at which aspect of the process things are going wrong and need to be adjusted. Besides the control of the negative energy balance and health status, other management factors that need to be maximized include heat detection, cow comfort, insemination technique, time of insemination during estrus and sperm quality. Only if management is on a very high level can high milk production and good fertility be a feasible combination!

Key words: dairy cow, milk production, reproductive disorders, management

INTRODUCTION

Before milk production starts, cows have to calve and each calving is followed by a milk production peak. This standard 'cow knowledge' clearly illustrates why reproduction is still of paramount importance in the modern dairy industry.

Recent studies both in the US as well as in Europe have indicated that in the last 35 years, the genetic potential for milk production in Holstein Friesian cows has increased by over 3000 kg per lactation, resulting in an actual genetic increase of about 100 kg/year. This is, however, only a part of the (success) story. The genetic potential for milk production sets the upper limit which an individual cow can achieve. How close she actually comes to reaching that limit is determined by the management conditions under which she has to produce.

During the last decades these conditions have been improved tremendously. There have been improvements in feeding practices, in the control and prevention of diseases and in other management practices such as housing. All together these improvements have contributed to the actual level of milk production, which on many farms has gone above 9000 kg per lactation (of 305 days).

Clearly, the aggressive genetic selection together with the fine tuning of the management has proven to be very successful. However, this

Corresponding author: Prof.dr. Geert Opsomer DVM, PhD,
Dipl ECAR, Dipl ECBHM
E-mail address: Geert.Opsomer@UGent.be
Present address: Department of Reproduction, Obstetrics and Herd Health
Faculty of Veterinary Medicine, Ghent University
Salisburylaan 133, B-9820 Merelbeke, Belgium

has not been without costs. When dairy farmers are currently asked what the principal health problems will be that their business will face in the near future, they invariably mention subfertility, mastitis and lameness. These diseases are known to be multifactorial and to a large extent dependent on management practices.

High yielding dairy cows produce well, but reproduce bad

The time period characterized by the steep increase in milk production, is unfortunately also characterized by a dramatic decline in reproductive performance. Both the average number of days open (interval from calving to the next conception) and the number of services per conception have increased substantially, while the conception rate has declined significantly (14, 15).

Worldwide, calving rates to first service are reported to have declined from 60% to 30-40% over the past 25 years. If this trend continues at its current rate, in a further 20 years only 20% of cows will conceive to first service. This conclusion has been confirmed independently in the UK (25, 26) and in the US (2), and subsequently in many other European countries.

Also in Flanders and The Netherlands, the increase in milk production per cow has been accompanied by a significant increase in the calving interval, from 395 days in 1987 to 419 days in 2007 while the 56 day non-return rate has remained relatively stable (6, 22, 23). Analyses of fertility data from local AI centres revealed that the prolongation of the calving interval was mainly due to a prolongation of the interval from parturition to first insemination, due to the inability of the farmers seeing their cows in heat at the moment they should inseminate them (21).

The main negative results of this decline in fertility are longer and hence 'inefficient' lactations and an increase in the number of cows that are culled for reproductive reasons. The significant waste of sperm and the retarded increase of young stock are also important contributors to a significant loss of income.

So why has reproductive performance declined so precipitously? This has proven to be a very difficult question to answer (33). However, a recurring theme is that for cows to reproduce successfully, a clean and healthy uterine environment is essential. Indeed, the uterus not only influences the resumption of normal ovarian cyclicity to a large extent, but also has to promote sperm transport and finally has to undergo considerable changes to support pregnancy.

The dilemma of the postpartum cow

A remarkable feature of cattle is the almost constant bacterial contamination of the uterine lumen within the first 2 weeks after parturition. However, cows have always been considered to be highly efficient in clearing this contamination, in contrast for example to horses. Present-day, high-yielding dairy cows obviously have more problems and do not quite live up to this reputation. As a result, we now see more cows with puerperal problems, such as retained placenta, acute metritis and abnormal vaginal discharge (Table 1).

Table 1. Average incidence of puerperal disturbances on 9 high-yielding dairy herds in Belgium (Opsomer et al., 2000a)

Puerperal disturbance	Incidence (n=463)
• abnormal calvings	16%
• retained placenta	18%
• acute (endo)metritis	15%
• abn vag discharge	20%
• perivaginitis	5%

Although it is very difficult to compare these data with those from earlier studies because of possible (historical) differences in the use of the terms 'endometritis' and 'metritis', it is clear that the overall incidence of uterine diseases in high yielding dairy cows has increased over time (Table 2). Besides the recurrent discussion about the definition of the words 'endometritis' and 'metritis', this large variation is also due to the differences in the diagnostic methods used to classify uterine infections. The use of modern techniques such as ultrasonography and the examination of endometrial aspirates for presence of inflammatory cells have obviously caused a steep increase in the reported incidence of endometritis.

Table 2. Evidence of an increasing trend in the incidence of (endo) metritis based on an extensive literature review.

Endometritis incidence	Year of the study	Authors
11%	1968	Tennant and Peddicord
10%	1977	Bouters and Vandeplassche
38%	1983	Oltenacu et al.
37%	1984	Markusfeld
20%	1986	Whitmore and Anderson
17% (clin) + 37% (subclin)	2002	LeBlanc/Kasimanickam
53%	2005	Gilbert et al.

Throughout the years however, authors always have agreed that the incidence of chronic endometritis (=localised infection of the superficial lining of the uterus occurring >3 weeks after calving), is significantly dependent on the incidence of acute metritis (= infection of the uterine cavity, and of the deeper layers of the uterus causing a sometimes life threatening disease shortly after calving). There is general agreement nowadays that up to 40% of animals have metritis within the first two weeks of calving and that in 10-15% of these animals infection persists for at least another three weeks causing the chronic uterine disease called endometritis (27).

As uterine inflammation occurs in all cows during uterine involution, the factors responsible for failure to resolve the endometrial inflammation at the start of the breeding period seem to be critical. The latter clearly emphasizes the need to detect and treat animals suffering from endometritis, efficiently and as soon as possible to avoid problems later on. On the average dairy farm however, disease detection is done by the veterinarian, but typically only during routine herd health checks. This means that in many cases, early warning signs of disease go unnoticed until such time that the disease is in its full clinical stage and becomes much more difficult to treat. As a result chronic endometritis may still be present at the moment cows should become pregnant.

Cows affected by retained placenta and/or acute metritis are furthermore at a significantly higher risk of other typical 'dairy cow diseases' as acetonaemia, left displaced abomasum and cystic ovarian disease. Large scale studies based on both American and European data showed, for example, that cows with retained placenta are 2.2 times more at risk of left displaced abomasum and 6.0 times more at risk of developing metritis. Metritis itself causes cows to be 2.0 times more at risk of ketosis; and ketosis makes cows significantly more sensitive to cystic ovarian disease and left displaced abomasum. Although there are some differences in the final numbers published among the different studies, there is an overall agreement that retained placenta and/or acute postpartum metritis is often, if not always, the key element in the disease history of recently calved high yielding dairy cows (4, 5, 24).

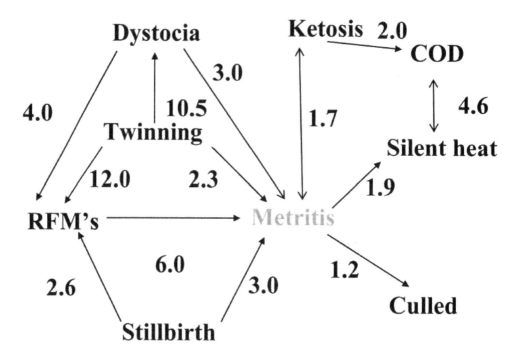

Figure 1. Results of risk factor analyses (odds ratios) for different postpartal diseases in high yielding dairy cows and underlying interactions. RFM= retained fetal membranes, COD= cystic ovarian disease

Although these relationships are clearly proven in large scale epidemiological studies, the underlying pathogenesis has not yet been fully elucidated. In a number of studies it has been demonstrated that the killing activity of neutrophils in high-yielding dairy cows is significantly reduced around the time of calving (11) (Fig. 2). This was further confirmed by *in vitro* studies in which a decreased killing activity of these cells was demonstrated when elevated amounts of ketone bodies were added to the culture medium. This finding probably explains the close relationship between infectious diseases and ketosis seen on present-day dairy herds.

Furthermore it has recently been shown that cows' going off feed is one of the most important risk factors for a left displaced abomasum after calving (32). In this case, the rumen is not able to act as a physical barrier against the gas filled enlarged abomasum which is hence able to change place in the abdomen. Cows suffering from acute metritis after calving have a distinct decrease in dry matter intake, which might explain the remarkably high incidence of left displaced abomasum in these patients.

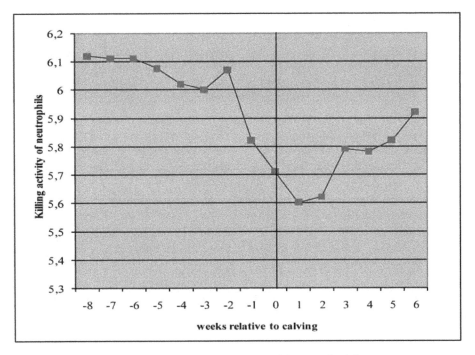

Figure 2. Killing activity of neutrophils around calving

A bad start usually ends up in a lot of costly troubles

Greater uterine bacterial contamination is associated with reduced ovarian follicular growth and function. Late resumption of regular ovarian cyclicity after parturition has, of course, long-term consequences for subsequent fertility. A comparison of ovarian activity in moderate yielding (4000-5000 kg milk per lactation) Friesian cows fed mainly grass and grass silage in Ireland (8), versus Belgian Holsteins producing 8000 to 9000 kg milk per lactation and fed high amounts of concentrates (18), revealed interesting differences. The Belgian cows not only had an increased number of puerperal disorders, but also a significantly elevated incidence of postpartum anoestrus, abnormal ovarian cycles and prolonged luteal phases (high progesterone for >20 days before breeding) (Table 3).

Table 3. A comparison of postpartum reproductive parameters based on measurement of progesterone in milk twice weekly in two different studies using moderate yielding Friesians (Fagan and Roche, 1986) or high-yielding Holsteins (Opsomer et al., 1998).

ResResults of studies based on progesterone analysis	Traditional herds (Fagan and Roche 1986)	High-yielding herds (Opsomer et al. 1998)
No. of cycles	448	463
Normal cyclical patterns (%)	78	53
Delayed cyclicity (%)	7	21
Temporary cessation of cyclicity (%)	3	3
Prolonged luteal phase (%)	3	20
Short cycles (%)	4	0,5
Other irregular patterns (%)	4	2,5

Large scale progesterone monitoring projects carried out in the UK over the last 30 years, have confirmed these striking data. Furthermore, a high number of puerperal disorders is significantly associated with an elevated number of postpartum aberrations of ovarian cyclicity, leading to an increased number of cows not seen in heat at the moment farmers should inseminate them.

Overt infection of the uterus will not only influence ovarian cyclicity (28), but also disrupt the establishment of pregnancy, both by the physiological presence of pus, as well by altered immune responses that are essential at the interface between the endometrium and the embryo. In this context, we can refer to cows discharging small amounts of pus in their mucus around the time of oestrus and insemination. While these cows are not clinically ill, they need veterinary attention because they may often end up as repeat breeders. Although it is quite obvious that pus reflects the presence of bacterial infection, in the majority of cases these small amounts of pus are just the remainders of the neutrophils which cleaned the uterus of bacterial contamination.

Based on the above, it is clear those difficulties during calving (dystocia) and immediately there after (e.g. retained placenta) predispose cows to endometritis and subfertility. Hence, all authors agree that the calculation of the total costs associated with uterine infections consists of a composition of both direct (such as treatment costs and the direct decrease in milk production), and indirect costs (such as increased number of inseminations, prolongation of the calving interval and increased culling rate). That's why depending on the source, calculated losses caused by puerperal disorders and endometritis vary between 160 to 420 euro per case.

Although a lot of authors mention that cows with puerperal disorders are at a significantly higher risk of other diseases, such as left displaced abomasum and ketosis, studies focusing on economic losses caused by endometritis often do not mention this. Therefore, it is clear that the figures mentioned are a serious underestimation of the real losses farmers have to face.

Negative energy balance

As NEB seems to be the ever-returning enemy of good fertility in high yielding dairy herds, the basic strategy to reduce the reproductive decline should definitely focus on keeping the NEB under control. While in modern dairy cows genetic progress in terms of milk yield has outstripped that for intake capacity, a certain degree of NEB is inevitable, certainly in early lactation (31). The extent of the NEB (both in depth as well as in duration) varies with the magnitude and rate of increase of milk yield compared to energy intake, however, and thus can be exacerbated if metabolic conditions, disease, housing or management practices impair nutrient intake.

Hence, management strategies by which the effect of a NEB can be limited must be targeted towards increasing nutrient intakes, especially energy. Immediately after calving, the paramount goal should be to maximize energy intake without disturbing rumen fermentation. The first aim of the management of a recently calved dairy cow is to optimize her general health status. Only when optimal health – including an excellent appetite – is achieved, can the focus shift towards achieving an optimal production level. In practice, in their enthusiasm to reach top production levels, farmers often forget this basic principle.

To optimize energy intake, all the while assuring optimal rumen fermentation, the intake of high quality forages in early lactation should be maximized. Once this has been achieved, the energy density of the ration may be increased by gradually raising the amount of concentrates. Generally, under Belgian circumstances, the maximum amount of concentrates given should not exceed 12 kg (9 kg in first lactation animals) and should only be reached at 3 weeks after calving (19). Increasing the amount of concentrates too fast may disturb ruminal fermentation, which in turn may give rise to ruminal acidosis and an increased incidence of left abomasal displacement.

Currently a lot of research is going on to study the effect of changing the proportion of the different ingredients of the ration. Increasing the amount of fat to maximize the energy content of the ration and hence the energy intake by the animal (16), or increasing the amount of glucogenic substances to temper the steep insulin decrease around the moment of calving (10) are excellent illustrations of such measures. For example, the ratio of n6:n3 fatty acids provided in the diet can influence the synthesis of the 2-series of prostaglandins, which are desirable after calving to speed up uterine involution, but undesirable after insemination as they can contribute to the breakdown of the corpus luteum of pregnancy. Hence, the practical implementation of our current knowledge needs to be a better timing of the introduction of rumen protected fats into the diet in accordance with the reproductive stage of the cow. Although primary results seem to be promising, these studies need further confirmation before definite conclusions can be drawn and the results transferred into practical recommendations.

Nutrient or dry matter intake is highly dependent on a lot of factors related both to the cow and to the environment. Among the cow factors, the general health status and body condition score are of major importance. Hence, transition cow programs should focus on maximizing general health and appetite and striving for the ideal body condition score of 3.5 (on 5-point scale) at calving. Aiming for optimal general health includes trimming of the claws at drying off, optimizing rumen health and avoiding metabolic and infectious diseases around calving. Besides this, the veterinarian should provide his herds with a specifically designed standard operating procedure for detecting ill cows as soon as possible and treating them properly.

Furthermore, efforts must be made to remove any environmental restrictions to feed intake, as the environment must be conducive to high intake. Cows need time and space for undisturbed feeding and rumination. There is clear evidence now that the design of food passages, barriers, troughs for water supply and cow traffic within the building definitely affect the intake cows will achieve (3). Intake can vary widely between individuals in a herd with a lot of competition for feeding space. Especially the intake of heifers is easily restricted by competition with older cows. The provision of adequate feeding space reduces this kind of competition largely. The grouping of cows and social behavior, also have their implications. A lot of attention should be paid to this point because during the transition period cows are transferred several times from one group to another. Each transfer or relocation implies another challenge for the cows as it brings them in contact with a new group and a new ration. All the energy that is spent in establishing a new social hierarchy is no longer available to produce or reproduce. At the same time, each change in the ration causes a serious drop in dry matter intake and should therefore also be avoided (3).

Although veterinary practitioners are currently not the only advisors on modern dairy herds, they have the advantage that they can use their "clinical eyes" to interpret what is happening in the herd (35). Besides the use of herd production data which are usually readily available, the use of clinical scoring systems has been proven to provide the veterinarian with an extra tool to evaluate the health status of the animals in relation to their production level. Hence, these scoring systems should be used to evaluate the management system used on the herds at a regular time interval. Furthermore, today's dairy cows may face a wide variety of environmental stressors. These may include overcrowding, infectious challenges, poor ventilation, poor footing or other forms of chronic or even acute pain, uncomfortable stables, rough handling, and frequent relocation in another group. Most of these stressors affect fertility and should therefore be avoided (7). Although stress is difficult to define and to show to the herd manager, a lack in cow comfort compromising the cows' health and fertility should be noticed and discussed during the regular herd health visits. While top managers have it at their finger-tips and do not need a lot of explanation to adapt their herd to the needs of their modern top producers, others definitely need to be confronted with some eye-openers.

CONCLUSIONS

In view of the complex nature of fertility, it is not surprising to find that ideal fertility criteria are extremely difficult to achieve. When infections are involved in a subfertility problem, this can be due either to specific (e.g. BVDV) or non-specific genital infections. The former often strike a whole herd, causing abortions and repeat breeding. The latter are opportunists of unsanitary conditions during calving, dystocia and abnormal puerperium. They often take an insidious course.

It is generally agreed, however, that the main negative influence on the fertility of a dairy herd stems not as much from specific or non-specific infections, but rather from the effects of a host of other factors. These factors seldom exert their effects individually but rather interact together, making it difficult to analyze infertility in a given herd. For example, the advancement of animal husbandry practices has increased both herd size and production, but man hours per cow have dwindled. The direct result of this decrease is that less time remains for detecting heats, instituting hygienic measures and trimming claws. Thus the final fertility status of a dairy herd is the result of interactions of a whole range of factors from environmental conditions such as season, herd size and age composition, to pure managerial factors such as breeding policy, nutrition and estrus detection. Breeding efficiency depends almost totally on whether or not the farmer is able to skillfully cope with these factors in his herd. By way of conclusion, subfertility has been proven to be a multifactorial disease and the optimization of herd fertility often requires the optimization of several interfering managerial factors. There is almost never a single solution. Although poor fertility is becoming more and more common in our top dairy herds, there is a wide variation between herds and sometimes between years within the same herd. This latter fact illustrates that the dairy herd acts as a dynamic structure and may need specific adaptations, depending on the specific situations the herd actually has to face.

Fertility of a dairy herd is thus a relative phenomenon, expressing what the cows have been able to achieve in the face of a host of interacting factors. To avoid a deterioration of fertility below the accepted standards, the advice given to the farmer should enable him to optimally manage his herd under the given environmental and management conditions. Such advice can best be given by paying regular visits to the farmer (Herd Health and Fertility Control Program) so as to impress upon him the relevant factors of management. Hence, the follow-up of the reproductive performance of a dairy herd should be continuous and not only be restricted to the curative interventions when things are really going wrong.

The cornerstone to improving the reproductive performance of lactating dairy cattle also involves the understanding of the biochemical and physiological principles controlling reproductive and lactational processes. The challenge is to integrate this knowledge into nutritional management, production medicine and reproductive management procedures, taking into account the specific obstacles each individual herd has to face, for the purpose of optimizing the fertility of the herd (30). In the absence of such a holistic approach, the response to traditional veterinary therapies and herd health programs may increasingly diminish.

REFERENCES

1. Bouters, R., Vandeplassche, M. (1977). Post partum infection in cattle: diagnosis and preventive and curative treatment. Journal of the South African Veterinary Association, 48, 237-239.

2. Butler, W.R. (2000). Nutritional interactions with reproductive performance in dairy cattle. Animal Reproduction Science, 60, 449-457.

3. Cook N, Nordlund K. (2004). Behavorial needs of the transition cow and considerations for special needs facility design. Vet Clin North Am, Food Anim Practi, 20, 495-520.

4. Curtis, C., Erb, H., Sniffen, C., Smith, R., Kronfeld, D. (1985). Path analysis of dry period nutrition, postpartum metabolic and reproductive disorders, and mastitis in Holstein cows. Journal of Dairy Science, 68, 2347-2360.

5. Correa M., Erb, H., Scarlett, J. (1993). Path analysis for seven postpartum disorders of Holstein cows. Journal of Dairy Science, 76, 1305-1312.

6. De Kruif, A., Leroy, J., Opsomer, G. (2008). Reproductive performance in high producing dairy cows: practical implicataions. Tierärztliche Praxis, 36 (Suppl 1), S29-S33.

7. Dobson, H., Smith, RF. (2001). What is stress, and how does it affect reproduction? Anim Repro Sci, 60-61, 743-752.

8. Fagan, J.G., Roche, J.F. (1986). Reproductive activity in post partum dairy cows based on progesterone concentrations in milk or rectal examination. Irish Veterinary Journal, 40, 124-131.

9. Gilbert, R., Shin, S., Guard, C., Erb, H., Frajblat, M. (2005). Prevalence of endometritis and its effects on reproductive performance of dairy cows. Theriogenology, 64, 1879-1888.

10. Gong, JG., Lee, WJ., Garnsworthy, PC., Webb, R. (2002). Effect of dietary-induced increases in circulating insulin concentrations during the early postpartum period on reproductive function in dairy cows. Repro, 123, 419-427.

11. Hoeben, D., Monfardini, E., Opsomer, G., Burvenich, C., Dosogne, H., de Kruif, A., Beckers, JF. (2000). Chemiluminescence of

bovine polymorphonuclear leucocytes during the periparturient period and relation with metabolic markers and bovine pregnancy-associated glycoprotein. Journal of Dairy Research, 67, 249-259.

12. Kasimanickam, R., Duffield, T., Foster, R., Gartley, C., Leslie, K., Walton, J. (2004). Endometrial cytology and ultrasonography for the detection of subclinical endometritis in postpartum dairy cows. Theriogenology, 62, 9-23.

13. LeBlanc, S.J., Duffield, T.F., Leslie, K.E., Bateman, K.G., Keefe, G.P., Walton, J.S., Johnson, W.H. (2002). Defining and diagnosing postpartum clinical endometritis and its impact on reproductive performance in dairy cows. Journal of Dairy Science, 85, 2223-2236.

14. Lucy, M.C. (2001). Reproductive loss in high-producing dairy cattle: where will it end? Journal of Dairy Science, 84, 1277-1293.

15. Leroy, J.L.M.R., de Kruif, A. (2006). Reduced reproductive performance in high producing dairy cows: is there actually a problem? Vlaams Diergeneeskundig Tijdschrift, 75, 55-60.

16. Mattos, R., Staples, CR., Thatcher, W.W. (2000). Effects of dietary fatty acids on reproduction in ruminants. Rev Repro, 5, 38-45.

17. Oltenacu, P.A., Frick, A., Lindhé, B. (1990). Epidemiological study of several clinical diseases, reproductive performance and culling in primiparous Swedish cattle. Preventive Veterinary Medicine, 9, 59-74.

18. Opsomer, G., Coryn, M., Deluyker, H., de Kruif, A. (1998). An analysis of ovarian dysfunction in high yielding dairy cows after calving based on progesterone profiles. Reproduction in Domestic Animals, 33, 193-204.

19. Opsomer, G., De Vliegher, S., de Kruif, A. (2004). Droogstand en transitieperiode van hoogproductieve melkkoeien: wat met de voeding? Vlaams Diergeneeskundig Tijdschrift, 73, 374-383.

20. Opsomer, G., Gröhn, Y.T., Coryn, M., Hertl, J., Deluyker H., de Kruif, A. (2000a). Risk factors for postpartum ovarian dysfunction in high producing dairy cows in Belgium. Theriogenology, 53, 841-857.

21. Opsomer, G., Laevens, H., Steegen, N., de Kruif, A. (2000b). A descriptive study of postpartal anoestrus in nine high-yielding dairy herds in Belgium. Vlaams Diergeneeskundig Tijdschrift, 69, 31-37.

22. Opsomer, G., Leroy, J., Vanholder T., Bossaert, P., de Kruif, A (2006a). High milk production and good fertility in modern dairy cows: the results of some recent research items. Slovenian Veterinary Research, 43, 31-39.

23. Opsomer, G., Leroy, J., Vanholder, T., Bossaert, P., de Kruif, A. (2006b). Subfertility in high yielding dairy cows: how te bring science into practice? Vlaams Diergeneeskundig Tijdschrift, 75, 113-119.

24. Peeler, E.J., Otte, M.J., Esslemont, R.J. (1994). Interrelationships of periparturient diseases in dairy cows. Veterinary Record, 134, 129-132.

25. Royal, M.D., Darwash, A.O., Flint, A.P.F., Webb, R., Wooliams, J.A., Lamming, G.E. (2000a). Declining fertility in dairy cattle: changes in traditional and endocrine parameters of fertility. Animal Science, 70, 487-501.

26. Royal, M.D., Mann, G.E., Flint, A.P.F. (2000b). Strategies for reversing the trend towards subfertility in dairy cattle. Veterinary Journal, 160, 53-60.

27. Sheldon, I.M., Dobson, H. (2004). Postpartum uterine health in cattle. Animal Reproduction Science, 64, 295-306.

28. Sheldon, I.M., Noakes, D.E., Rycroft, A.N., Pfeiffer, D.U., Dobson, H. (2002). Influence of uterine bacterial contamination after parturition on ovarian dominant follicle selection and follicle growth and function in cattle. Reproduction, 123, 837-845.

29. Tennant, B., Peddicord, R.G. (1968). The influence of delayed uterine involution and endometritis on bovine fertility. Cornell Veterinarian, 58, 185-192.

30. Thatcher, W., Bilby, T., Bartolome, J., Silvestre, F., Staples, C., Santos, J. (2006). Strategies for improving fertility in the modern dairy cow. Theriogenol, 65, 30-44.

31. Thomas, C., Leach, KA., Logue, DN., Ferries, C., Phipps, RH. (1999). Management options to reduce load. In: JD Oldham, G. Simm, AF Groen, BL Nielsen, JE Pryce, TLJ. Lawrence (Eds.), Metabolic stress in dairy cows (pp 129-139). Occasional publication No. 24., British Society of Animal Science.

32. Van Winden, S., Jorritsma, R., Müller, K., Noordhuizen, J. (2003). Feed intake, milk yield and metabolic parameters prior to left displaced abomasum in dairy cows. Journal of Dairy Science, 86, 1465-1471.

33. Vanholder, T., Leroy, J.L.M.R., Opsomer, G., de Kruif, A. (2006). Interactions between energy balance and ovarian activity in high yielding dairy cows early postpartum: A review. Vlaams Diergeneeskundig Tijdschrift, 75, 79-85.

34. Whitmore, H., Anderson, K. (1986). Possible adverse effects of antimicrobial treatments of uterine infections. In: Morrow D.A., W.B. (Ed.), Current therapy in theriogenology; Vol 2. (pp.42-44). Saunders, Philadelphia.

35. Zaaijer, D., Noordhuizen, JPTM. (2003). A novel scoring system for monitoring the relationship between nutritional efficiency and fertility in dairy cows. Irish Vet J, 56, 145-151.

6

DEVELOPMENT AND VALIDATION OF CONFIRMATORY METHOD FOR ANALYSIS OF NITROFURAN METABOLITES IN MILK, HONEY, POULTRY MEAT AND FISH BY LIQUID CHROMATOGRAPHY-MASS SPECTROMETRY

Fatih Alkan[1], Arzu Kotan[1], Nurullah Ozdemir[2]

[1]Pendik Veterinary Control Institute, Department of Pharmacology, Laboratory of Residue. 34890 Pendik, Istanbul, Turkey
[2]Namik Kemal University, Veterinary Faculty, Department of Pharmacology and Toxicology, Degirmenalti Mevkii, 59030 Tekirdag, Turkey

ABSTRACT

In this study we have devoloped and validated a confirmatory analysis method for nitrofuran metabolites, which is in accordance with European Commission Decision 2002/657/EC requirements. Nitrofuran metabolites in honey, milk, poultry meat and fish samples were acidic hydrolised followed by derivatisation with nitrobenzaldehyde and liquid-liquid extracted with ethylacetate. The quantitative and confirmative determination of nitrofuran metbolites was performed by liquid chromatography/electrospray ionisation tandem mass spectrometry (LC/ESI-MS/MS) in the positive ion mode. In-house method validation was performed and reported data of validation (specificity, linearity, recovery, CC_α and CC_β). The advantage of this method is that it avoids the use of clean-up by Solid-Phase Extraction (SPE). Furthermore, low levels of nitrofuran metabolites are detectable and quantitatively confirmed at a rapid rate in all samples.

Key words: fish, honey, LC-MS/MS, milk, nitrofuran metabolites, poultry meat

INTRODUCTION

Nitrofurans are broad spectrum antibacterial agents known as Schiff's bases, which are derivates of nitrofuraldehyde. In veterinary medicine, it were used in the treatment of gastrointestinal and dermatological infections in beef, pork, poultry, fish and shrimp, and also applied as a contribution to the systemic and feed as growth promoters. In addition, nitrofurans were used in the treatment of bacterial infections in bee colony health (1).

Nitrofurans have been prohibited from use in food-producing animals in the European Union and most countries due to public health and safety concerns, particularly in relation to the carcinogenic potential of either the parent compounds or their metabolites (2). The use of nitrofurans in food-producing animal was prohibited in Turkey (3).

A minimum required performance limit (MRPL) for nitrofurans is set in European Union for the metabolites in poultry meat and aquaculture products at the level of 1 µg kg^{-1} for all metabolites (4).

Analytically, residues are checked only for marker metabolites of the 4 nitrofuran chemicals, in particular: 3-amino-2-oxazolidinone (AOZ) for furazolidone, 3-amino-5-methylmorpholino-2-oxazolidinone (AMOZ) for furaltadone, 1-aminohydantoin (AHD) for nitrofurantoin and semicarbazide (SEM) for nitrofurazone (5).

Several methods have been reported in the analysis of nitrofuran metabolite in food samples. These include thin-layer chromatography (TLC) (6), high performance liquid chromatography diode-array detector (HPLC DAD) (7) and UV detector (8, 9), liquid chromatography-mass

Corresponding author: Assist. Prof. Nurullah Ozdemir, PhD
E-mail address: nozdemir@nku.edu.tr
Present address: University of Namik Kemal, Faculty of Veterinary Medicine, Department of Pharmacology and Toxicology 59030 Tekirdag, Turkey

spectrometry (LC-MS/MS) (10, 11, 12). LC-MS/MS analyses were considered very sensitive and commonly used the confirmatory analysis.

In the current study, a method was devoloped and validated for quick confirmatory analysis of nitrofuran metabolites (AOZ, AMOZ, AHD and SEM). All samples were acidic hydrolised followed by derivatisation with nitrobenzaldehyde and liquid-liquid extracted with ethylacetate. The quantitative and confirmatory determination of nitrofuran metabolites was performed by liquid chromatography/electrospray ionisation tandem mass spectrometry (LC/ESI-MS/MS) in the positive ion mode.

MATERIAL AND METHODS

Reagents and standards

3-amino-2-oxazolidinone (AOZ), 1-aminohydantoin (AHD), AMOZ-d5, $(C^{13})_3$-AHD, $C^{13}N^{15}$-N^{15}-SEM, 2NP-AOZ, 2NP-AMOZ, 2NP-AHD and 2-nitrobenzaldehyde (2-NBA), 3-amino-5-morpholinomethyl-2-oxazolidinon (AMOZ), semicarbazide hydrochloride (SEM), AOZ-d4, 2NP-AOZ-D4, 2NP-AMOZ-D5, 2NP-$(C^{13})_3$–AHD and 2NP-$C^{13}N^{15}$-N^{15}-SEM were obtained from Dr. Ehrenstorfer and Witega. The purity of all compounds was greater than 99%.

Methanol (MeOH) and ethylacetate (LC grade), hydrochloric acid (HCl), dimethylsulphoxide (DMSO), *n*-hexane and potassium hydrogen phosphate were supplied by Merck. The water was purified with a from a Milli-Q purifying system (Elga PureLab Prima).

Individual standart stock solutions of 1 mg/mL were prepared in methanol, but SEM was prepared in DMSO. Working solutions of 10 ng/mL were diluted by methanol. All standard stock soutions were stored -20 °C, and the working solutions were stored in refrigerator.

The concentration and content of mix standard solution were used to spiked samples with AMOZ, AOZ, AHD and SEM at a 8, 16, 20 and 20 ng/mL respectively. The concentration and content of internal mix standard solutions were used AOZ-d4, AMOZ-d5, $(C^{13})_3$-AHD and $C^{13}N^{15}$-N^{15}-SEM at a 40, 40, 100 and 100 ng/mL, respectively.

Sample preparation

Collected samples for validation were known to be negative in the screening analysis within the national program for residues control in Turkey. Only, the milk samples were centrifuged at 3500 g, +4°C, 15 min and upper the fat layer was removed before extraction.

Two grams or 2 mL homogenised samples (milk, honey, poultry meat and fish) were weighed into 50 mL polypropylene centrifuge tubes. Standard spiking solution mix (50, 100, 150 and 200 µL), internal standard solution mix (100 µL) and 5 mL of 0.1 M HCl were added. The extraxtion tube was shaken for 2 min by vortex. 2-nitrobenzaldehyde (2-NBA) (50 mM, 300 µL) were added and the mixture shaken for 2 min by vortex. The tube were capped and incubated overnight (16 h) in the 37°C temperature. After derivatization, the samples were cooled in room temperature and neutralized by addition 1 mL of 1 M K_2PO_4 and mixed for 2 min by vortex. Ethylacetate (5 mL) and n-hexane (3 mL) was added and mixed for 15 min by vortex and centrifuged at 4000 g for 15 min. The organic phase (6 mL) was collected into a 15 mL graduated glass tubes. The organic fraction was evaporated to dryness under a stream of nitrogen in a water bath at 42°C.

The dry residue was reconstituted with n-hexane (2 mL) and mixed for 2 min by vortex and methanol/water (5/95) (0.7 mL) was added and mixed for 2 min by vortex. 0.5 mL samples were taken from the lower phase with the help of syringe or automatic pipette and filtered using a 0.2 µm syringe filter into an autosampler vial.

Instrumentation

Chromatographic analyses were performed on a LC-MS/MS equipment consisted of a Thermo Electron TSQ Quantum Access Max, mass spectrometer controlled by the Xcalibur (2.2 SP1) software.

Chromatographic separations were achieved on Phenomenex Synergy Hydro RP (150x2.00 mm 80Å 4 µm), protected with a C18 guard column. The mobile phase was deionised water/methanol (80/20) (A) and methanol acidified with 0.1% acetic acid. The linear gradient was: 0-2 min 100% A, 2-9 min 10% A and 9-15 min 100% A and flow rate of 0.25 mL/min. Injection volume was 50 µL. The column was thermostated at 40 °C. The analysis of samples were carried in the positive ESI-MS-MS ion mode.

Mass spectrometry

MS/MS parameters and precursor-product ions of each compound were tuned by direct infusion in the SRM mode and 0.25 mL/min flow rate of the mobile phase A and B) (50:50).

The concentration and content of mix standards derivatizes and internal standards used for control of the MS-detector, were 25 µg kg^{-1} for 2-NP-SEM-$C^{13}N^{15}$-N^{15} and 2-NP-$(C^{13})_3$-AHD and other standards at 10 µg kg^{-1} .

MS/MS detector parameters are given in Table 1. The precursor-product ions of each compound and their collision energy are given in Table 2.

Table 1. MS detector parameters

Ionization Mode	ESI +	
Spray Voltage	3000	
Vaporizer Temperature	300 °C	
Capillary Temperature	300 °C	
Sheath Gas	35 psi	
Ion Sweep Gas	0,5 psi	
Aux Gas	15 psi	
Skimmer Offset	3	
Q2 CID Gas	1,3 psi	
Data Proses	5	
Mass peak width in amu	Q1=0,7	Q3=0,7

RESULTS

Specificity/Selectivity

Specificity/selectivity were evaluated via analysis of blank matrix samples fortified with mixed benzimidazole and nitroimidazole standards (concentration of 1 µg kg^{-1} each) and with standards of nitrofuran metabolites. According to analysis no significant peaks with an S/N (signal to noise) ratios of 3 or more and chromatographic interference were being observed at the retention times of the targeted nitrofuran metabolites.

Linearity

The matrix calibration curves were at four levels: 0.4, 0.8, 1.2 and 1.6 µg kg^{-1} for AOZ, AMOZ, AHD and SEM, which is in accordance with the MRPL levels. For each compound we made three matrix calibration curves, using blank samples, over three days with 6 replicates at four concentration levels. No significant differences were found between the different matrix curves (r^2>0.9941) shown in Table 3.

Table 2. LC–MS/MS confirmation parameters for the analytes

Analyte	MS MH+ (m/z)	MS-MS (m/z)	Collision Energy	Width	Tube Lens	Dwell Time
2-NP-SEM	209.0	166.0*	11	0,05	98	0,1
		192.0	13	0,05	98	0,1
2-NP-SEM-$C^{13}N^{15}$-N^{15}	212.0	168.0	10	0,05	115	0,1
2-NP-AHD	249.0	134.0	12	0,05	71	0,1
		104.1*	22	0,05	71	0,1
2-NP-$(C^{13})_3$-AHD	252.0	134.0	12	0,05	71	0,1
2-NP-AOZ	236.0	134.0	13	0,05	64	0,1
		104.0*	22	0,05	64	0,1
2-NP-AOZ-D4	240.0	133.9	12	0,05	65	0,1
2-NP-AMOZ	335.0	291.0	12	0,05	70	0,1
		261.9*	17	0,05	70	0,1
2-NP-AMOZ-D5	340.0	296.0	12	0,05	71	0,1

*Confirmation ion

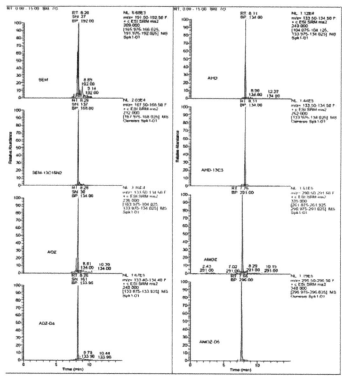

Figure 1. Chromatograms of blank milk samples fortified at 0.2 µg kg⁻¹ for AMOZ, 0.3 µg kg⁻¹ for AOZ and AHD, 0.4 µg kg⁻¹ for SEM

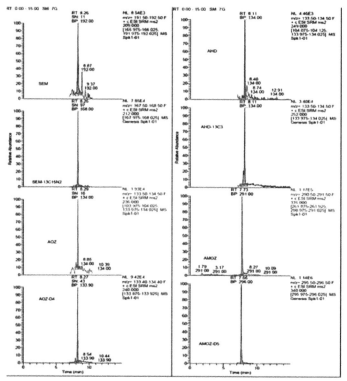

Figure 2. Chromatograms of blank honey samples fortified at 0.2 µg kg⁻¹ for AMOZ, 0.4 µg kg⁻¹ for AOZ and SEM, 0.5 µg kg⁻¹ for AHD

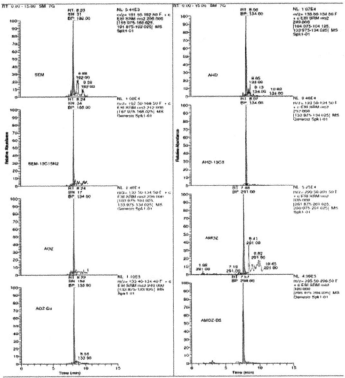

Figure 3. Chromatograms of blank poultry meat samples fortified at 0.2 µg kg⁻¹ for AMOZ, 0.4 µg kg⁻¹ for AOZ, 0.5 µg kg⁻¹ for SEM and AHD

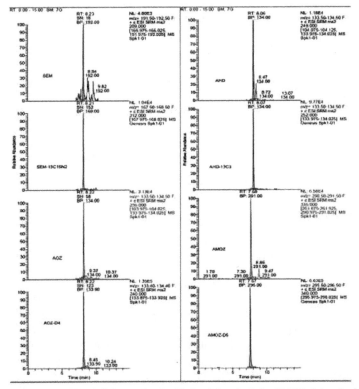

Figure 4. Chromatograms of blank fish samples fortified at 0.2 µg kg⁻¹ for AMOZ, 0.4 µg kg⁻¹ for AOZ, 0.5 µg kg⁻¹ for SEM and AHD

Decision limit (CC$_\alpha$) and detection capability (CC$_\beta$)

The CC$_\alpha$ and CC$_\beta$ for banned substances were calculated with the application of the following formula;

$$CC\alpha = C_1 + 2.33 \times SD_{wIR}$$

where in C$_1$ is lowest concentration level of the validation study (MRPL) and SD$_{wIR}$ is the standard deviation from within-laboratory reproducibility.

$$CC\beta = CC\alpha + 1.64 \times SD_{wIR,CC\alpha}$$

where in SD$_{wIR,CC\alpha}$ is standard deviation at CC$_\alpha$ concentration.

For each compound of CC$_\alpha$ and CC$_\beta$ were calculated from the linearity study. The mean value CCα and CCβ were presented in Table 3.

ESI-MS conditions. Figure 1, 2, 3 and 4 show LC/MS/MS extracted-ion chromatograms obtained from analysis of a spiked samples.

This method has been developed and in-house validated in four different matrices (milk, honey, poultry meat and fish) according to the European Commission Decision 2002/657/EC requirements (13). Also, all four matrices have been accredited according to ISO 17025 by TURKAK (Agency of Accreditation in Turkey).

The majority of the method for nitrofuran metabolites in food then employ a solid phase extraction (SPE) step in order clean-up. Barbosa et al. (7), determinated of nitrofurans in animal feeds by liquid chromatography-UV photodiode

Table 3. Summary of Linearity, CC$_\alpha$, and CC$_\beta$

Analyte	Calibration range ($\mu g\ kg^{-1}$)	Linearity (r^2)				CC$_\alpha$ ($\mu g\ kg^{-1}$)				CC$_\beta$ ($\mu g\ kg^{-1}$)			
		Honey	Milk	Poultry Meat	Fish	Honey	Milk	Poultry Meat	Fish	Honey	Milk	Poultry Meat	Fish
AOZ	0.4-1.6	0.999	0.998	0.994	0.997	0.44	0.33	0.45	0.45	0.46	0.35	0.48	0.48
AMOZ	0.2-0.8	0.999	0.998	0.998	0.996	0.21	0.22	0.22	0.23	0.22	0.23	0.23	0.24
AHD	0.5-2.0	0.998	0.999	0.995	0.996	0.54	0.34	0.56	0.59	0.57	0.37	0.60	0.65
SEM	0.4-0.6	0.996	0.995	0.994	0.995	0.44	0.47	0.59	0.61	0.47	0.51	0.65	0.69

Recovery

The method recoveries and RSDs were determined from 6 replicates at four concentration levels spiking blank samples over three days. The recovery results were observed in acceptable range of 70-110%. All the data relating to method recovery and precision were summarisedin Table 4; mean recoveries ranging and CV% values were satisfactory, required by Decision 2002/657/EC.

Evaluation

In order to evaluate this method, it eventually participating in the Food Analysis Performance Assessment Scheme (FAPAS), the test of "Nitrofuran Metabolites in Prawns" (FAPAS 02229, 12/05/2014, Lab No:75). AOZ total assigned value were 0.934 µg kg^{-1} , the results of our laboratory 0.8 µg kg^{-1} . Z-score were -0.7. The result is good and satisfactory.

DISCUSSION

To measure nitrofuran metabolites using the selective reaction-monitoring (SRM) mode, full scan and product ion spectra of the analytes were investigated under the LC conditions described in mass Spectrometry section. Nitrofuran metabolites could be detected under positive ionization mode

array detection and liquid chromatography-ionspray tandem mass spectrometry. Following ethyl acetate extraction at mild alkaline conditions and purification on NH$_2$ column (SPE), the nitrofurans are determined using liquid chromatography with photodiode-array detection (LC-DAD).

Mottier et al. (11) quantitative determinated of four nitrofuran metabolites in meat by isotope dilution liquid chromatography–electrospray ionisation–tandem mass spectrometry. This study, was used a method liquid–liquid extraction and clean-up on a polymeric solid phase extraction cartridge (SPE) are then performed before LC–MS/MS analysis by positive electrospray ionisation (ESI).

Consequently this LC–ESI–MS–MS method allows the simultaneous determination of nitrofuran metabolites in four matrix. The method avoids the use of clean-up by SPE and could be performed quickly. The obtained validation results indicate the accordance of the method with Decision 2002/657/EC (13). The repeatability and within-laboratory reproducibility (precision) of the method are less than 9.86 % for all analytes. The CC$_\alpha$ and CC$_\beta$ are below the MRPL of 1 µg kg-1. This method has been used for confirmatory analysis of nitrofuran metabolites in honey, milk, poultry meat and fish sample.

Table 4. Recovery of nitrofuran metabolites: between-day repeat measures

	Honey				Milk				Poultry Meat				Fish			
	Added Amount µg kg⁻¹	Mean Amount Calculated µg kg⁻¹	Rec %	CV %	Added Amount µg kg⁻¹	Mean Amount Calculated µg kg⁻¹	Rec %	CV %	Added Amount µg kg⁻¹	Mean Amount Calculated µg kg⁻¹	Rec %	CV %	Added Amount µg kg⁻¹	Mean Amount Calculated µg kg⁻¹	Rec %	CV %
AOZ	0.4	0.40	100.50	5.27	0.3	0.30	98.96	4.69	0.4	0.40	99.75	3.98	0.4	0.41	102.08	1.23
	0.8	0.80	100.25	1.42	0.6	0.60	99.67	2.13	0.8	0.78	97.54	4.88	0.8	0.79	98.13	4.22
	1.2	1.19	99.22	0.82	0.9	0.91	101.81	0.64	1.2	1.24	103.61	1.57	1.2	1.21	100.42	2.33
	1.6	1.61	100.35	0.67	1.2	1.19	99.14	0.62	1.6	1.58	98.60	0.40	1.6	1.60	100.10	1.46
AMOZ	0.2	0.20	101.00	3.09	0.2	0.20	100.50	1.99	0.2	0.20	99.33	3.64	0.2	0.20	100.00	1.80
	0.4	0.39	98.58	1.30	0.4	0.40	100.75	1.55	0.4	0.40	99.58	1.82	0.4	0.40	100.33	1.70
	0.6	0.61	100.83	0.29	0.6	0.59	98.33	1.48	0.6	0.61	101.28	1.53	0.6	0.60	99.44	1.37
	0.8	0.80	99.79	1.25	0.8	0.81	100.71	1.26	0.8	0.80	99.46	0.62	0.8	0.80	100.25	1.07
AHD	0.5	0,50	99.33	4.42	0.3	0.31	102.00	3.32	0.5	0.52	103.93	2.90	0.5	0.48	96.40	5.24
	1.0	1,00	99.70	3.12	0.6	0.59	98.56	2.02	1.0	0.98	97.70	4.88	1.0	1.01	101.13	4.81
	1.5	1.52	101.00	1.44	0.9	0.90	99.93	1.01	1.5	1.49	99.07	4.04	1.5	1.53	102.11	1.15
	2.0	1.99	99.53	0.98	1.2	1.20	100.31	0.43	2.0	2.02	100.85	1.76	2.0	1.97	98.73	0.82
SEM	0.4	0.40	100.00	2.50	0.4	0.39	97.67	6.84	0.5	0.49	97.73	6.29	0.5	0.49	98.73	9.86
	0.8	0.80	100.29	3.25	0.8	0.80	99.67	3.93	1.0	1.00	99.97	3.88	1.0	0.99	98.57	0.06
	1.2	1.20	99.64	4.00	1.2	1.23	102.67	1.25	1.5	1.54	102.33	3.94	1.5	1.55	103.11	1.83
	1.6	1.60	100.13	1.58	1.6	1.58	98.73	1.84	2.0	1.98	98.83	2.40	2.0	1.97	98.68	1.89

CONCLUSION

A rapid and sensitive method described in this paper provides reliable, simultaneous quantitative analysis for nitrofuran metabolites residues in milk, honey, poultry meat and fish samples. The optimized procedure provides significant advantages including simplicity, low operation cost, avoids the use of clean-up by SPE.

Thus should be performed quickly confirmative analysis for nitrofuran metabolites residues in milk, honey, poultry meat and fish samples and used as a routine analysis.

REFERENCES

1. Barbosa J., Ferreira S., Pais A.C., Silveria M.I.N. Ramos F. (2011). Nitrofuran in poultry: use, control and residue analysis. In: Hendricks B.P, editor. Agricultural researche updates volume 1. (p 1-50). Hauppauge, New York: Nova Science Publishers, Inc.

2. Commission Decision 1995/1442/EC, 1995 of 26 June 1995, amending of Annexes I, II, III and IV to Regulation (ECC) No 2377/90, laying down a Community Procedure for the establishment of maximum residue limits of veterinary medicinal products in foodstuffs of animal origin. Off. J. Eur. Union, L143;26-30.

3. Commission Decision 2003/181/EC, 13 March 2003, amending decision 2002/657/EC as regards the setting of minimum performance limits (MRPLs) for certain residues in food animal origin, Off. J. Eur. Union, L71/17, 2003.

4. Turkish Food Codex. 2012/23856.

5. European Food Safety Authority (2015). Scientific opinion on nitrofurans and their metabolites in food. EFSA Journal 2015, 13(6): 4140.

6. Harry S.V., George W.H. (1981). Highly specific and sensitive detection method for nitrofurans by thin-layer chromatography. J Chromatogr A, 208 (1), 161-163.
http://dx.doi.org/10.1016/S0021-9673(00)87980-7

7. Barbosa J., Moura S., Barbosa R., Ramos F. Silveria M.I.N. (2007). Determination of nitrofurans in animal feeds by liquid chromatography-UV photodiode array detection and liquid chromatography-ionspray tandem mass- spectrometry. Anal Chim Acta, 586, 359–365.
http://dx.doi.org/10.1016/j.aca.2006.11.053
PMid:17386735

8. McCracken R.J., Kennedy D.G. (1997). Determination of furazolidone in animal feeds chromatography with UV and thermospray mass detection. J Chromatogr A, 771, 349-354.
http://dx.doi.org/10.1016/S0021-9673(97)00178-7

9. Cooper K.M., Mulder P.P.J., Van Rhijn J.A., Kovacsics L., Mccracken R.J., Young P.B. Kennedy D.G. (2005). Depletion of four nitrofuran antibiotics and their tissue-bound metabolites in porcine tissues and determination using LC-MS/MS and HPLC-UV. Food Addit Contam, 22(5): 406–414.
http://dx.doi.org/10.1080/02652030512331385218
PMid:16019811

10. Rodziewicz L. (2008). Determination of nitrofuran metabolites in milk by liquid chromatography–electrospray ionization tandem mass spectrometry. Journal of Chromatography B, 864 156–160.
http://dx.doi.org/10.1016/j.jchromb.2008.01.008
PMid:18280226

11. Mottier P., Khong S.P., Gremaud E., Richoz J., Delatour T., Goldman T Guy P.A. (2005). Quantitative determination of four nitrofuran metabolites in meat by isotope dilution liquid chromatography–electrospray ionisation–tandem mass spectrometry. J Chromatogr A, 1067 85–91.
http://dx.doi.org/10.1016/j.chroma.2004.08.160

12. Szilagyi S., Calle B. (2006). Development and validation of an analytical method for the determination of semicarbazide in fresh egg and in egg powder based on the use of liquid chromatography tandem mass spectrometry Analytica Chimica Acta, 572, 113–120.
http://dx.doi.org/10.1016/j.aca.2006.05.012
PMid:17723467

13. Commission Decision 2003/181/EC, 13 March 2003, amending decision 2002/657/EC as regards the setting of minimum performance limits (MRPLs) for certain residues in food animal origin, Off. J. Eur. Union, L71/17, 2003.

7

THE EFFECTS OF L-CARNITINE IN BUDD-CHIARI SYNDROME IN A DOMESTIC CAT

Aliye Sağkan Öztürk[1], Nuri Altuğ[2], Serkan İrfan Köse[1], Oktay Hasan Öztürk[3]

[1]Department of Internal Medicine, Faculty of Veterinary Medicine,
Mustafa Kemal University, 31040, Hatay, Turkey
[2]Department of Internal Medicine, Faculty of Veterinary Medicine,
Namık Kemal University, 59030, Tekirdağ, Turkey
[3]Department of Biochemistry, Faculty of Medicine, Akdeniz University,
07985, Antalya, Turkey

ABSTRACT

This paper describes a thrombosis in the vena cava caudalis of a 15 year-old cat with ascites. Trauma and eventually feline enteric corona virus infection in the cat were not detected. In the intrahepatic region, a blockage of vena cava caudalis was brought to light by ultrasonographic imaging. An aspirate of abdominal fluid revealed modified transudate. Liver enzyme levels were increased in the serum sample of the cat. The levels of total oxidant status (TOS) and total antioxidant status (TAS) were elevated in the peritoneal fluid. Liver protection diet with L-carnitine, diuretic therapy and antimicrobial drugs were administrated for treatment of the cat. During the continuous treatment, the amount of abdominal fluid decreased, but never completely absorbed. L-carnitine was administered to the cat during the time of treatment, and subsequently the levels of liver enzymes decreased. However, the cat died because of recurrent ascites and persistent thrombosis. In conclusion, ultrasonographic examination was very reliable, non-invasive and highly useful diagnostic method for BCS and L-carnitine has crucial effects on the quality of life, energy metabolism and liver enzyme levels. However, the blockage of the vena cava caudalis could not completely respond to medical treatment and thrombosis should be eliminated by surgical intervention.

Key words: Budd-Chiari syndrome, cat, L-carnitine, peritoneal fluid

INTRODUCTION

Budd-Chiari syndrome (BCS) is a clinical condition resulting from the blockage of the main hepatic veins or vena cava caudalis (1, 2). Nakamura et al. (3) determined membranous obstructions affected both vena cava caudalis and the hepatic veins. In 18% of cases, only the vena cava caudalis was affected, while the hepatic veins were affected in 10% of the cases. The blockages in the vena cava caudalis can be severe and may cause hepatocellular necrosis, hepatic failure, cirrhosis, and encephalopathy (4, 5). BCS is very rare in the literature and practice in domestic animals. Therefore, the aim of this case report was to describe Budd-Chiari syndrome in a cat, with mild clinical, ultrasonographic and laboratory findings, as well as treatment of affected cat. Laboratory findings were used to evaluate the effects of L-carnitine on liver and oxidative status of the cat.

Corresponding author: Asst. Prof. Serkan İrfan Köse, PhD
E-mail address: srknirfn@gmail.com
Present address: Department of Internal Medicine,
Faculty of Veterinary Medicine, Mustafa Kemal University,
31040, Hatay, Turkey

CASE REPORT

A 15 year-old female cat, with clinical sings of vomiting and severe abdominal distension was admitted at the clinic (Fig. 1).

There was no history data of any trauma and infection with feline enteric coronavirus (FCoV). Polymerase Chain Reaction (conventional-PCR) on corona virus was negative. The clinical and the

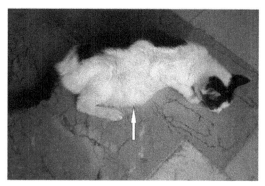

Figure 1. A 15 year-old female cat with abdominal distension (white arrow)

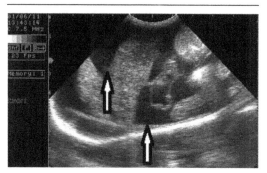

Figure 2. The ascites is seen in the anechoic area

ultrasonographic examination revealed abdominal pain, hepatomegaly, ascites, and increased liver echogenicity (Fig. 2).

After the aspiration of abdominal fluid, a cytology smear was prepared and the fluid was described as modified transudate. Cytology findings in the cell population of the aspirated abdominal fluid described mesothelial cells, macrophages, non-degenerate neutrophils and small lymphocytes. A blockage of the vena cava caudalis at the intrahepatic region called Budd-Chiari syndrome was found with ultrasonographic examination. The location

of the thrombus was confirmed by longitudinal and transversal cross-section. The thrombus was 0.87 cm in diameter at the junction of the hepatic vein and the vena cava caudalis (Fig. 3 and Fig. 4).

During this study, we proposed a hepatoprotective and lower salt diet (easy digestible foods with high quality protein and highly digestible protein; Prescription Diet® h/d®, l/d® feline-Hill's Pet Nutriton). The following medical therapy was recommended: cefuroxime axetyl 25 mg/kg/ body weight 10 days, furosemide 2 mg/kg body weight 10 days, and total 330 mg dosage L-carnitine. After fortnight of therapy, the cat's appetite was increased and laboratory results got better as well. Obtained biochemical results are presented in Table 1. The amount of abdominal fluid in the cat was reduced as a result of the diuretic therapy; but the serum concentration of urea was elevated. A small amount of fluid was detected in the abdomen at the beginning of the therapy. After antibiotics and furosemide treatment, the L-carnitine administration was continued. In the following period, the amount of abdominal fluid increased again and unfortunately the cat died three months after the onset of the disease. The animal owner did not allow the necropsy.

A total of 5 ml blood samples were collected with venipuncture of vena cephalica antebrachi externa. Some biochemical (serum tubes with clot factor) and hematological (tubes for whole blood with EDTA) analyses were performed, such as liver transaminases alanine aminotransferase (ALT) and aspartate aminotransferase (AST), further gamma glutamyl transferase (GGT), total bilirubin, albumin, total protein, direct bilirubin levels, total antioxidant capacity status (TAS) and total oxidant status (TOS), in the serum samples. Furthermore, TAS and TOS in ascites fluid were examined.

Total antioxidant and oxidant capacities were determined colorimetrically (PowerWave XS, BioTek Instrument, Bedfordshire/UK) using a

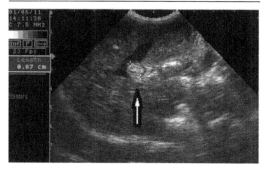

Figure 3. Enlarged vena cava caudalis from thrombosis (ventradorsal position-transversal cross-section)

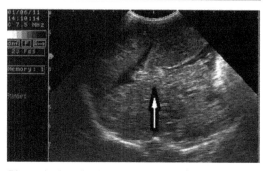

Figure 4. Thrombosis of vena cava caudalis (ventradorsal position-longutidinal cross-section)

commercial kit (Rel Assay Diagnostic, Gaziantep, Turkey) as previously described by Durgut et al. (6). Serum TAC was determined using a novel automated measurement method developed elsewhere (7). The results are expressed as μmol of Trolox equivalent/liter. Total oxidant status levels were measured using commercially available kits (Rel Assay Diagnostic, Gaziantep, Turkey). The assay was calibrated with hydrogen peroxide (H_2O_2), and the results were expressed in terms of micromolar H_2O_2 equivalent per liter (μmol H_2O_2 equivalent/L) (8).

The levels of ALT and AST, total bilirubin and direct bilirubin in the serum sample were marked increased, with regards to the serum albumin and total protein concentration. Serum levels of urea and creatinine were in physiological range at the beginning of the therapy. There were no marked changes in the hematological parameters (Table 1).

of hepatic vein stenosis, causing ascites and mild anemia in a cat was described by Schrope (9).

Humans with BCS, have a thin fibrous band or segmental fibro muscular membrane, formed in both supra hepatic areas (entrance of the hepatic veins and from the right atrium), as well as intrahepatically (in the liver) and in the vena cava inferior (1, 3, 10). A membranous obstruction of the inferior vena cava known as idiopathic Budd-Chiari syndrome in humans is a rare clinical condition (11, 12). In this study, we determined full obstruction in both vena cava caudalis and hepatic vein in the intrahepatic region (Fig. 2 and Fig. 3), called the Budd-Chiari syndrome, by ultrasonographic examination similarly as other studies (3, 9).

Liver damage may be increased by oxidative stress. Oxidative stress has an important role in the pathogenesis of viral hepatitis, sepsis and bacterial infections (13, 14). Liver enzymes (ALT, AST,

Table 1. Hematological findings in blood samples

Parameters	Blood samples			
	First week	Second week	Third week	Fourth week
RBC (x10^{12}g/L)	7.41	6.60	6.82	6.16
HGB (g/L)	96.0	81.0	89.0	75.0
HCT (%)	24.59	22.30	22.70	21.03
MCV (fL)	33	34	33	34
MCHC (g/L)	389.0	364.0	393.0	356.0
Total Bilirubin (μmol/L)	15.39	42.75	17.1	*
Direct Bilirubin(μmol/L)	15.39	34.2	13.68	*
Urea (mmol/L)	10.353	24.99	16.422	13.209
Creatinine (μmol/L)	96.356	109.616	101.66	61.88

*Not detected

Concentrations of TAS and TOS were higher in the peritoneal fluid compared with the serum samples (Table 2 and Table 3). Concentration of enzymes was increased, particularly gamma glutamyl transferase (GGT).

DISCUSSION

This clinical case describes the ultrasonographic and laboratory examinations of BCS. The first case

GGT), oxidative stress index-OSI and TOS increases are marked in animals with fasciolosis, while TAS decreases in serum and plasma samples (15). In this study, the levels of TAS and TOS were increased in the peritoneal fluid compared with serum samples (Table 3) and some data supported our findings (14, 16). On the other hand, the level of enzymes was increased at the beginning of treatment, particularly parenchymal enzymes, reported by Braun (17).

The response to medical therapy in the case of BCS is generally poor. The effect of diuretic therapy

Table 2. Biochemical findings in blood samples and peritoneal fluid

Parameters	Blood samples				Peritoneal fluid
	First week	Second week	Third week	Fourth week	
AST (U/L)	654	409	273	139	48
ALT (U/L)	1534	674	666	143	22
GGT (U/L)	<4	>4	>4	33	<4
Total Protein (g/l)	59.0	67.0	*	66.0	17.0
Albumin (g/l)	24.0	28.0	*	21.0	6.0

is uncertain (18). We used L-carnitine as liver-protection, a low salt diet and diuretic treatment. Prescribed therapy improved the condition and the quality of life of the cat, but for a short time, until the end of the therapy.

Table 3. TAS and TOS findings in blood samples and peritoneal fluid

Parameters	Blood	Peritoneal Fluid
TAS (mmolTrolox eq./L)	0.042	0.12
TOS (μmol H2O2/L)	6.542	9.318

L-carnitine metabolism is impaired in patients with hepatic impairment. Deficiency of L-carnitine might be a secondary factor for liver injuries (19, 20). It is reported that L-carnitine has protective effects on liver with its potent free radical scavenging and antioxidant actions against oxidative damage in hepatic ischemia-reperfusion injury (21). L-carnitine was administered during the time of treatment, and weekly liver enzyme analysis was performed. The liver enzyme concentrations were decreased during the time of treatment. L-carnitine might improve liver damage, and might prolong the survival time with liver protection effect.

CONCLUSION

In summary, thrombosis of vena cava caudalis, also known as BCS, was described for the first time in a domestic cat in Turkey. Ultrasound can be used as reliable non-invasive diagnostic method for detecting BCS. Furthermore, in the cat with BCS, the use of L-carnitine which has hepatoprotective effects was beneficial as supportive treatment. Medical treatment for BCS was not completely effective, only surgical removing of occlusion ensured normal bloodstream in vena cava caudalis. This study will be of great importance for future studies, diagnosis and "treatments" of BCS in animals.

ACKNOWLEDGEMENT

The authors would like to thank Prof. V. Soydal Ataseven, DVM, PhD. from Department of Virology, Faculty of Vet. Medicine, Mustafa Kemal Univ., Hatay, Turkey for his help with the PCR analysis.

REFERENCES

1. Simpson, I.W. (1982). Membranous obstruction of the inferior vena cava and hepatocellular carcinoma in South Africa. Gastroenterol. 82, 171-178.

2. Stanley, P. (1989). Budd-Chiari syndrome. Radiol. 170, 625-627.
   http://dx.doi.org/10.1148/radiology.170.3.2644657
   PMid:2644657

3. Nakamura T., Nakamura S., Aikawa T., Suziki, O., Onodera, A., Karoji, N. (1968). Obstruction of the inferior vena cava in the hepatic portion and the hepatic veins. Angiol. 19(8): 479-500.
   http://dx.doi.org/10.1177/000331976801900805

4. Amesur, N.B., Zajko, A.B. (2006). Interventional radiology in liver transplantation. Liver Transpl Surg. 12, 330-351.
   http://dx.doi.org/10.1002/lt.20731
   PMid:16498660

5. Zhang, X., Qing-Le, L. (2007). Etiology, treatment, and classification of Budd-Chiari syndrome. Chin Med J. 120, 159-161.
   http://dx.doi.org/10.3901/JME.2007.04.159

6. Durgut, R., Ataseven, V.S., Sagkan-Ozturk, A., Ozturk, O.H. (2013). Evaluation of total oxidative stress and total antioxidant status in cows with natural bovine herpesvirus-1 infection. J Anim Sci. 91, 1–5.
   http://dx.doi.org/10.2527/jas.2012-5516
   PMid:23798525

7. Erel, O. (2004). A novel automated method to measure total antioxidant response against potent free radical reactions. Clin Biochem. 37, 112-119.
   http://dx.doi.org/10.1016/j.clinbiochem.2003.10.014
   PMid:14725941

8. Erel, O. (2005). A new automated colorimetric method for measuring total oxidant status. Clin Biochem. 38, 1103-1111.
   http://dx.doi.org/10.1016/j.clinbiochem.2005.08.008
   PMid:16214125

9. Schrope, D.S. (2010). Hepatic vein stenosis (Budd-Chiari syndrome) as a cause of ascites in a cat. J Vet Cardiol. 12, 197-202.
   http://dx.doi.org/10.1016/j.jvc.2010.05.002
   PMid:21078565

10. Okuda, K., Kage, M., Shrestha, S.M. (1998). Proposal of a new nomenclature for Budd-Chiari syndrome: hepatic vein thrombosis versus thrombosis of the inferior vena cava at its hepatic portion. Hepatology 28, 1191-1198.
    http://dx.doi.org/10.1002/hep.510280505
    PMid:9794901

11. Okuda, K. (2001). Membranous obstruction of the inferior vena cava (obliterative hepatocavopathy, Okuda). J Gastroenterol Hepatol. 16, 1179-1183.
    http://dx.doi.org/10.1046/j.1440-1746.2001.02577.x
    PMid:11903732

12. Takayasu, K., Muramatsu, Y., Moriyama, N., Wakao, F., Makuuchi, M., Takayama, T., Kosuge, T., Okazaki, N., Yamada, R. (1994). Radiological study of idiopathic Budd-Chiari syndrome complicated by hepatocellular carcinoma: a report of four cases. Am J Gastroenterol. 88, 249-253.

13. Horoz, M., Bolukbas, C., Bolukbas, F.F., Aslan, M., Koylu, A.O., Selek, S., Erel, O. (2006). Oxidative stres in hepatitis C infected end-stage renal disease subjects. BMC Infect Dis. 6, 114.
http://dx.doi.org/10.1186/1471-2334-6-114
PMid:16842626 PMCid:PMC1543638

14. Karaagac, L., Koruk, S.T., Koruk, I., Aksoy, N. (2011). Decreasing oxidative stress in response to treatment in patients with brucellosis: could it be used to monitor treatment. Int J Infect Dis. 15(5): 346-349.
http://dx.doi.org/10.1016/j.ijid.2011.01.009
PMid:21376649

15. Karsen, H., Sunnetcioglu, M., Ceylan, R.M. (2011). Evaluation of oxidative status in patients with Fasciola hepatica infection. Afr Health Sci. 11(1): 14-18.
http://dx.doi.org/10.4314/ahs.v11i3.70064

16. Maden, M., Ozturk, S.A., Bulbul, A., Avci, G., Yazar, E. (2012). Acute phase proteins, oxidative stress and enzyme activities of blood serum and peritoneal fluid in abomasal displacement cases. J Vet Intern Med. 26, 1470–1475.
http://dx.doi.org/10.1111/j.1939-1676.2012.01018.x
PMid:23113812

17. Braun, U. (2008). Clinical findings and diagnosis of thrombosis of the caudal vena cava in cattle. The Vet J. 175, 118–125.
http://dx.doi.org/10.1016/j.tvjl.2006.11.013
PMid:17239635

18. Fisher, N.C., Mccafferty, I., Dolapci, M., Wali, M., Buckels, J.A.C., Olliff, S.P., Elias, E. (1999). Managing Budd-Chiari syndrome: a restrospective review of percutaneous hepatic vein angioplasty and surgical shunting. Gut 44, 568-574.
http://dx.doi.org/10.1136/gut.44.4.568
PMid:10075967 PMCid:PMC1727471

19. Lin, X.H., Jiao, L.L., Xu, G.B., Tian, G.S. (2006). Significance of serum carnitine in patients with liver diseases. Zhonghua Gan Zang Bing ZaZhi, 14(5): 367-369.

20. Malaguarnera, M., Vacante, M., Giordano, M., Motta, M., Bertino, G., Pennisi, M., Neri, S., Malaguernera, M., Li Volti, G., Galvano, F. (2011). L-carnitine supplementation improves hematological pattern in patients affected by HCV treated with Peg interferon-α 2b plus ribavirin. World J Gastroenterol. 17(39): 4414-4420.
http://dx.doi.org/10.3748/wjg.v17.i39.4414
PMid:22110268 PMCid:PMC3218156

21. Cekin, AH., Gur, G., Turkoglu, S., Aldemir, D., Yılmaz, U., Gursoy, M., Taskoparan, M., Boyacıoğlu, S. (2013). The protective effect of L-carnitine on hepatic ischemia-reperfusion injury in rats. Turk J Gastroenterol. 24 (1): 51-56.
PMid:23794344

8

PRACTICAL USE OF REGISTERED VETERINARY MEDICINAL PRODUCTS IN MACEDONIA IN IDENTIFYING THE RISK OF DEVELOPING OF ANTIMICROBIAL RESISTANCE

Velev Romel[1], Krleska-Veleva Natasa[2]

[1]*Department of Pharmacology and Toxicology, Faculty of Veterinary Medicine, University "Ss. Cyril and Methodius", Skopje, R. Macedonia;*
[2]*Replek Farm, Kozle 188, 1000 Skopje, R. Macedonia*

ABSTRACT

The use of antimicrobial agents is the key risk factor for the development and spread of antimicrobial resistance. It is therefore generally recognized that data on the usage of antimicrobial agents in food-producing animals are essential for identifying and quantifying the risk of developing and spreading of antimicrobial resistance in the food-chain. According to the WHO guidelines, the Anatomical Therapeutic Chemical system for the classification of veterinary medicines (ATC-vet) is widely recognized as a classification tool. The aim of this work is to analyze the list of registered veterinary medicinal products in R. Macedonia and to evaluate the quality and practical use of this list according to the ATC-vet classification in order to identify the risk of developing and spreading of antimicrobial resistance.

Key words: antimicrobial agents, antimicrobial resistance, veterinary medicinal products, ATCvet classification system

INTRODUCTION

Antimicrobials are valuable tools in the preservation of animal health and animal welfare, and must be cherished as they may save lives and prevent animal suffering (1). But the use of antimicrobial agents is the key risk factor for the development and spread of antimicrobial resistance (AMR). It is therefore generally recognized that data on the usage of antimicrobial agents in food-producing animals (and companion animals) are essential for identifying and quantifying the risk of developing and spreading of AMR in the food-chain (2). The World Health Organization has indicated the follow up of antimicrobial resistance as one of the three top priorities (1). Antimicrobial resistance is defined as the ability of a microorganism to grow or survive in the presence of an antimicrobial at a concentration that is usually sufficient to inhibit or kill microorganisms of the same species. Antimicrobial consumption in animals selects for antimicrobial resistant bacteria in animals, leading to therapy failure of bacterial infections. Yet it might also endanger human health through either transfer of resistant bacteria or their resistance genes from animals to humans. The magnitude of this risk still needs to be quantified while increasing evidence of resistance transfer between environments is found (1). This was also acknowledged by the European Council in 2008 through the Council Conclusions on Antimicrobial Resistance, which called upon the Member States to strengthen surveillance systems and improve data quality on antimicrobial resistance and on use of antimicrobial agents within both human and veterinary sectors (3). Having this in mind we decided to respond to the latest and to estimate the use of antimicrobial agents in veterinary sector in the Republic of Macedonia (RM) by analyzing the List of Registered Veterinary Medicinal Products (VMPs) and evaluating of the quality and practical use of this list according to the

Corresponding author: Prof. Romel Velev, PhD

e-mail: vromel@fvm.ukim.edu.mk
Present address: Ss. Cyril and Methodius University in Skopje
Faculty of Veterinary medicine - Skopje
Department of Farmacology and Toxicology
Lazar Pop-Trajkov 5-7 1000, Skopje, R. of Macedonia

Anatomical Therapeutic Chemical System for the Classification of Veterinary Medicines, with the aim of identifying the risk of development and spread of antimicrobial resistance.

ATCvet classification system

To harmonize the veterinary antimicrobial agents to be included in the material, the Anatomical Therapeutic Chemical System for the Classification of Veterinary Medicines (ATCvet) was applied. According to the WHO guidelines, the ATCvet is widely recognized as a classification tool. This system is based on the same overall principles as the ATC system for substances used in human medicine (4). In most cases an ATC code exists which can be used to classify a product in the ATCvet system. The ATCvet code is created by placing the letter Q in front of the ATC code. In some cases, however, specific ATCvet codes are created, e.g. Immunologicals (QI) and Antibacterials for intramammary use (QJ51) (4). In both the ATC and the ATCvet systems, medicinal products are divided into groups, according to their therapeutic use (1st level) (see the Table below).

ATCvet	Anatomical groups (1st level)	ATC
QA	Alimentary tract and metabolism	A
QB	Blood and blood forming organs	B
QC	Cardiovascular system	C
QD	Dermatologicals	D
QG	Genito-urinary system and sex hormones	G
QH	Systemic hormonal preparations, excl. sex hormones and insulins	H
QI	Immunologicals	-
QJ	Anti-infectives for systemic use	J
QL	Antineoplastic and immunomodulating agents	L
QM	Musculo-skeletal system	M
QN	Nervous system	N
QP	Antiparasitic products, insecticides and repellents	P
QR	Respiratory system	R
QS	Sensory organs	S
QV	Various	V

ATCvet ▶   **◀ ATC/DDD**

Within most of the 1st level groups, medicinal products are subdivided into different therapeutic main groups (2nd level), coded for example as QA01, QA02, QA03 etc. Two levels of chemical/therapeutic/pharmacological subgroups (3rd and 4th levels), e.g. QA02A, QA02B etc. at the 3rd level and QA02AA, QA02AB etc at the 4th level, provide further subdivisions. At a 5th level, e.g. QA02AA01, chemical substances are classified. This subdivision does not apply to QI – Immunologicals (4).

Distribution of veterinary medicines in RM

The first step in setting up surveillance of veterinary antimicrobial agents in some country is to identify and describe of the distribution system for veterinary antimicrobial agents (8). In our country, all VMPs containing antimicrobial agents are prescription-only medicines. This includes medicated premixes containing pharmaceutically active substances like antimicrobial agents. VMPs containing antimicrobial agents are provided by Wholesaler Distributors (WD) to retailers of veterinary medicinal products (veterinary pharmacies) and veterinary organizations. Wholesaler-distributors obtain the VMPs from a wholesaler or from the Marketing Authorization Holder (MAH)/manufacturers.

Antimicrobial VMPs are only available to animal owners/farmers by delivery from a pharmacy on veterinary prescription or directly from the veterinary organizations. Only veterinarians are entitled to sell VMPs to animal owners/farmers. Veterinarians have to confirm the distribution of veterinary drugs to owners of food-producing animals if used for food production. Sales of VMPs by pharmacies account for a negligible amount of sales for farm animals. Medicated feeds have to be prescribed by veterinarians and manufactured either by authorized feed mills or by authorized farms. They are also may be imported to Macedonia. Medicated feeds containing antimicrobials are prepared from authorized premixes that are distributed through wholesaler-distributors. From feed mills, only farmers are receivers. Medicated feeds are used primarily for pig and poultry production.

Legal basis for the monitoring of sales of VMPs in RM

The collection of sales data by MAH/WDs is based on the national Law on veterinary medicinal products (Official Gazette of the Republic Macedonia No. 42/2010- article 37)(10). MAH/WDs are obliged to keep records of all sales and to deliver these records (by template for the amount of sold out VMPs) to the Sector for Public Veterinary Health in Food and Veterinary Agency (FVA) on a yearly basis (11). The fact that many antimicrobial products are registered for use in different animal species and that there are currently no data available on the proportions of products used in the different species makes extrapolation up to animal species level unachievable at this very moment. The MAH of the products do provide estimated proportions to be included in the periodic safety update reports, yet these estimates are not always at hand, and are often based on limited data. For these reasons it was not feasible to use these data.

MATERIALS AND METHODS

Data of all registered/renewed VMPs on the Macedonian market are collected from the web site of FVA (12), pharmaceutical companies (n=37) producing or importing VMPs and from MAH/WDs (n=16) that are assigned by the FVA to distribute them. The registered/renewed VMPs in last five years in Macedonia are classified according to composition of active component/s and main therapeutic indications regarding to the system of organs to which are intended to act on. An appropriate code from ATCvet Index 2013 provided from WHO Collaborating Centre for Drug Statistics Methodology at Norwegian Institute of Public Health (4) was designated to each VMP. On this way we have created a list of registered/renewed VMPs with appropriate ATCvet code and made a detailed analysis of the number of registered VMPs classified by the system of organs and qualitative analysis of specific groups of VMPs. In particular, we analyzed groups of antimicrobial agents in different therapeutic main groups (see Table 3) in order to estimate the use of antimicrobial agents in veterinary sector in the RM and to identify the risk of developing and spreading of antimicrobial resistance.

RESULTS AND DISCUSSION

In Macedonia, 318 VMPs were registered or renewed during the period from 01.01.2008 to 31.12.2012. Figure 1 shows the number of registered/renewed VMPs per year and manufacturers. All registered VMPs are from import, mainly from 37 manufacturers from 16 European countries (Holland 18.2%, Serbia 17.0%, Croatia 15.0 %, Bulgaria 7.2 %, Slovenia 7.2 %). In the period of 15 years, about 850 VMPs were registered/renewed or approximately 45 – 50 per year. In 2009 and 2012, a little reduction in the number of registered/renewed VMPs on the Macedonian market is observed, largely due to newly adopted legislation for registration and the impossibility of MAH/WD in quick time to adjust to the new regulations.

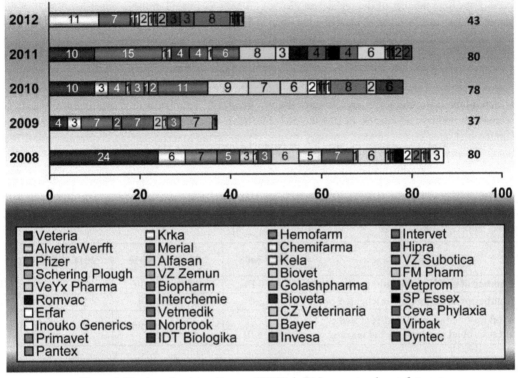

Figure 1. Number of registered/renewed VMPs in RM per year and manufacturers

Table 1 shows the number of registered/renewed VMPs on the Macedonian market this moment according to their therapeutic use. The largest number of registered VMPs are from group QJ – Anti-infectives for systemic use (n = 93), while on the other hand there are no VMPs registered for primary therapeutic effect on cardiovascular system (group QC), for treatment of neoplasm (group QL-Antineoplastic and immunomodulating agents) and for treatment of diseases of eyes and ears (group QS - Sensory organs). Some of the anatomical groups like a group QB - Blood and blood forming organs, group QM - Musculo-skeletal system and group QR - Respiratory system were represented by insignificant number of VMPs.

Table 1. Number of registered VMPs in RM according to their therapeutic use

	Anatomical groups (1st level)	No. of VMPs
QA	Alimentary tract and metabolism	38
QB	Blood and blood forming organs	4
QC	Cardiovascular system	0
QD	Dermatologicals	9
QG	Genito-urinary system and sex hormones	17
QH	Systemic hormonal preparations, excl. sex hormones and insulins	13
QI	Immunologicals	74
QJ	Antiinfectives for systemic use	93
QL	Antineoplastic and immunomodulating agents	0
QM	Musculo-skeletal system	2
QN	Nervous system	11
QP	Antiparasitic products, insecticides and repellents	53
QR	Respiratory system	2
QS	Sensory organs	0
QV	Various	2
	Total:	318

From the total number of the registered VMPs, pharmaceuticals are 76.7% (n=244) while immune-preparations are 23.3% (n=74). The amount of antimicrobial agents and their combinations is 32.7% (n=104), while the amount of antiparasitic is 16.7% (n=53). From the total number of registered immune-preparations greater number are vaccines for poultry and swines. In RM the use of antimicrobial agents is expanded, contrary to the immune-preparations. The above mentioned data are partly in coordination with the data for the registered

VMPs in other European countries (5,6,7). Small market for specific VMPs results in lack of interest of the pharmaceutical companies to register VMPs with low or no commercial value, creating serious problem for the veterinary practitioners. Table 2 provides an overview of the number of registered/renewed antimicrobial pharmaceuticals and the number of antimicrobial medicated premixes per year on the Macedonian market for the period 2008 - 2012.

Table 2. Overview of the number of registered/renewed antimicrobial products on the Macedonian market in period 2008 - 2012

	2008	2009	2010	2011	2012
Number of antimicrobial pharmaceuticals	18	8	30	17	15
Number of antimicrobial medicated premixes	7	2	4	2	1
Total number of registered/renewed antimicrobial products on the market	25	10	34	19	16

In the period of 5 years, 104 antimicrobial products were registered and renewed or approximately 20 per year. In RM the use of parenteral forms of antimicrobial products (inj. sol.; inj. susp.) is expanded 51% (n=53), contrary to antimicrobial medicated premixes 15.4% (n=16). The amount of intramammary products is 6.73% (n=7), while the amount of intrauterine products is 2.9% (n=3). With exception of macrolide antibiotics tulathromycin and tilmicosin (since 2009 and

2012) and third generation cephalosporin ceftiofur (since 2009), no additional active substances were registered on the market in the reported years. Thus the observed number in available products is largely due to the marketing of new formulations or new generic products based on existing active substances. Table 3 provides an overview of the number of antimicrobial agents from different therapeutic main groups available on the Macedonian market this moment.

Table 3. Groups of antimicrobial agents and corresponding ATCvet codes available on the Macedonian market this moment

Groups of antimicrobial agents	ATCvet codes	Total
Antimicrobial agents for intestinal use	QA07AA; QA07AB	4
Antimicrobial agents for dermatological use	QD06AA; QD06BA	4
Antimicrobial agents for intrauterine use	QG51AA; QG51AC; QG51AE; QG51AX QG51BA; QG51BC; QG51BE	3
Antimicrobial agents for systemic use	QJ01	86
Antimicrobial agents for intramammary use	QJ51	7
Antimicrobial agents for use in sensory organs	QS01AA; QS01AB QS02AA QS03AA	0
Antimicrobial agents for use as antiparasitic	QP51AG	0

Antimicrobial products which are used as antiparasitic agents (group QP51AG) and for use in sensory organs were not registered. Some group of the antimicrobial agents like a group QA07 – Antibacterials for intestinal use, group QD06 - Antimicrobial agents for dermatological use, group QG51- Antibacterials for intrauterine use and group QJ51 - Antibacterials for intramammary use were represented by insignificant number of VMPs. The ATCvet codes (ATC level 3 or 4) included in each antimicrobial class are listed in Table 4.

Table 4. ATCvet codes included in the different classes of antimicrobials

Class of antimicrobials	ATCvet codes included	Total
Aminoglycosides	QA07AA01 (1) QJ01GA01 (1), GB03 (1), GB04 (1)	4
Cephalosporins	QG51AA05 (1) QJ01DA90 (3); DB01 (1) QJ51DA01 (1)	6
Amphenicols	QJ01BA52 (1); BA90 (3)	4
Macrolides	QJ01FA90 (1), FA91 (1), FA94 (1)	3
Penicillins	QJ01CA04 (5); CE30 (4); CR02 (3) QJ51RC (1)	13
Polymyxins	QA07AA10 (1)	1
Quinolones	QJ01MA90 (12) QJ01MB07 (1)	13
Sulfonamides and trimethoprim	QA07AB (2) QJ01EQ (4); EW (6)	12
Tetracyclines	QD06AA (3) QD07C (1) QG51AA01 (1); AA08 (1) QJ01AA02 (1), AA03 (2); AA06(9)	18
Pleuromutilins	QJ01XQ01 (7)	7

Combinations of antibacterials	QJ01RA01(penicillins)/QJ01RA95(polymyxins)(1)
	QJ01RA01(penicillins)/QJ01RA97(aminoglycosides) (8)
	QJ01RA02 (sulfonamides)/QJ01RA90(tetracyclines) (1)
	QJ01RA02/QJ01RA90/QJ01RA97 (2)
	QJ01RA90 (tetracyclines + tiamulin) (3)
	QJ01RA94 (lincosamides + spectinomycin) (1)
	QJ01RV01 (penicillin+polymyxin+corticosteroid) (1)
	    (penicillin+aminoglycos+corticosteroid) (1)
	QJ51RC23 (penicillin+aminoglycosides) (2)
	QJ51RV01 (cephalosporin+corticosteroid) (1)
	    (penicillin+aminoglycosides+ corticosteroid)(1)
	tetracyclin+aminoglycosid+bacitracin+corticosteroid)(1)
		23

Tetracyclines (n=25), penicillins (n=27) and quinolones (n=13) are the top three antimicrobial classes, comprising approximately 62.5 % of all registered antimicrobial agents. Generally, tetracyclines and/or penicillins accounted for the highest proportion of the use in the reporting period. For antimicrobial agents considered to be critically important antimicrobials in human medicine, such as the 3rd and 4th-generation cephalosporins, macrolides and the fluoroquinolones, an overall increase in usage is observed. These classes of compounds are used for food producing animals and could potentially influence the prevalence of resistance. 3rd and 4th-generation cephalosporins and fluoroquinolones are considered as particularly important in human medicine because they are among the only alternatives for the treatment of certain infectious diseases in humans. Measures to counter a further increase and spread of resistance in animals should therefore be considered.

Although there is a legal basis for the collection of sales data on VMPs on an annual basis from MAH/WDs to the FVA in this moment the data is not available to us. It should be emphasized that sales of antimicrobial agents (mg per population correction factor - PCU) are not indicators for the level of exposure (9). The main goal of calculating the amount of antimicrobial agents is to adjust trends in the use within a country for possible changes in the size of animal livestock population and number of slaughtered animals (7). Also, the sales data on veterinary antimicrobial agents cover all species, while the population correction factor does not include companion animals or minor species.

DISCUSSION

The use of antimicrobial agents is an important risk factor for the development of antimicrobial resistance. Monitoring of use of antimicrobials is one of the important sources of information used for the assessment and management of risks related to antimicrobial resistance. Our work provides the first data on the usage of antimicrobial drugs in animals in Macedonia for the given period and shows a high usage of antimicrobials in veterinary sector. Many European countries have been reporting these already for several years. Moreover it has recently become a European engagement from member states to report on the level of antimicrobial consumption in animal production (7). Also in the context of methicillin resistant Staphylococcus aureus, extended spectrum beta-lactamase, and other emerging resistance traits, comparable and evolutionary data on antimicrobial consumption are needed. This work can thus also be seen as a starting point for continuous monitoring of using the antimicrobial agents in future. The reported table will also be used as a reference for comparison and to evaluate effects of policy measures.

As the data presented in this work are aggregated per antimicrobial class, they do not allow for more in-depth analysis. The types and incidences of infectious diseases vary considerably between animal species and production category (e.g. veal versus dairy cattle), and consequently the sales of veterinary antibacterial agents are thought to be influenced by animal species demographics. To identify the factors underlying the differences

observed, there is a need for detailed sales data of each antimicrobial VMPs. As a first step, the use of the standardized ESVAC template for the collection of data (9) will provide detailed data at package level, including information on administration form and herd treatment versus individual treatment, allowing for more detailed analysis than can be done using the aggregated data. As some agents are administered in much higher dosages than others (e.g. tetracyclines versus cephalosporins), there is a need to continue to refine the tools for analyzing the data on sales of antimicrobial agents. The next steps should be to analyze the data taking into account variance in the dosing and the treatment duration of each antimicrobial VMPs.

CONCLUSIONS

The extended and uncontrolled use of antimicrobial agents in Macedonia is representing the main risk factor for the development of antimicrobial resistance. Data on the usage of antimicrobial agents particularly in food producing animals is essential for identifying and quantifying this risk in the food-chain. The ATCvet classification gives a detailed view on the real quantity of the different classes of registered VMPs. It is practical tool for identification of different groups of VMPs for the veterinary practitioners as well as all subjects involved in production, trade and distribution of VMPs. The results obtained given an overall picture of trends in the use of veterinary antimicrobial agents in R. Macedonia. Currently data indicate a high use of antimicrobials indicating that this class of VMP should be monitored closely to avoid the appearance of antimicrobial resistance and possible consequences for animal and human health. Nevertheless, such data should be interpreted with caution, with further analysis to assess exposure trends and the effect of policy measures for prudent use.

REFERENCES

1. BelVetSac - Belgian Veterinary Surveillance of Antimicrobial Consumption - National consumption report 2007– 2008 – 2009. http://www.belvetsac.ugent.be/pages/home/BelvetSAC_report_2007-8-9%20 finaal.pdf

2. ESVAC (2011). European Medicines Agency. Trends in the sales of veterinary antimicrobial agents in nine European countries. Reporting period: 2005-2009 (EMA/238630/2011). In the European Medicines Agency web page (http://www.ema.europa.eu/).

3. Council of the European Union (2007). Council Conclusions on Antimicrobial Resistance. Luxembourg, 10 June 2008 (http://cpme.dyndns.org:591/database/2008/Info.2008-124.enonly.Council.conclusions.AMR.pdf)

4. WHO Collaborating Centre for Drug Statistics Methodology. Guidelines for ATCvet classification (2012). Oslo, 2012.(http://www.whocc.no/atcvet/)

5. Chevance, A., Moulin, G. (2011). Sales survey of Veterinary Medicinal Products containing Antimicrobials in France – 2010. Volumes and estimated consumption of antimicrobials in animals. ANSES-ANMV, Fougères. In ANSES http://www.anses.fr/Documents/ANMV-Ra-749 Antibiotiques2010EN.pdf.

6. Moulin, G., Chevance, A. (2010). Sales Survey of Veterinary Medicinal Products Containing Antimicrobials in France - 2009 /February 2010, Anses-ANMV, Fougères (www.anses.fr/Documents/ANMV-Ra-Antibiotiques2009EN.pdf).

7. Grave K., Torren-Edo J., Mackay D. (2010). Comparison of the sales of veterinary antibacterial agents between 10 European countries. Journal of Antimicrobial Chemotherapy, 65: 2037 - 2040.

8. EMA/76066/2010. European Surveillance of Veterinary Antimicrobial Consumption (ESVAC). Data Collection Protocol (www.ema.europa.eu/docs/en GB/document library/Other/2010/04/WC500089584.pdf).

9. EMA/790974/2010. ESVAC Data Collection Form (www.ema.europa.eu/docs/en GB/document library/Template or form/2010/04/WC500089585.xls).

10. Official Gazette of the Republic Macedonia 42/2010. Law on Veterinary Medicinal Products.

11. Food and Veterinary Agency of R. Macedonia. Template for the amount of sold out VMPs (http://www.fva.gov.mk/images/stories/1112_04_Obrazez.pdf)

12. Food and Veterinary Agency of R. Macedonia. Register on Veterinary Medicinal Products.(http://www.fva.gov.mk/images/stories/1010.01_REGISTER_VMP_Vs_021_05.03.201397-2003_English.pdf)

LIGHT AND TRANSMISSION ELECTRON MICROSCOPICAL CHANGES ASSOCIATED WITH *LEIURUS QUINQESTRIATUS* VENOM IN RABBITS

Salah H. Afifi[1], Reham El-Kashef[2], A. Sh. Seddek[2], Diefy A. Salem[1]

*[1]Department of Pathology, Faculty of Veterinary Medicine,
Assiut University, Assiut, Egypt
[2]Department of Forensic Medicine and Toxicology, Faculty of Veterinary Medicine,
South Valley University, Kena, Egypt*

ABSTRACT

Thirty California female rabbits were obtained from the Animal Care Center, College of Agriculture, South Valley University and acclimated to laboratory conditions for one week. The *Leiurus quinquestriatus* (LQ) venom was collected from mature scorpions by electrical stimulation of the telson. A single dose of crude venom of 0.4 ml/kg (diluted in normal saline with a ratio of 1:1) was injected into a peripheral ear vein. The lungs, brains, hearts, kidneys, were sampled and fixed in 10% formalin from rabbits sacrificed at zero, 30 minutes, 1hr, and 4hrs, post-envenomation (three animals at each sacrifice). Respiratory distress and neurological manifestations were the main clinical signs. Congestion of the lungs was started at one hour post-envenomation. Vascular changes including hyperemia and hemorrhage were also observed till 24 hours post-envenomation. The main histopathological changes of the lungs were edema, hemorrhage, emphysema, and eosinophilic bronchitis. Transmission electron microscopy revealed several eosinophils with abundant granules and breakdown of their membranes suggesting degranulation. The cerebrum showed malacia and edema. Myocardial damage expressed by focal area of myolysis at half-hour post-envenomation and interstitial edema by at 1, and 4 hour post-envenomation was also evident. In conclusion, scorpion venom induced consistent and relevant histopathological changes in all examined organs.

Key words: *Leiurus quinqestriatus* venom, rabbits, light and transmission electron microscopy

INTRODUCTION

Scorpion stings are a major public health and veterinary problem in tropical and sub-tropical countries. Most of the scorpions that are dangerously venomous to humans and animals belong to the buthidae. The reported LD_{50} of *Leiurus quinquestriatus* (L.Q.) venom is ranged from 0.16 - 0.5mg/kg in different animals (1). The voltage dependent ion channels, sodium, potassium and calcium channels are the main targets of scorpion venom action. The symptoms of scorpion envenomation result from a complex interaction of parasympathetic and sympathetic stimulation along with the release of a variety of endogenous compounds i.e. catecholamines, angiotensin II, glucagon, corticosteroids, bradykinins. Fatalities are primarily the result of cardiovascular and respiratory dysfunction and failure (2). L. Q. scorpion is one of the most important members of the buthidae family. It is reported as one of the most dangerous scorpions in the world. This is because its venom is a powerful cocktail of neurtoxins with a low LD_{50} (3). The reported LD_{50} of L.Q. venom is ranged from 0.16 - 0.5 mg/kg in different animals which confirm the severity of this species of scorpion (1).

The objective of this study is to investigate *in vivo* the pathological changes associated with *Leiurus quinquestriatus* crude venom injection on female rabbits.

Corresponding author: Dr. Salah H. Afifi, PhD
E-mail address: afifi_s_4@hotmail.com
Present address: Department of Pathology, Faculty of Veterinary Medicine, Assiut University, Assiut, Egypt

MATERIAL AND METHODS

A number of 30 California female rabbits (1.5-2.4 kg) were obtained from the Animal Care Center, College of Agriculture, South Valley University.

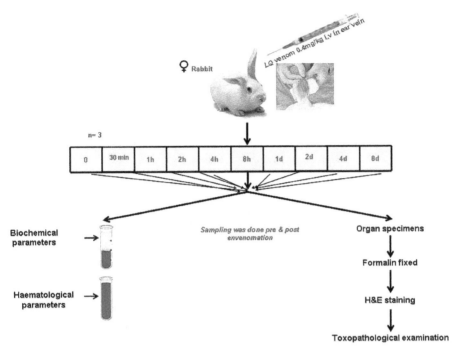

Figure 1. Experimental design in the current study

Animals were housed under specific pathogen free condition with water and feed ad libitum. The animals were kept under observation for one week prior to the start of treatment for acclimatization.

A single dose of crude L.Q. venom of 0.4 mg/kg was injected i.v. in the peripheral ear vein. The venom was diluted in normal saline with a ratio 1:1. Samples collected in a time course started from 0 up to 8 days post injection as shown in Fig. 1.

Rabbits were anaesthetized by chloroform and post mortem examination was carried out. For histopathological examination 3 animals were used per time point (n=3) and sampling done pre and post envenomation.

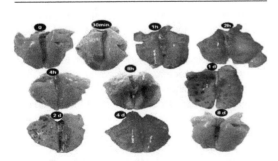

Figure 2. Gross appearance of rabbit's lungs at different intervals of envenomation, as well as the non-exposed rabbits

RESULTS

Grossly, wide spread of congestion all over the body organs was observed including lungs, heart, brain, liver, stomach, intestine, kidneys, spleen, ovary and fallopian tube. The lung and brain appeared to be the most affected organs. The lungs showed time dependent congestion and petechial hemorrhage with peak at Day 1. By Day 8 post injection, the lungs look similar to the control (Fig. 2).

The lungs exposed to administration of scorpion poison via I.V. route and collected at 0.5h showed marked alveolar emphysema and damage of the bronchiolar epithelium (Fig. 4) compared to the control at zero time (Fig. 3). The lungs at 1h post exposure had the previous changes observed at 0.5h beside interstitial hemorrhage (Fig. 5). Moreover, focal area of consolidation was observed. The lungs collected at 4 h showed more advanced changes of the lung tissues which were observed in this time interval. This change was expressed by peri-vascular inflammatory cellular reaction mainly of eosinophils (Fig. 6).

Transmission electron microscopy proved these eosinophils with abundant dense granules in their cytoplasm, as well as the breakdown of its membranes (Fig. 7 and Fig. 8).

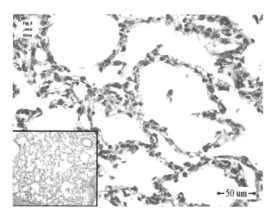

Figure 3. Lung of rabbits collected at Zero hour post-exposure showing the normal appearance of alveoli. Bar = 50um.

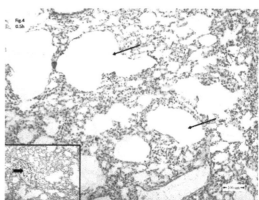

Figure 4. Lung of rabbits collected at half hour post-exposure to Scorpion poison showing well expressed alveolar emphysema (arrow) and damage of bronchiolar epithelium. H&E; bar=100µm

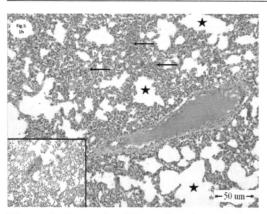

Figure 5. Lung of rabbits collected at 1 hour post-exposure to Scorpion poison showing alveolar emphysema (star) and interstitial hemorrhage (arrow). H&E; bar=50µm

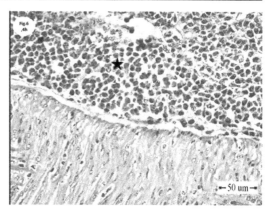

Figure 6. Lung of rabbits collected at 4 hours post-exposure to Scorpion poison showing eosinophilic bronchitis (star). H&E; bar=50µm

The brain collected at 0.5h post-envenomation had focal area of malacia. This area showed the feature of liquefactive necrosis (Fig. 10). The brains of rabbits at 1h post-exposure showed marked edema which is expressed by vacuolation (Fig. 11). While, the brains collected at 4h had well-defined edema (Fig. 12) compared to the brains collected at zero time (Fig. 9).

The hearts of rabbits collected at half hours showed severe myocardiolysis (Fig. 14). While at 1, and 4 hours, the hearts showed marked interstitial edema (Fig. 15) compared to the hearts collected at zero time (Fig. 13).

The kidneys collected at half and 1 hour showed focal necrosis of tubular epithelium (Fig. 17). While kidneys of rabbits collected at 4 hours post-exposure to Scorpion poison showed well expressed interstitial hemorrhage and necrosis of the tubular epithelium (Fig. 18) compared to the kidneys collected at zero time (Fig. 16).

DISCUSSION

Leiurus quinquestriatus was recorded to be the most dangerous scorpion in the world. This is due to complex venom composition particularly the potent neurotoxins:chlorotoxin and charbydotoxin (4). Scorpion venom is known to be fatal and produces several alterations in different organs of the body. Alterations in respiratory system components lead to altered lung mechanics, characterized by histological abnormalities, edema, hemorrhage, inflammation and increased deposition of matrix extra-cellular proteins (5). There are several reports indicating that the venom caused well-expressed morphological changes in the lung. These changes were mainly lung edema, hemorrhage, and pneumonia (6, 7).

In the present study, the lung lesions start with emphysema and damage of bronchiolar epithelium at 0.5 hours followed by hemorrhage at one-hour. The lung edema and the perivascular eosinophilic

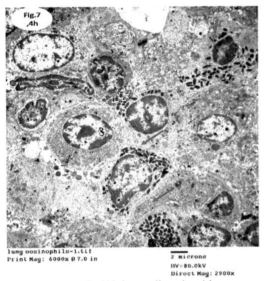

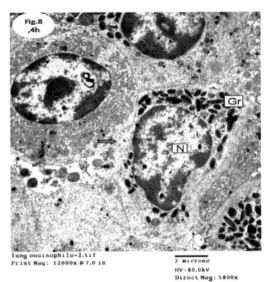

Figure 7. TEM of rabbit lung collected at 4 hours post-exposure showing eosinophils with abundant dark granules. Lead citrate and uranyl acetate. Magnification 6000 x.

Figure 8. TEM of rabbit lung collected at 4 hours post-exposure showing breakdown of eosinophil membranes. Lead citrate and uranyl acetate. Magnification 12000 x.

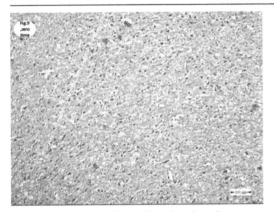

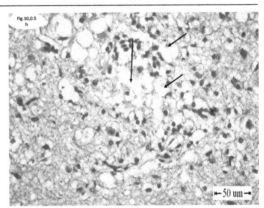

Figure 9. Brain of rabbit collected at Zero hour post-exposure showing the normal appearance of cerebrum. H&E; bar=100μm

Figure 10. Brain of rabbits collected at half hour post-exposure to Scorpion poison showing liquefactive necrosis (arrow). H&E; bar=100μm

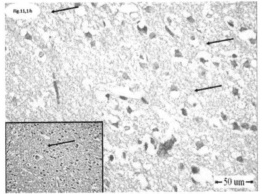

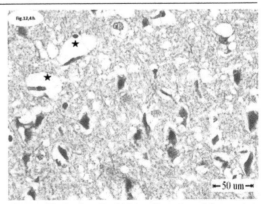

Figure 11. Brain of rabbits collected at 1 hour post-exposure to Scorpion poison showing marked edema which appeared as clear well defined vacuoles (Mouth-eaten, arrow). H&E; bar=100μm

Figure 12. Brain of rabbits collected at 4 hour post-exposure to Scorpion poison showing well-defined edema. H&E; bar=100μm

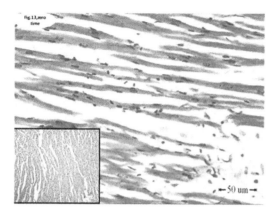

Figure 13. Heart of rabbit collected at Zero hour post-exposure showing the normal appearance of myocardium. H&E; bar=100µm

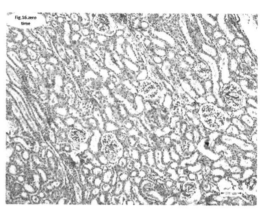

Figure 16. kidney of rabbit collected at Zero hour post-exposure showing the normal appearance of glomeruli, tubules, and interstitial tissues. H&E; bar=100µm

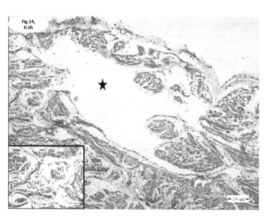

Figure 14. Heart of rabbits collected at half hour post-exposure to Scorpion poison showed focal area of sever myocardiao- lysis (star). H&E; bar=100µm

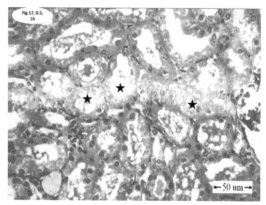

Figure 17. kidney of rabbit collected at half & 1 h post-exposure to Scorpion poison showing focal necrosis of tubular epithelium (stars). H&E; bar=100µm

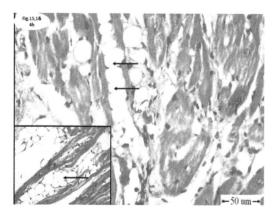

Figure 15. Hearts of rabbits collected at 1 and 4 hours post-exposure to Scorpion poison showed marked Interstitial edema (arrows). H&E; bar=100µm

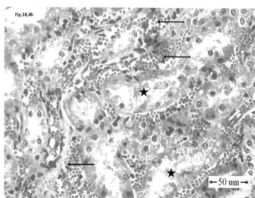

Figure 18. Kidneys of rabbits collected at 4 hours post-exposure to Scorpion poison showing well expressed interstitial hemorrhage (arrow) and necrosis of tubular epithelium (star). H&E; bar=100µm

accumulation in the lung tissue were observed at four hours. These changes were previously described (6, 7). The lung edema is considered to be the main morphological change due to the venom of scorpion such as *Tityus serrulatus,* one of the most venomous scorpions. Its venom is made up of water-soluble and water-insoluble proteins, among which tityus toxin are the most toxic component (8). Transmission electron microscopy in the present study proved the appearance of eosinophils and suggested degranulation of its content had occurred and attributed to the respiratory distress observed clinically.

The present study showed a focal area of malacia characterized by liquifactive necrosis at 0.5 hour. This result may suggest that the toxin of this species has a strong effect within short time, especially with the route of inoculation (i.v). It is known that the scorpion toxins bind to neurotoxin receptor sites blocking sodium channel inactivation or potassium channels. The binding to these channel receptors increases the depolarization time of the channel and consequently, induces excessive neurotransmitter release resulting in the brain damage (9).

Myocardial toxicity is considered one of the major causes of death beside respiratory failure, especially in children stung by the scorpion venom. Scorpion venoms is known to stimulate branches of autonomic nerves with subsequent release of catecholamines (10). Reversible myocardial injury has been attributed to the release of a marker known as Cardiac Tropnin I (CT1), while irreversible injury of the heart may be attributed to the release of CT1 resulting from the damaged myocardial cells (10, 11, 12, 13). In the present study, irreversible myocardial damage expressed by necrosis was observed only at half-hour. This result may suggest an immediate effect of the venom (toxins produced by the species used in the study).

The nephrotoxic effect of scorpion venoms has been documented. Mansour et al. (14) described the microscopic appearance of renal tissues of rats envenomed with the toxin of L.Q scorpion. The study revealed dose and time-dependent pathological changes including glomerular congestion at early stages of envenoming developing to glomerular hypertrophy and hypercellularity followed by mesangiolysis. The epithelial cells of the renal tubules were severely swollen and suffered from necrobiotic changes or cellular damage and their lumina contained eosinophilic masses or hyaline casts.

The present study at half-hour showed necrosis of the glomerular tuft, which is expressed by disappearance of most of the lining epithelium namely mesengial, endothelial, and pericytes cells.

Focal area of severe necrosis of the kidney tubular epithelium, sever inter-tublar hemorrhage by one-hour post-evenomnation, interstitial hemorrhage of the kidney was noticed as well as necrosis of the tubular epithelium lining by four-hours. These results were similar to those reported by Mansour et al. (14).

CONCLUSION

In conclusion, respiratory distress could be due to eosinophilic bronchitis observed by both light and transmission electron microscope. Irreversible myocardial damage expressed by necrosis and edema was evident in this study. Nephrotoxicity was also evident. Scorpion venom is a hazard to human beings due to its effect on the lungs, brains, hearts and kidneys.

REFERENCES

1. Gueron, M., Ilia, R., Sofer, S. (1992). The cardiovascular system after scorpion envenomation. A review. J Toxicol Clin Toxicol. 30 (2): 245 – 258.
http://dx.doi.org/10.3109/15563659209038636
PMid:1588674

2. Cupo, P., Figueiredo, A. B., Filho, A. P., Pintya, A. O., Tavares, G.A., Caligaris, F. (2007). Acute left ventricular dysfunction of severe scorpion envenomation is related to myocardial perfusion disturbance. Int J Cardiol. 116 (1): 98 – 106.
http://dx.doi.org/10.1016/j.ijcard.2006.02.015
PMid:16828898

3. Ross, L. K. (2008). Leiurus quinquestriatus (Ehrenberg, 1828). The Scorpion Files.
http://www.ntnu.no/ub/scorpion-files/l_quinquestriatus_info.pdf

4. Debin, J. A., Strichartz (1991). Chloride channel inhibition by the venom of the scorpion Leiurus quinquestriatus. Toxicon. 29, 1403 – 1408.
http://dx.doi.org/10.1016/0041-0101(91)90128-E

5. Santos, F. B., Nagato, L. K., Boechem, N. M., Negri, E. M., Guimara˜ es, A., Capelozzi, V. L., Faffe, D. S., Zin, W. A., Rocco, P. R. (2006). Time course of lung parenchyma remodeling in pulmonary and extra-pulmonary acute lung injury. J Appl Physiol (1985) 100(1): 98 –106.
http://dx.doi.org/10.1152/japplphysiol.00395.2005
PMid:16109834

6. De Matos, I. M., Rocha, O. A., Leite, R., Freire-Maia, L. (1997). Lung oedema induced by Tityus serrulatus scorpion venom in the rat. Comp Biochem Physiol C Pharmacol Toxicol Endocrinol. 118 (2): 143 - 148.
http://dx.doi.org/10.1016/S0742-8413(97)00086-8

7. Paneque Peres, A. C., Nonaka, P. N., de Carvalho, T., Toyama, M. H., Silva, C. A., Vieira, R. P., Dolhnikoff, M., Zamuner, S. R., de Oliveira, L. V. (2009). Effects of Tityus serrulatus scorpion venom on lung mechanics and inflammation in mice. Toxicon. 53 (7 - 8): 779 - 785.

8. Nunan, E. A., Arya, V., Hochhaus, G., Cardoso, V. N., Moraes-Santos, T. (2004). Age effects on the pharmacokinetics of tityustoxin from Tityus serrulatus scorpion venom in rats. Braz. J. Med. Biol. Res. 37, 385 – 390.
http://dx.doi.org/10.1590/S0100-879X2004000300016
PMid:15060708

9. Carvalho, F. F., Nencioni, A. L., Lebrun, I., Sandoval, M. R., Dorce, V. A. (1998). Behavioral, electroencephalographic, and histopathologic effects of a neuropeptide isolated from Tityus serrulatus scorpion venom in rats. Pharmacol Biochem Behav. 60 (1): 7 - 14.
http://dx.doi.org/10.1016/S0091-3057(97)00407-3

10. Bakir, F., Ozkan, O., Alcigir, M. E., Vural, S. A. (2012). Effects of Androctonus crassicauda scorpion venom on the heart tissue. Journal of animal and veterinary advances 11, 2594 - 2599.
http://dx.doi.org/10.3923/javaa.2012.2594.2599

11. Chue, W. W., Dieter, R. S., Stone, C. K. (2002). Evolving clinical applications of cardiac markers: A review of the literature. WMJ. 101, 49 - 55.

12. Correa, M. M., Sampaio, S. V., Lopes, R. A., Mancuso, L. C., Cunha, O. A., Franco, J. J., Giglio, J. R. (1997). Biochemical and histopathological alterations induced in rats by Tityus serrulatus scorpion venom and its major neurotoxin Tityustoxin-I. Toxicon. 35, 1053 - 1057.
http://dx.doi.org/10.1016/S0041-0101(96)00219-X

13. Ibrahim, H. A., Nabil, Z. I., Abdel-Rahman, M. S. (1996). Effect of scorpion Leiurus quinquestriatus (H&E) venom on the electrophysiology of mammalian heart. III-Blood biochemical studies. J. Egypt Ger. Soc. Zool. 21, 309 - 312.

14. Mansour, N. M., Tawfik, M. N., Rahmy, T. R., Yaseen, A. E. (2007). Protective effect of Ambrosia maritima plant extract against renal alterations induced by Leiurus quinquestriatus scorpion envenoming. Egyptian journal of natural toxins 4 (2): 101 -130.

10

MYXOMATOUS MITRAL VALVE DISEASE
IN DOGS - AN UPDATE AND PERSPECTIVES

Aleksandra Domanjko Petrič

Clinic for Surgery and Small Animal Medicine, Veterinary Faculty,
University of Ljubljana, Cesta v Mestni log 47, 1000 Ljubljana, Slovenia

ABSTRACT

Myxomatous mitral valve disease is a common cause of congestive heart failure in geriatric dogs. Many studies have been done in terms of epidemiology, pathology, associated neurohormonal changes in the disease progression, prognostic factors, and survival and treatment modalities. The presented paper presents a review of some of the studies in the mitral valve disease story.

Key words: mitral valve disease, review, dog

INTRODUCTION

When discussing myxomatous valve disease in dogs, one has in mind atrioventricular valves, in particular the mitral valve, which is affected the most commonly and followed by the tricuspid, aortic valve and pulmonic valve, the last being seldom degenerated.

Myxomatous mitral valve disease (MVD) is the most common cause of heart failure in dogs (1). In literature it can be found under various names, such as chronic valve disease, degenerative valve disease, endocardiosis, and chronic myxomatous valvular disease. It is dealt with a chronic degenerative disease with a progressive valve thickening that starts at the valve edges and causes valve insufficiency (Fig. 1). Over time, the degeneration progresses, as does the insufficiency of the valve.

Epidemiology
The disease is typically found in many small-breed dogs, although there are some large breeds

Corresponding author: Assoc. Prof. Aleksandra Domanjko Petrič, PhD.
E-mail address: aleksandra.domanjko@vf.uni-lj.si
Present address: Clinic for Surgery and Small Animal Medicine
Veterinary Faculty, University of Ljubljana
Cesta v Mestni log 47, 1000 Ljubljana, Slovenia

that are also predisposed. Breeds such as small mixed breed dogs, Poodles, Yorkshire Terriers, Chihuahuas, Cavalier King Charles Spaniels, Miniature and Standard Schnauzers, Cocker Spaniels, Miniature Pinschers, Pekingese, Shi-Tzu, Dachshunds and Dobermans are most commonly reported (1, 2, 3, 4, 5, 6). Males predominated in most of these studies. Prevalence was strongly associated with breed, age and body size (1, 5).

This disease is very rare in cats, although the actual prevalence in this species is not known.

Natural history of the disease
The disease is characterized by a systolic murmur at the mitral area, which increases in intensity as the disease progresses, and radiates to the right side and to the pulmonary areas. The murmur is a hallmark of the disease and can be found in middle-aged to aged dogs, although Cavalier King Charles Spaniels (CKCS) can be affected as early as from one to two years of age (7). Cavalier King Charles Spaniels seem also to have a higher prevalence of MMVD in comparison to other breeds (8). Murmurs can provide valuable information regarding disease severity; the intensity of the murmur correlates with the severity of MMVD and heart failure class. An increase in the intensity of the S1 sound and a decrease of the S2 sound with the presence of S3 sound are signs of moderate to severe MMVD (9). A right-side murmur can indicate the radiation of a loud mitral murmur to the right side or concomitant tricuspid regurgitation and possible pulmonary hypertension (PHT).

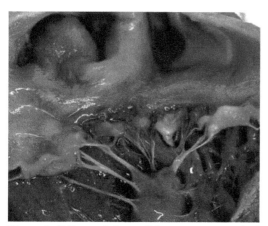

Figure 1. Pathomorphology of the myxomatous mitral valve disease

A loud systolic right-apical murmur was significantly associated with a tricuspid regurgitant pressure gradient (TR) of ≥ 35 mmHg. A stronger right-than-left apical-murmur had a positive predictive value (PPV) of 83% and was 96% specific for TR≥35 mmHg; when combined with syncope, it had a PPV of 92% and was 92% specific (10). Pedersen's study revealed that 82% of CKCSs aged one to three years and 97% of dogs aged more than three years had various degrees of mitral valve prolapse, which is one of the predisposition factors for MMVD (7). Other factors that may contribute to the disease are physical, physiological and other types of stress. In addition, endothelial dysfunction further promotes thickening of the valve leaflets due to shear stress (11). Recently, it has been determined that neurotransmitter serotonin concentrations might be associated with MMVD. The study of Ljungvall et al. revealed that dogs with severe MMVD had lower serum serotonin concentrations than healthy dogs (P = .0025) and dogs with mild MMVD (P = .0011). It was found also that serum serotonin concentrations decreased with increasing left-atrial-to-aortic-root ratio (LA/Ao) (12).

In the pathogenesis of the disease, genetic factors play a very important role, which is supported by the fact that the disease is more prevalent in certain breeds of dogs (13).

Direct evidence of genetic influence in MMVD was studied by Swenson in CKCSs and Olsen in Dachshunds (3, 14), although the exact mode of inheritance was not given.

It seems that in dogs that are genetically more burdened the disease progresses more rapidly and at a younger age. The course of the disease can have a few typical courses of progression: 1) It can start at an older age, progress slowly and never end in heart failure; 2) It progresses slowly and then suddenly after chordal rupture progresses rapidly and ends in acute heart failure; 3) It progresses

slowly and eventually ends in heart failure; 4) It can progress subclinically and end in sudden death. One reason for sudden death is left atrial rupture, which occurs rarely (Fig. 2). Most commonly, dogs with MMVD die or are euthanized because of progressive heart failure and pulmonary edema (Fig. 3) or worsening of clinical signs (Fig. 4) (4, 5, 15). The majority of dogs with MMVD do not develop congestive heart failure (8) and those dogs have a favorable prognosis, while dogs that develop congestive heart failure have high morbidity. The median survival times of dogs with moderate and severe congestive heart failure (CHF) was 33 and 9 months, respectively (5). Dogs receiving pimobendan instead of benazepril hydrochloride, additionally to diuretics, have significantly longer survival times (16). The quality of life was similar in dogs receiving pimobendan or benazepril, but the time to increase the treatment regime was longer in pimobendan group, heart size was smaller and water retention was less in the pimobendan group (17).

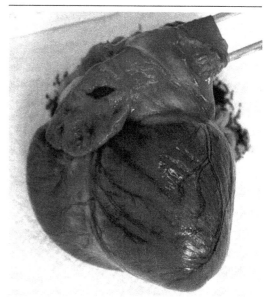

Figure 2. Rupture of the left atrium (LA) between the body of LA and its auricle. A distinct watery sound was heard during systole "in this dog"

Dogs with atrial fibrillation had significantly shorter survival (median 195 days) than dogs without this arrhythmia (median survival 632 days) (4). Arrhythmias are seen in dogs in all stages of MMVD; however, supraventricular and other arrhythmias did not appear associated with the level of severity of MMVD (18). Arrhythmias seem to be a rare cause of syncope in MMVD dogs (18). Dogs with a history of syncope and MMVD tend to have decreased heart rate variability (HRV) and sinus arrhythmia compared to dogs without a history of syncope (18).

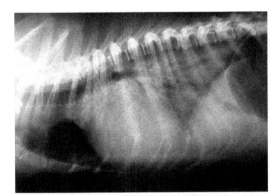

Figure 3. Severe cardiogenic pulmonary edema due to MMVD. Mostly left heart enlargement with left atrium elevating trachea at the hilar region. Air bronchograms are evident

Despite the fact that this is a disease of the mitral valve, the whole heart undergoes changes that cause its remodeling. The triggering event of these geometrical and structural changes is the increase of end-diastolic pressure and hence end-diastolic wall stress due to the volume overload (19). The leaking valve causes regurgitation of the stroke volume into the low-pressure atrium during systole. The consequence of this wall stress is degradation of the collagen weave between cardiomyocytes. With the progression of mitral valve degeneration, the mitral regurgitation increases, and then the atrio-ventricular annulus dilates and worsens the regurgitant orifice. The LV end-diastolic (EDV) and end-systolic volume (ESV) increase, and the total stroke volume (SV) increase, but the forward stroke volume decreases. The increased wall stress initiates a continuation of collagen loss and myocyte stretch (19). The result is increased end-diastolic LV diameter, and cardiac output is up to 30% less than the baseline output. A recent study revealed that the most cardiac enlargement occurs in the year proceeding congestive heart failure (20).

Increasing end-diastolic volume, increasing wall stress, cardiomyocyte stretch, thinning of the cardiac wall, rounding of the LV apex, and decreased systolic function of the LV despite normal to increased measured shortening fraction (SF%) contribute to the development of the clinical manifestation of the disease.

Pathomorphology and pathohystologic changes in MMVD

The mitral valve leaflets consist of four distinct layers. The atrial side is called "atriallis" and the ventricular side is called "ventricularis"; both layers consist of endothelial cells. Below these endothelial layers lies a thin layer consisting of collagen fibers, elastic fibers and fibroblasts; on the atrial side there

is also smooth muscle. Between the two layers are the spongiosa and the fibrosa layers (19). With the progression of the disease, the endothelium proliferates, and the number of fibroblasts increases; there are areas where the endothelial layer is damaged, exposing the basement membrane or the collagen matrix. The spongiosa proliferates, and the fibrosa degenerates in the course of the disease. The thickened spongiosa has the appearance of mesenchymal tissue, thus, the name "myxomatous" (21). In the spongiosa, myofibroblasts proliferate

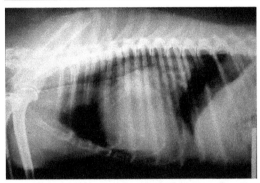

Figure 4. Extremely enlarged left atrium elevating and compressing the trachea and causing an almost uncontrollable cough in a 13-year-old Fox Terrier

and form small nodules. In the fibrosa layer, the collagen fibers become swollen and hyalinized, fragmented and vanish. In the region of high velocity, regurgitant jets in the left atrium jet lesions occur and can cause left atrial tear with haemopericard and acute tamponade and/or sudden death (Fig. 5).

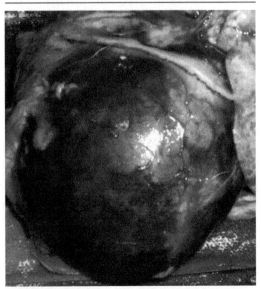

Figure 5. Left atrial tear with haemopericard and acute tamponade

Symptomatology and diagnosis

As mentioned above, the characteristic systolic plateau-shaped murmur can be heard in the predisposed breeds of dogs, and the disease can have a long asymptomatic course. The symptoms usually begin with the development of left heart failure. The dog is usually presented for tachypnea/dyspnea, cough or syncope. The cough is harsh and dry, can gradually increase in frequency and can be a sign of pulmonary edema or main stem bronchus compression due to enlarged left atrium. A similar cough can also be caused by pulmonary disease such as chronic bronchitis that is common in the small sized dogs and can be mistaken for pulmonary edema. The latter is usually accompanied by tachypnea and/or dyspnea (22). The owner can be asked if the dog has had an increased respiratory rate lately. Normally, the respiratory rate does not exceed 30 breaths per minute in dogs regardless of body weight, age or geographic location (23).

Dyspnea can also be caused by pleural effusion or ascites due to right heart failure. Right heart failure in MMVD is a sign of progressive mitral valve disease and pulmonary hypertension that can be accompanied by tricuspid valve degeneration. Clinical signs may develop gradually and progress or they may come acutely due to sudden worsening of the disease. The owner may not have noticed the gradual declining of the dog's physical activity, or acute disease may be caused by a rupture of chordae tendinae, the onset of arrhythmia (usually atrial fibrillation) or some kind of stress that puts the animal over the edge (separation from the owner, new environment, exertion). Hearing the typical murmur over the mitral area can determine the diagnosis of MMVD, and heart failure can be confirmed by thoracic radiography (Fig 3). Echocardiography further documents the individual chamber enlargement, the magnitude of regurgitant flow, the severity of mitral degeneration, valve prolapse, chordal rupture and pulmonary hypertension (Fig 6). Systolic function is difficult to assess in MMVD due to the enhanced sympathetic tone (24).

In an acute setting, which is rare, the cardiac chambers may not be enlarged. In the more common chronic mitral regurgitation, the dilated left ventricular end-diastolic diameter and normal end-systolic diameter, which can also dilate in the late stages of the disease, are usually seen. Therefore, the shortening fraction is increased (over 50%) and comes to normal with advanced disease. Left ventricular end-diastolic diameter, left atrium to aorta ratio (LA/Ao) are echocardiographic measures that independently predict the risk of heart failure (22). The same study confirmed that a radiographically estimated vertebral heart score > 12 and plasma N terminal pro B-type natriuretic peptide (NT pro-BNP) > 1500 pmol/L are measures of threatened heart failure (22).

Electrocardiography serves to identify rhythm disturbances, which are more common in the advanced stages of the disease. The most commonly seen ECG changes are of chamber enlargement, atrial premature complexes, atrial fibrillation, sinus tachycardia, and less commonly ventricular arrhythmias.

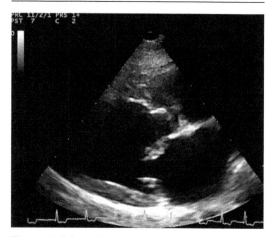

Figure 6. Echocardiographic image showing thickened mitral valve

Radiographically, stages of left ventricular and left atrial enlargement with more or less or no pulmonary edema (Fig. 4) are perceived as interstitial and alveolar patterns. The latter is seen in severe pulmonary edema.

Treatment options for MMVD

1. Pharmacological management of MMVD

The new treatment recommendations for the MMVD rely on the new ACVIM (American College of Veterinary Internal Medicine) classification of cardiac disease that was adapted from the American College of Cardiology and uses an A-through-D categorization scheme. The novel element of this scheme is that it does not rely heavily on exercise tolerance, as the previous scheme did, and also includes dogs in Category A that do not yet have a cardiac disease but have a risk of developing it, i.e. predisposed breeds such as Cavalier King Charles Spaniels. Category B includes dogs with mild heart disease; B1 being reserved for dogs without and B2 with cardiomegaly, but no history of present or past heart failure. Category C includes dogs in heart failure, either one with need of hospitalization (C1) or treated at home (C2). Category D is reserved for dogs in refractory heart failure and divided in D1 and D2 similar to category C. Categorized dogs can be moved from one to another category, depending on the stage of the disease (25).

Class A dogs are those that are predisposed to MMVD, such as specific breeds, and geriatric dogs, and have no signs of disease at the point of diagnosis. The consensus is that these dogs at risk should be screened regularly for the disease (auscultation and additional echocardiography for certain breeds like Cavalier King Charles Spaniels).

Class B patients are divided into two groups. B1 patients have cardiac disease but do not have clinical signs or cardiomegaly. For this group of dogs, there is no recommended treatment at this time that would prolong this asymptomatic period. At this stage, only periodic assessment is recommended in order to identify dogs that have a progression of the disease.

B2 patients have mitral regurgitation and cardiomegaly, but no clinical signs. As mentioned above, the disease in these dogs progresses in a non-linear manner; the most rapid change is observed during the last six to twelve months prior to the onset of CHF and during CHF (20, 22, 30, 31). There is no consensus for this group of patients regarding whether or not a therapy might be beneficial. Two studies showed that long-term treatment with enalapril in asymptomatic dogs with MVD and MR did not or modestly delayed the onset of heart failure regardless of whether or not cardiomegaly was present at initiation of the study (27, 28). Despite the lack of consensus, some use angiotensin-converting enzyme inhibitors (ACE-I) in this period of the disease, as it was shown in some studies in dogs and people to have some beneficial effect (28, 29).

Other drugs that might be used at this stage of the disease, such as inodilators (i.e. pimobendan), mineralocorticoid receptor blocker (i.e. spironolactone), or beta-adenergic receptor blockers, have no proven beneficial effect on reducing progression of the disease; therefore, there is no consent of using any of these drugs (26).

Class C is reserved for dogs having signs of heart failure at present or in the past, such as signs of congestion and edema or low output signs (exercise intolerance, weakness, syncope).

C1 class represents dogs having an acute episode of heart failure, secondary to severe MMVD, and needing to be hospitalized for stabilization. This may be the first episode of presenting heart failure signs or is a worsening of an already treated dog for CHF. This crisis may be due to a chordal rupture, the onset of arrhythmia, atrial rupture or a stressful event. The ACVIM panel suggested the following

pharmacological management: beside the oxygen supplementation and nursing care, furosemide 1–4 mg/kg IV, IM or SC as bolus or 1 mg/kg CRI (constant rate) infusion, the latest being reserved for dogs not responding to a bolus injection (32). My personal experience is to use higher doses of furosemide such as 4–8 mg/kg in severe pulmonary edema cases; the dose depends on the kidney status of the animal, the amount of water taken and age. Monitoring respiratory rate, ECG, urine output and drinking is essential. The crucial note here is if the animal is too stressed because of dyspnea and it is obvious that cardiogenic edema is most likely, I do not stress the dog with radiography, but rather wait until it is at least stable to do a dorso-ventral view. The ACVIM panelists suggest also using pimobendan at 0.25–0.3 mg/kg q12 h (26). Other drugs, such as ACE-I, dobutamine, and hydralazine, did not meet consensus by the group at this stage of the disease (26).

Class C2 represents dogs that have clinical signs of CHF, but are stable enough to go home on therapy. The most common and suggested therapy by panelists is furosemide (1–2 mg /kg q12 h to 4–6 mg/kg q8 h orally), ACE-I (dose depends of the drug used), pimobendan (0.25–0.3 mg/kg q12 h) (26). For the following drugs, no consensus has been reached but many cardiologists use spironolactone for its diuretic, potassium-sparing and presumably anti-fibrotic properties, digoxin (0.22 mg/m²) for rate control, beta adrenergic blockers in cases of atrial fibrillation to control the ventricular rate, or ventricular arrhythmias. Diltiazem can be used as well for the rate control in atrial fibrillation. Other drugs that can be utilized and are used by some veterinarians are amlodipine (up to 0.1 mg/kg q12 h, needs to be titrated and monitor blood pressure), hydrochlorthiazide (2–4 mg/kg q12 h) and torsemide (0.2mg/kg q12-24 h) instead of furosemide. These last three drugs are usually reserved for refractory heart failure cases. Care should be taken not to use beta-blockers until the patient is stable, because these agents can exacerbate the signs of overt heart failure.

Class D patients are those that have more than one episode of heart failure and have been treated with relapses or are refractory to conventional treatment, or have signs of low output failure (weakness, syncope or exercise intolerance).

Class D1 represents dogs with acute worsening of CHF and needing hospitalization. They have clinical signs of congestive and or/low output heart failure. These patients require optimal care in terms of stabilizing their hemodynamic status. Usually they need pleural or abdominal centesis, oxygen, nursing care. They need furosemide, in the already mentioned doses in C1 patients and pimobendan for inotropic an afterload reducing support. Amlodipine may be used for afterload reduction with careful arterial pressure monitoring.

Class D2 patients are similar to D1, they have signs of congestion or low output failure, and have had relapses of it but are suitable for home treatment. The recommended pharmaceutical treatment is furosemide (1–6 mg/kg q8-12 h) with careful monitoring of renal parameters; mild azotemia is unavoidable and well tolerated. Diuresis can be increased by higher dosage or increased frequency of application, also in refractory cases furosemide can be given by SQ injection by the owner instead of a tablet. In these cases, additional diuretics are added like hydrochlorthiazide (1–2 mg q12–24 h), spironolactone (2 mg /kg q24h) or torsemide (0.1 × dose of furosemide) (26, 32). To this drug regimen, other drugs can be added, such as digoxin, beta-blockers, cough suppressants, bronchodilators, sildenafil, but no consensus has been reached on them (26).

With this polypharmacological management, patients can be supported for quite some time, depending of the state at the first presentation, age, kidney status and owner care.

Prognostic information can be gained also from the serial measurements of high-sensitivity cardiac troponin I and NT-proBNP (N-terminal pro B-type natriuretic peptide). High-sensitivity cardiac troponin I, left-ventricular end-systolic diameter normalized to body weight, heart rate and age were independently associated with decreased survival time (33).

2. Surgical management of MMVD

Dogs with severe mitral regurgitation have poor prognosis even with all the pharmacological options that currently exist. Recent improvements in cardiopulmonary bypass techniques have enabled its use in small breed dogs (34, 35). In the case of prosthetic valves, matching the size of the valve and conquering thrombosis is essential for long-term prognosis (36). Recently, successful techniques for mitral valve repair with annuloplasty and chordal replacement have been utilized, which enables long-term survival for severe MMVD patients (37). Costs and availability are the major drawbacks of this option.

Future perspectives

There are still more questions than answers in this disease (38).

More studies regarding the effect of various therapies on the disease progression and outcome are in progress. Disease pathways are studied to help understand molecular pathophysiology and discover possible drug interactions. Genetic studies are evolving for uncovering hereditary aspects of the disease and suggesting possible breeding perspectives that would both help to produce more healthy individuals and combat the disease with means of gene replacement therapy.

CONCLUSION

Mitral valve disease has become a widely recognized disease that enables early diagnosis and treatment. A wide range of pharmacological options for treatment of MMVD provide reasonable quality of life and survival. Surgical repair of the mitral valve provides an option for severely ill animals.

REFERENCES

1. Borgarelli, M., Buchanan, J.W. (2012). Historical review, epidemiology and natural history of degenerative mitral valve disease. J. Vet. Cardiol. 14, 93-101.
   http://dx.doi.org/10.1016/j.jvc.2012.01.011

2. Buchanan, J. W. (1999). Prevalence of cardiovascular disorders: Prevalence of cardiovascular diseases. In: P. Fox, D. Sisson and S. Moise (Eds). Textbook of Canine and Feline Cardiology. 2nd ed. (pp 457-470). WB Saunders, Philadelphia

3. Olsen, L.H., Fredholm, M., Pedersen, H.D. (1999). Epidemiology and inheritance of mitral valve prolapse in Dachshunds. J. Vet. Intern. Med. 13(5):448-456.
   http://dx.doi.org/10.1111/j.1939-1676.1999.tb01462.x

4. Domanjko Petrič, A., Hozjan, E., Blejec, A. (2007). Predisposition and survival of different breeds with chronic valvular disease. Proceedings of 17th European College Veterinary Internal Medicine – Companion Animals Congress, pp. 239, 13th -15th September, Budapest, Hungary.

5. Borgarelli, M., Savarino, P., Crosara, S., Santilli, R.A., Chiavegato, D., Poggi, M., Bellino, C., La Rosa, G., Zanatta, R., Haggstrom, J., Tarducci, A. (2008). Survival characteristics and prognostic variables of dogs with mitral regurgitation attributable to myxomatous valve disease. J. Vet. Intern. Med. 22, 120-128.
   http://dx.doi.org/10.1111/j.1939-1676.2007.0008.x

6. Garncarz, M., Parzeniecka-Jaworska, M., Jank, M., Łój, M. (2013). A retrospective study of clinical signs and epidemiology of chronic valve disease in a group of 207 Dachshunds in Poland. Acta Vet. Scand. Jul 11, 55:52.

7. Pedersen, H.D, Lorentzen, K.A., Kristensen, B.Ø. (1999). Echocardiographic mitral valve prolapse in Cavalier King Charles Spaniels: epidemiology and prognostic significance for regurgitation. Vet. Rec. 144, 315-320.
http://dx.doi.org/10.1136/vr.144.12.315

8. Serfass, P., Chetboul, V., Sampedrano, C.C., Nicolle, A., Benalloul, T., Laforge, H., Gau, C. Hébert, C., Pouchelon, J.L., Tissier, R. (2006). Retrospective study of 942 small-sized dogs: Prevalence of left apical systolic heart murmur and left-sided heart failure, critical effects of breed and sex. J. Vet. Cardiol., 8(1): 11-18.
http://dx.doi.org/10.1016/j.jvc.2005.10.001

9. Hägström, J., Kvart, C., Hansson, K. (1995). Heart sounds and Murmurs: Changes related to severity of chronic valvular disease in the Cavalier King Charles Spaniel. J. Vet. Intern. Med. 9, 75-85.
http://dx.doi.org/10.1111/j.1939-1676.1995.tb03276.x

10. Ohad, D.G. Lenchner, I. Bdolah-Abram, T., Segev, G. (2013). A loud right-apical systolic murmur is associated with the diagnosis of secondary pulmonary arterial hypertension: Retrospective analysis of data from 201 consecutive client-owned dogs (2006–2007). Vet. J. 198, 690–695.
http://dx.doi.org/10.1016/j.tvjl.2013.09.067

11. Pedersen, H.D. (2000). Mitral valve prolapse in the dog. Pathogenesis, pathophysiology and comparative aspects or early myxomatous mitral valve disease. PhD thesis, Copenhagen

12. Ljungvall, I., Höglund, K., Lilliehöök, I., Oyama, M.A., Tidholm, A., Tvedten, H., Hägström, J. (2013). Serum serotonin concentration is associated with severity of myxomatous mitral valve disease in dogs. J. Vet. Intern. Med. 27, 1105–1112.
http://dx.doi.org/10.1111/jvim.12137

13. Detweiler, DK., Patterson, DF. (1965). The prevalence and types of cardiovascular disease in dogs. Ann N Y Acad Sci. Sep 8; 127(1): 481-516.

14. Swenson, L., Hägström, J., Kvart, C., Juneja, R.K. (1996). Relationship between parental cardiac status in Cavalier King Charles Spaniels and prevalence and severity of chronic valvular disease in offspring. J. Amer. Vet. Med. Assoc. 208, 2009-2012.

15. Domanjko Petrič, A., Blagus, R., Mlakar, N. (2013). Survival characteristics in the myxomatous mitral valve disease. Proceedings of the 23rd European College Veterinary Internal Medicine – Companion Animals Congress, September 12-15th, Liverpool

16. Hägström, J., Boswood, A., O'Grady, M., et al. (2008). Effect of pimobendan or benazepril hydrochloride on survival times in dogs with congestive heart failure caused by naturally occurring myxomatous mitral valve disease: the QUEST study. J Vet. Intern. Med. 22(5):1124-1135.
http://dx.doi.org/10.1111/j.1939-1676.2008.0150.x

17. Hägström, J., Boswood, A., O'Grady, M., Jöns, O., et al. (2013). Longitudinal analysis of quality of life, clinical, radiographic, echocardiographic, and laboratory variables in dogs with myxomatous mitral valve disease receiving pimobendan or benazepril: the QUEST study. J Vet. Intern. Med. Nov-Dec; 27(6):1441-1451.

18. Rasmussen, C.E., Falk, T., Domanjko Petrič, A., et al. (2014). Holter monitoring of small breed dogs with advanced myxomatous mitral valve disease with and without a history of syncope. J. Vet. Intern. Med. 28(2): 363-370.
http://dx.doi.org/10.1111/jvim.12290

19. Dillon, R., Dell'Italia, L.J., Tillson, M., Killingsworth, C., Denney, T., Hathcock, J., Botzman, L. (2012). Left ventricular remodeling in preclinical experimental mitral regurgitation of dogs. J Vet. Cardiol. 14, 1, 73-92.
http://dx.doi.org/10.1016/j.jvc.2012.01.012

20. Lord, P., Hansson, K., Kvart, C., Hägström, J. (2010). Rate of change of heart size before congestive heart failure in dogs with mitral regurgitation. J. Small Anim. Pract. 51(4):210-218.
http://dx.doi.org/10.1111/j.1748-5827.2010.00910.x

21. Kittleson, M.D. (2005). Myxomatous mitral valve disease. In: Kittleson, M.D. and Kienle R.D. Small Animal Cardiovascular Medicine.
http://www.vin.com/members/cms/project/defaultadv1.aspx?pid=5928&catId=8440&perlredir=1

22. Reynolds, C.A., Brown, D.C., Rush, J.E., Fox, P.R., Nguyenba, T.P., Lehmkuhl, L.B., Gordon, S.G., Kellihan, H.B., Stepien, R.L, Lefbom, B.K., Meier, C.K., Oyama, M.A. (2012). Prediction of first onset of congestive heart failure in dogs with degenerative mitral valve disease: The PREDICT cohort study. J. Vet. Cardiol. 14, 1, 193-202.
http://dx.doi.org/10.1016/j.jvc.2012.01.008

23. Rishniw, M., Ljungvall, I., Porciello, F., Hägström, J., Ohad, D.G. (2012). Sleeping respiratory rates in apparently healthy adult dogs.Res. Vet. Sci. 93(2):965-9.
http://dx.doi.org/10.1016/j.rvsc.2011.12.014

24. Bonagura, JD, Schober, KE. (2009). Can ventricular function be assessed by echocardiography in chronic canine mitral valve disease? J Small Anim. Pract. Sep; 50 Suppl. 1, 12-24.

25. Atkins, C., Bonagura, J., Ettinger, S., Fox, P., Gordon, S., Haggstrom, J., Hamlin, R., Keene, B., Luis-Fuentes, V., Stepien, R. (2009). Guidelines for the diagnosis and treatment of canine chronic valvular heart disease. J Vet. Intern. Med. 23(6):1142-50.
http://dx.doi.org/10.1111/j.1939-1676.2009.0392.x

26. Atkins, C. E., Hägström, J. (2012). Pharmacologic management of myxomatous mitral valve disease in dogs. J Vet. Cardiol., 14, 1, 165-184.
http://dx.doi.org/10.1016/j.jvc.2012.02.002

27. Kvart, C., Häggström, J., Pedersen, HD., Hansson, K., et al. (2002). Efficacy of enalapril for prevention of congestive heart failure in dogs with myxomatous valve disease and asymptomatic mitral regurgitation. J Vet Intern Med. Jan-Feb; 16(1): 80-88.

28. Atkins, C., Keene, B., Brown, W., Coats, J., Crawford, M., et al. (2007). Results of the veterinary enalapril trial to prove reduction in onset of heart failure in dogs chronically treated with enalapril alone for compensated, naturally occurring mitral valve insufficiency. J. Am. Vet. Med. Assoc. 23, 1061–1069. http://dx.doi.org/10.2460/javma.231.7.1061

29. The SOLVD Investigators. (1992). Effect of enalapril on mortality and the development of heart failure in asymptomatic patients with reduced left ventricular ejection fractions. New Eng. J. Med. 327, 725–727.

30. Tarnow, I., Olsen L.H., Kvart, C., Höglund, K., Moesgaard, S.G., Kamstrup, T.S., Pedersen, H.D., Häggström, J. (2009). Predictive value of natriuretic peptides in dogs with mitral valve disease. Vet. J. 180, 195–201.
http://dx.doi.org/10.1016/j.tvjl.2007.12.026

31. Ljungvall, I., Höglund, K., Carnabuci, C., Tidholm, A., Häggström, J. (2011). Assessment of global and regional left ventricular volume and shape by real-time 3-dimensional echocardiography in dogs with myxomatous mitral valve disease. J. Vet. Intern. Med. 25, 1036–1043.
http://dx.doi.org/10.1111/j.1939-1676.2011.0774.x

32. Atkins, J., Bonagura, S., Ettinger, P., Fox, S., Gordon, J., Häggström, R., Hamlin, B., Keene (Chair), V., Luis-Fuentes, Stepien, R. (2009). Guidelines for the diagnosis and treatment of canine chronic valvular heart disease. J. Vet. Intern. Med. 23: 1142–1150. http://dx.doi.org/10.1111/j.1939-1676.2009.0392.x

33. Hezzell, M.J, Boswood, A., Chang, Y.M., Moonarmart, W., Souttar, K., Elliott, J. (2012). The combined prognostic potential of serum high-sensitivity cardiac troponin I and N-terminal pro-B-type natriuretic peptide concentrations in dogs with degenerative mitral valve disease. J Vet Intern Med. Mar-Apr; 26(2):302-311.

34. Kanemoto, D., Taguchi, S., Yokoyama, M., Mizuno, H., Suzuki, T Kanamoto (2010). Open heart surgery with deep hypothermia and cardiopulmonary bypass in small and toy dogs. Vet. Surg. 39, 674–679.

35. Yamano, S., Uechi, M., Tanaka, K., Hori, Y., Ebisawa, T., Harada, K., Mizukoshi, T. (2011). Surgical repair of a complete endocardial cushion defect in a dog. Vet. Surg. 40, 408–412.
http://dx.doi.org/10.1111/j.1532-950X.2011.00797.x

36. Orton, E.C., Hackett, T.B., Mama, K., Boon, J.A. (2005). Technique and outcome of mitral valve replacement in dogs. J. Am. Vet. Med. Assoc. 226, 1508–1511. http://dx.doi.org/10.2460/javma.2005.226.1508

37. Masami Uechi. (2012). Mitral valve repair in dogs. J. Vet. Cardiol. 14, 185-192. http://dx.doi.org/10.1016/j.jvc.2012.01.004

38. Orton, C.E. (2012). Mitral valve degenerations: still more questions than answers. J. Vet. Cardiol. 14, 3-5. http://dx.doi.org/10.1016/j.jvc.2012.02.003

11

STUDY OF THE EFFECTS OF BREED ON SOME INNATE IMMUNITY PARAMETERS IN RAMS

Genova Krasimira[1], Dimitrova Ivona[2], Stancheva Nevyana[1], Angelov Geno[1],
Nakev Jivko[3], Mehmedov Tandju[1], Georgieva Svetlana[4]

[1]*Faculty of Veterinary Medicine, University of Forestry, Sofia, Bulgaria*
[2]*Agronomy Faculty, University of Forestry, Sofia, Bulgaria*
[3]*Agricultural Institute, Shumen, Bulgaria*
[4]*Faculty of Agriculture, Trakia University, Stara Zagora, Bulgaria*

ABSTRACT

Investigations were carried out on 26 rams from the breeds Karakachan and Copper-Red Shoumen. The non-specific immune parameters, phagocytic activity of leukocytes, bactericidal activity of phagocytes systems (oxygen-dependent and oxygen independent) and total plasma protein level were evaluated. Phagocytic response was evaluated against *S. aureus* 209-P with a certain percentage of active phagocytes (phagocytic index) and the number of absorbed particles per one phagocytic cells (phagocyte number). Phagocytosis completion index was defined as the percentage of the microbial cells that have been destroyed by phagocytes after incubation. State of the oxygen-dependent bactericidal systems of phagocytes was assessed in vitro using the NBT test, which reflects the ability of superoxide restore NBT in diphormazane. NBT test was evaluated by the degree of reduction in spontaneous and stimulated reactions, taking into account the intracellular deposits diphormazane. Our studies and results shows that the rams from the two local Bulgarian breeds have a high activity of innate immune parameters and that's may be useful and important in the breeding programs as an indicator of resistance and highly tolerance to oxidative stress.

Key words: sheep, indigenous breeds, phagocytic activity, NBT test, total plasma protein

INTRODUCTION

The problem of providing the population with high-grade and organic food is recognized as the second largest problem among the ten closest global problems of mankind, formulated by leading experts in the WHO.

The efficiency of livestock development depends on many factors. Fundamental of these is genetically based level of productivity.

It is known now that the immune system is the most sensitive indicator system that responds to changes in environmental factors. The external effects of impact is on the performance of innate immune resistance and specific immune system (6). In this connection, when acclimatizing highly productive animals, it becomes very important to study the state's natural resistance factors.

The problem of increasing non-specific resistance of farm animals is still relevant today. Breeding for improvement of natural resistance plays a primary role in the problem of disease control, as well as in the creation of animals that are suitable to the conditions of industrial technology (7, 13).

The present study was undertaken to investigate the effects of breed on PMN phagocytic activity, metabolic activity of neutrophils and on the total plasma protein level.

Corresponding author: Prof. Genova Krasimira, PhD
E-mail address: dr_kig@abv.bg;
Present address: Faculty of Veterinary Medicine,
University of Forestry, Sofia, Bulgaria

MATERIALS AND METHODS

Animals
The study was conducted on 18 rams from the breed Karakachan and 8 rams from the breed Copper Red Shoumen.

Blood collection
Venous blood was collected From each normal animal with Vacutainer tubes containing heparin as an anticoagulant.

Bacteria
In these experiments we used an alive culture of the *Staphylococcus aureus* strain 209P. Bacterial cultures were grown in standard media at 37 °C during 18h and then taken for our investigations.

Absorptive and metabolic activity of peripheral blood neutrophils
A modified method of Gordienko et al., (5) was used to study the absorptive phagocytosis phase with bacterial cells and oxygen-depended metabolism of peripheral blood neutrophiles in NBT-reactions. Briefly, a18h microbial suspension of *Staphylococcus aureus* strain 209P with a density of $2 \times 10^9/cm^3$ was used. Phagocytosis was measured by the phagocytosis index (PI) - (% phagocytosis) and phagocyte number (PN). Oxidative metabolism was measured by the nitroblue tetrazolium (NBT) reduction test. In conical tubes 0.1 ml whole heparinized blood, 0.1 ml medium 199, and 0,1 ml 1% NBT solution were mixed. The samples were incubated at 370C for 40 minutes, blood smears were performed and Giemsa stained. We counted, at the optical microscope, the proportion of positive NBT polymorphonuclear leukocytes which had included and reduced NBT dye to nitroformazan - a dark-blue precipitate (3). Stimulated NBT test - leukocytes were stimulated with 0,1 ml suspension *St. aureus*.

Total serum proteins
The level of total serum protein was examined with the semi-automatic biochemical analyzer Screen master LIHD-113 (Hospital Diagnostic, Germany).

Statistics
The significance of differences for all parameters was estimated by Student's T-test.

RESULTS

Phagocytic activity of the blood neutrophils in rams from two breeds is shown on Figure 1. The animals from Karakachan breed had lower phagocytic index and phagocytic number compared to the rams from Copper-Red Shoumen breed (p<0,01).

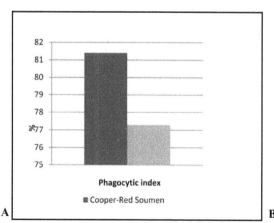
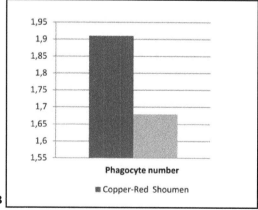

Figure 1 A, B. Phagocytic activity of neutrophils of rams

The capacity of the non-stimulated neutrophils of Cooper–Red Shumen rams to reduce NBT was found to be not significantly increased in comparison to rams from the other breed.

The stimulation of polymorphonuclear and mononuclear cells was accompanied by the significantly higher capacity of leukocytes to reduce NBT in rams from the Karakachan breed (Fig. 2)

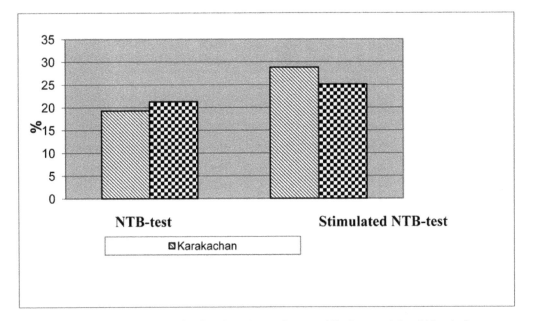

Figure 2. Spontaneous and stimulated NBT-test of neutrophils from peripheral blood of rams

Serum values of total proteins in rams from two breeds are presented in Table 1.

Serum levels of the total proteins were within the normal parameters, but they were about 12% higher in the Karakachan rams, when comparing the rams .

Table 1. Serum values of proteins in Karakachan and Copper-Red Shoumen rams

		Rams	
		Karakachan	Copper-Red Shoumen
Parameters	**Normal values**		
Total protein g/dL	6.8-8.2	8.05±1.31	7.15±1.9

Values are mean±standard error of mean (p<0.05)

DISCUSSION

The natural resistance of the body is essential for animal life. It is caused by humoral factors and by the ability of specific cellular components - phagocytosis. These nonspecific reactions are labile and they depend on various factors, like stress and on the breed. In this regard, the study of non-specific immunity, related with the breed is of great

scientific and practical importance, if we consider the contradictory scientific results (1, 8, 12).

Phagocytosis is an important mechanism of nonspecific immunity. In the blood, polymorphonuclear and mononuclear leukocytes act as "professional" phagocytes. In our study, the pattern of phagocytic activity of the leukocytes was determined by the phagocytic number and index. As a test system we use *St.aureus* 209 P, while other authors used different particles and crystals (2). The phagocytic activity in rams was determined by Semerjiev (11), who observed tendency for changes of PI and PN depending on the season. Variations of leukocyte phagocytic activity due to the season and breed were found out in goat kids, goats and bucks (9,10). As shown by presented results, the rams from the Cooper–Red Shumen breed had higher phagocytic activity than the animals from the Karakachan breed. In contrast Semerjiev et al. (8) observed lower values of PI and PN in rams from both breeds.

NBT test is used for studies of ability of the innate immune system to kill the bacteria. Statement of the NBT test in two versions helped us to calculate the functional reserve of cells.

The values of the stimulated NBT test characterized the activity of phagocytic cells in the presence of antigenic stimulus. They are considered as criteria for the complete phagocytosis. Spontaneous NBT-test is used to evaluate the degree of activation of intracellular phagocytic systems. Our results indicate a good phagocytic activity, which is in correlation with the results of Deptula et al. (4) .

Blood proteins reflect on the state of the metabolic processes in the rams. At the level of blood total protein affect the nature of nutrition and metabolic disorders. Changes in the metabolic rate are reflection of the adaptation processes. The data obtained can serve as a rationale for identifying the productive and breed potential of the rams, as well as of the work aimed to regulate these processes.

CONCLUSION

It was concluded that there are breed-related difference in the innate immune parameters in rams. The phagocytic activity of Cooper–Red Shumen rams was higher than in the animals from Karakachan breed.

ACKNOWLEDGMENT

Research was part of the project 501/22- 05.12.2012 (2012-2014) "Development of DNA markers (CAST, MSTN) for fattening ability and meat quality in Synthetic population Bulgarian Milk, Karakachan and Copper Red Shumen sheep breeds" financed by the Ministry of Education, Youth and Science, Republic of Bulgaria.

REFERENCES

1. Akhmadiev, G.M. (2013). Evaluation and stress sensitivity and stress resistance inruminants and their offspring. Modern directions of theoretical and applied researches'2013, 19-30 march, 1-13

2. Benda V., J. Hoiipes. (1991) Phagocytic Activity of Leukocytes in Sheep and Goats. Acta vet. Brno, 60: 149-152.

3. Cocarla, D., S. Gotia. (2000). In vitro effect of Felodipin on leucocyte phagocytosis and ROS formation in peripheral blood of the patients with chronic metabolic hepatitis. TMJ, XLI-VII, 1: 75-78.

4. Deptula, W., P. Miedźwiedzka, J. Śliwa, M. Kaczmarczyk,B.Tokarz-Deptuła,B..Hukowska -Szematowicz, Pawlikowska, M. (2008). Values of selected immune indices in healthy rabbits. Centr Eur J Immunol, 33, 4: 190-192.

5. Gordienko,G., Samsygina, G., Dudina T., Borodin T. (2003). Method for the detection the absorbency of metabolic activity of neutro-phils in peripheral blood by phagocytosis and NBT test. Patent of the Russian Federation RU 2249215.

6. Haitov, R., Pinegin B., Istamov, H. (1995). Ecological immunology, (pp.18-37) Moscow, VNIRO press.

7. Mescheryakov, O. (1995). Economic efficiency in veterinary care of cattle farms. Veterinariya, 12: 16-18.

8. Semerdjiev V., Maslev, T., L. Sotirov, L., N. Sandev, N., Iliev, M., Gercev, G., Yankov, I. Hristova, T. (2008). Breed-, age- and gender-related features of phagocytic activity in sheep duringthe autumn. J. Mount. Agricult. Balk., 1: 1-12.

9. Semerdjiev, V. (2010). Seasonal and breed-related features of blood phagocytic activity in goats and bucks, Journal of Mountain agricul-ture on the Balkans, 13, 2: 367-380.

10. Semerdjiev V., Zunev, P., Maslev, Ts., Sandev, N., Sotirov, L., Bochukov, A., Atanasov, A., Koinarski. Ts., (2010). Bloodphagocytic activity in goat kids depending on the season,

breed, age and gender. Journal of Mountain agriculture on the Balkans, 13, 3: 633-646.

11. Semerdjiev, V. (2011). Breed, gender and seasonal variations of blood phagocytic activity in local sheep breeds reared in Bulgaria., Trakia Journal of Sciences, 9, 2, 69-75.

12. Tunikov, G. (1983). Enhancing the natural resistance of cows at inbreeding. Genetic resistance to diseases of farm animals, 3, 23.

13. Warner, C., D., Meeker D., Rothsild, M. (1992). Genetic control of immune responsiveness: A. review of the use as a tool for selecion for disease resistense. J. Anim. Sc., 64, 2: 394-406.

12

OPTIMIZATION, VALIDATION AND APPLICATION OF UV-VIS SPECTROPHOTOMETRIC-COLORIMETRIC METHODS FOR DETERMINATION OF TRIMETHOPRIM IN DIFFERENT MEDICINAL PRODUCTS

Goran Stojković[1], Elizabeta Dimitrieska-Stojković[2], Marija Soklevska[1], Romel Velev[2]

[1]University "Ss. Cyril and Methodius", Faculty of Natural Sciences and Mathematics, Institute of Chemistry, Skopje, Republic of Macedonia
[2]University "Ss. Cyril and Methodius", Faculty of Veterinary Medicine – Skopje, Institute for Food, Skopje, Republic of Macedonia

ABSTRACT

Two simple, sensitive, selective, precise, and accurate methods for determination of trimethoprim in different sulfonamide formulations intended for use in human and veterinary medicine were optimized and validated. The methods are based on the trimethoprim reaction with bromcresol green (BCG) and 2,4-dinitro-1-fluorobenzene (DNFB). As extraction solvents we used 10 % N,N-dimethylacetamide in methanol and acetone for both methods, respectively. The colored products are quantified applying visible spectrophotometry at their corresponding absorption maxima. The methods were validated for linearity, sensitivity, accuracy, and precision. We tested the method applicability on four different medicinal products in tablet and powder forms containing sulfametrole and sulfamethoxazole in combination with trimethoprim. The results revealed that both methods are equally accurate with recoveries within the range 95-105 %. The obtained between-day precision for both methods, when applied on four different medicinal products, was within in the range 1.08-3.20 %. By applying the F-statistical test ($P<0.05$), it was concluded that for three medicinal products tested both methods are applicable with statistically insignificant difference in precision. The optimized and validated BCG and DNFB methods could find application in routine quality control of trimethoprim in various formulation forms, at different concentration levels, and in combination with different sulfonamides.

Key words: medicinal products, trimethoprim, UV/Vis spectrophotometry, validation

INTRODUCTION

Trimethoprim (2,4-diamino-5-(3'4'5'-trimethoxy benzyl)pyrimidine) (Scheme 1) is a well known biological agent, employed as a potent metabolic inhibitor of bacterial dihydrofolic acid reductase (1). This drug is exhibiting high antibacterial activity against strains resistant to other antibiotics frequently used, e.g. β-lactams. The therapeutic activity of trimethoprim could be attributed to the pyrimidine ring system (see Scheme 1), also present

in other biologically active substances such as nucleic acids, several vitamins, and coenzymes (2). The introduction of combination of trimethoprim (TMP) and sulfamethoxazole (SMX) in the middle of the 1970s resulted in increased use of sulfonamides for treatment of specific microbial infections (3). Due to their synergistic activity, sulfonamides potentiated with trimethoprim are one of the most widely used antimicrobial compounds against gram-negative and gram-positive bacteria.

The optimal combination of the two agents for their synergistic activity was found to be 5:1 (4). Pharmacologically, this ratio is optimal for satisfactory reduction of both the toxicity of the individual agents and possible resistance of the organism to them, thus enhancing the therapeutic effect.

The mixture of sulfonamides and TMP in pharmaceutical preparations was studied in a number of investigations and the latter provide several analytical methods for the determination

Corresponding author: Assoc. Prof. Goran Stojković, PhD
E-mail address: goranst@pmf.ukim.mk
Present address: University "Ss. Cyril and Methodius",
Faculty of Natural Sciences and Mathematics,
Institute of Chemistry, Skopje, Republic of Macedonia

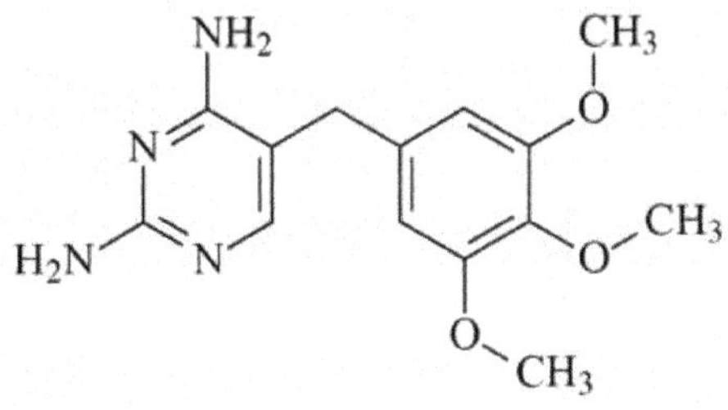

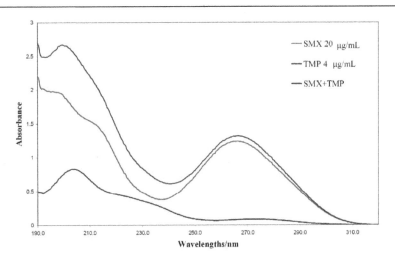

Scheme 1. Structural formula of trimethoprim

thereof. Such methods include different analytical techniques mostly ultraviolet and visible (UV-Vis) spectrophotometry (3, 5-8), derivative spectrophotometry (9-11), high performance liquid chromatography (HPLC) (12-14) and chemometric methods applying multivariate calibrations (7). Other more rarely reported methods for TMP determination are titrimetric (16), voltametric (17), polarographic (18). Even though the Official pharmacopeia method includes HPLC determination (19), still, there are numerous UV-Vis methods proven as satisfactory alternative to the liquid chromatography (3, 8, 10, 11, 15). The main advantage thereof is their simplicity, rapidity, and low cost-effectiveness.

formulations, are based on direct (7, 9, 10) and colorimetric spectrophotometry (5, 8, 15). Regarding the colorimetric spectrophotometry, the first publication (5), describes application of several reagents as π-acceptors for obtaining adduct products: bromothymol blue, bromocresol green, and alizarin red S. As extraction solvents the authors have proposed chloroform, methylene chloride and chlorobenzene. Adekoge et al. (8) have developed a method for spectrophotometric determination of TMP following charge-transfer complexation with chloranilic acid. The published study by Al-Sabha et al. (15), describes spectrophotometric determination of TMP based on the reaction of the amine group with 2,4-dinitro-1-fluorobenzene (DNFB) reagent in acetone medium. The main advance of these colorimetric methods is the significant difference in the absorption maxima of the compounds obtained, in comparison to the neat compounds, towards higher wavelengths in the visible spectra.

In this work, we have focused on optimization and validation of two colorimetric spectrophotometric methods with bromocresol green (BCG) and DNFB, for determination of TMP in pharmaceutical products intended for use in human and veterinary medicine. In terms of improving the method performances

Figure 1. UV spectra of SMX (20 µg mL⁻¹), TMP (4 µg mL⁻¹) and SMX+TMP

The UV absorption spectra of SMX and TMP show overlapping with each other (Fig. 1), creating a serious problem for their analysis in the pharmaceutical products. Therefore, various sample preparation techniques for the simultaneous determination of SMX and TMP in pharmaceuticals have been developed. The first order UV-Vis spectrophotometric methods to determinate TMP, in pure form and pharmaceutical

and applicability, we have introduced some modifications in both methods such as different extraction solvents, experimental conditions and extended method ranges. With such modifications performed, we tested the methods reliability in terms of sensitivity, accuracy, and precision. Over more, we tested the methods applicability on real samples i.e. different formulations, different sulfonamides present in two formulation forms

– tablets and powder. So far, there is insufficient literature data regarding method validation for TMP according to the internationally accepted criteria (20), when applied on formulations intended for use in veterinary medicine. The validation parameters obtained from the method applicability studies were analyzed for significance using suitable statistical tests.

MATERIAL AND METHODS

Apparatus

The solutions were sonificated in VWR Ultrasonic cleaner (HF40 kHz, 60 W). The UV spectra of the blanks, standard and sample solutions, were recorded on a Varian Carry 50 UV/Visible Spectrophotometer, at room temperature in 1 cm quartz cell. The wavelength range was from 190 to 800 nm, with resolution 0.5 nm and scan rate of 300 nm/min. For spectral data acquisition and processing Varian Cary WinUV 2002 Software (Varian, Mulgrave, Victoria, Australia), was used.

method, we prepared a series of calibration standards with concentrations of 1, 5, 10, 15, 20, 25, 30 and 35 μg/mL. The series of calibration standards for the DNFB method were prepared in the range 20, 30, 40, 50, 60, 70, 80, and 90 μg/mL.

Samples

The method validation and applicability was tested on four different medicinal products containing sulfonamides and TMP. The detailed description of each formulation is presented in Table 1.

Optimization of the bromcresol green and 2,4-dinitro-1-fluorobenzene method

The previously published BCG method (5) was modified and optimized towards obtaining the best linearity and recovery. For this purpose, first, different solvents were tested in different media: methanol, ethanol, 10 % N,N-dimethylacetamide in methanol, obtaining the best achievable method performances. The next step was the optimization of the sonification time; therefore, the samples were

Table 1. Content of sulfonamides and trimethoprim in medicinal products

Formulation ID	Form	Sulfonamide content*	Trimethoprim content*	Field of application
Formulation 1	tablet	sulfametrole 400 mg/tablet	80 mg/tablet	human medicine
Formulation 2	tablet	sulfametoxazole 400 mg/tablet	80 mg/tablet	human medicine
Formulation 3 (producer A)	powder	sulfametoxazole 100 mg/g	20 mg/g	veterinary medicine
Formulaion 4 (producer B)	powder	sulfametoxazole 100 mg/g	20 mg/g	veterinary medicine

*nominal content according to the producers specifications

Reagents

Bromocresol green (Kemika, Zagreb, Croatia) was dissolved in 10 % N,N-dimethylacetamide (Sigma-Aldrich, St Louis, USA) in methanol, at concentration of 0.001 mol/L, and DFNB (Sigma-Aldrich, St Louis, USA) was dissolved in methanol at concentration of 0.01 mol/L. Methanol HPLC grade and acetone with purity ≥99.5 % used were supplied from Sigma-Aldrich (St Louis, USA). For pH adjustment, a NaOH solution with concentration of 0.1 mol/L was applied. The analytical standard of TMP (Vetranal) purchased from Fluka (St. Gallen, Switzerland), was used for preparation of stock solution containing 1.00 mg/mL in HPLC grade methanol (Sigma-Aldrich, Bellafonte, USA). From this stock applying suitable dilutions, for the BCG

treated for 30, 45, and 60 minutes in the ultrasonic bath.

The DNFB assay was performed on the basis of the previously published method by Al-Sabha and Hamody (15). Thus, some modifications were necessary towards the optimal heating temperature and time, as well as use of different filtration means. By monitoring the linearity and trueness performances, we chose the most appropriate experimental conditions.

Standard and sample preparation and measurement

Bromcresol green method

Adequate mass portions of the tested formulations (0.0356 g, 0.0312 g, 0.250 g and 0.250 g, for Formulation 1, 2, 3 and 4, respectively) were transferred in 50 mL volumetric flasks and filled up to 2/3 with 10 % solution of N,N-dimethylacetamide in methanol. The solutions were sonificated at room temperature for 30 and 45 minutes for human and veterinary formulations, respectively. In the next step they were filled up with 10 % solution of N,N-dimethylacetamide in methanol to a volume of 50 mL. Afterwards they were filtered through quantitative filter (ashless, grade 41, by Whatman). A suitable aliquot of the initial solutions (equal to TMP concentration of ~100 µg/mL) was taken obtaining a TMP concentration of 20 µg/mL in 10 mL

and 0.375 g for for Formulation 1, 2, 3 and 4, respectively) were transferred in 25 mL volumetric flask and filled up to 2/3 with in acetone. We sonicated the samples for 30 min, filled up with acetone to the final volume, and consequently filtered them through quantitative filter (ashless, grade 41, by Whatman) and 0.45 µm syringe filters. Afterwards, suitable aliquots of the initial solution with concentration of ~300 µg/mL of TMP was taken obtaining a TMP concentration of 60 µg/mL in 10 mL volumetric flasks. Two mililiters of DNFB reagent were added and the solution was heated for 40 min at 50 °C and additionally for 10 min at 60 °C.

Scheme 2. TMP-BCG adduct

volumetric flasks. In the following step, 1 mL of the BCG solution was added, and the pH value of the media was adjusted with 20-25 µL of the 0.1 M NaOH solution to a value of approximately 7.5. Finally, the samples were filled up to volume with 10% N,N-dimethylacetamide. Before performing the spectrophotometric measurement, the samples were filtered through 0.45 µm syringe filters. The suitably prepared series of standards were processed as described for the samples. The standard and sample solutions prepared are with green color and exhibit absorption maxima around 620 nm, as a result of the TMP-BCG adduct formed (Scheme 2). The absorbance was measured against reagent blank prepared following the same procedure.

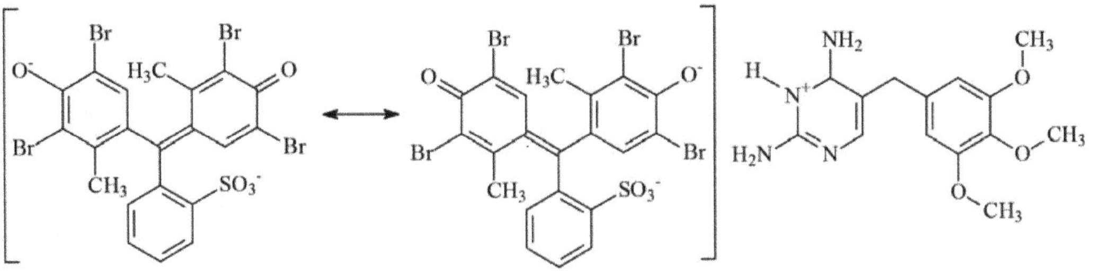

2,4- Dinitro-1-fluorobenzene method

For DNFB method, the measured mass portions of the formulations (0.0536 g, 0.0469 g, 0.375 g

The heating time and temperature were somewhat modified in comparison to the previously published method (15), thus avoiding acetone evaporation. After cooling the samples to room temperature, we filled them up with acetone and measured on the spectrophotometer, against similarly prepared regent blank. The series of standards for the DNFB method mentioned above were processed following the same procedure. The product of reaction of nucleophilic substitution of TMP with DNFB (Scheme 3) is with pale red color and exhibit absorption maxima around 540 nm.

Method validation

The validation for both methods applied for TMP determination in investigated formulations was conducted according to the ICH requirements (20). The methods were tested for linearity, limit of detection (LOD), limit of quantification (LOQ),

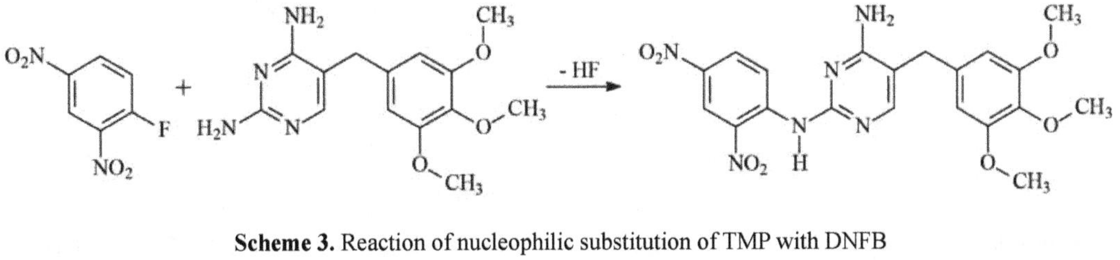

Scheme 3. Reaction of nucleophilic substitution of TMP with DNFB

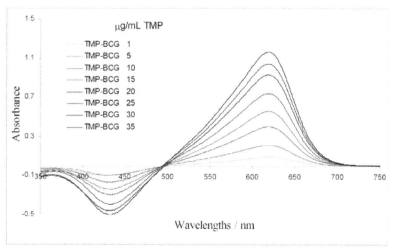

Figure 2. UV/Vis spectra of standard solutions of trimethoprim (1–35 µg mL^{-1}) obtained with BCG method

accuracy estimated through recovery experiments, and precision. LOD and LOQ were estimated through the standard errors of the calibration curves (21). For recovery assessment for BCG method each formulation was spiked with TMP standard of 10 µg mL^{-1} in triplicates, equal to final concentration of 30 µg mL^{-1}. Precision for BCG method was estimated performing six individually measured replicates for each formulation at level of 20 µg mL^{-1}. Regarding the DNFB method, the solution formulations containing 60 µg mL^{-1} were spiked with TMP solution containing 30 µg mL^{-1} of the analyte. Precision assessment was performed on six replicates in two different days for each formulation. The adjusted TMP concentration was 20 and 60 µg mL^{-1}, for the BCG and DNFB method, respectively.

Statistical analysis

The statistical analysis of the validation data obtained was performed using Microsoft Office Excel 2003. The recovery and precision data obtained for investigated formulations were tested applying *t*-test and *F*-test for significance, at a confidence level of 95 % ($P < 0.05$).

RESULTS

Method validation
Linearity of the BCG and DNFB method

For the BCG method, the linearity observed was within the range 1–35 µg mL^{-1}, from eight calibration points measured in five replicates.

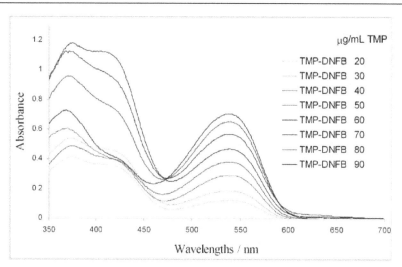

Figure 3. UV/Vis spectra of standard solutions of trimethoprim (20–90 µg mL^{-1}) obtained with DNFB method

Table 2. Linearity, sensitivity and accuracy of BCG and DNFB method

Parameters	Testing method	
	BCG	DNFB
Range/μg mL^{-1}	1–35	20–90
Calibration curves	y=0.0326x+0.0687	y=0.0086x-0.0572
Linearity (R^2)	0.9976	0.9981
LOD/μg mL^{-1}	2.72	4.90
LOQ/μg mL^{-1}	9.09	16.31
Recovery*/% (Formulation 1)	97.57±3.45[†]	97.53±2.68[†]
Recovery*/% (Formulation 2)	98.31±2.15[†]	103.13±0.39[†]
Recovery*/% (Formulation 3)	99.49±1.27[†]	99.33±2.13[†]
Recovery*/% (Formulation 4)	100.91±3.56[†]	99.46±2.33[†]
Average recovery	99.07±1.46[†]	99.86±2.35[†]

* n=3, spiking level 10 μg mL^{-1} for BCG method and 30 μg mL^{-1} for DNFB method
[†] ±relative standard deviation (%)

Calibration curve was determined from the signals of the absorbances maxima at 618 nm (Fig. 2).

Negative absorbance values in spectra occur due to the higher presence of BCG in the blank in comparison to the solutions where TMP is present. By increasing the TMP concentration, the amount of BCG decreases due to adduct formed. The correlation coefficient value (R^2) was 0.9976 (Table 2). For the DNFB method, the linearity was determined in the range 20–90 μg mL^{-1}, with R^2 of 0.9981 (Table 2), on the basis of the signals measured at 538 nm from eight calibration points in five replicates (Fig. 3).

Sensitivity and accuracy of the BCG and DNB method

Even though the method sensitivity is not a crucial parameter when analytes in sufficiently high concentrations are analyzed, yet, we wanted to determine the LODs and LOQs for the modified methods. These parameters are estimated through the standard deviation of the calibration curve slope (21). The obtained sensitivity parameters for the BCG method are within the method range, while for the DNFB method they were estimated to be below the lowest calibration standard (Table 2).

To test the method suitability in term of accuracy, recovery experiments were conducted by

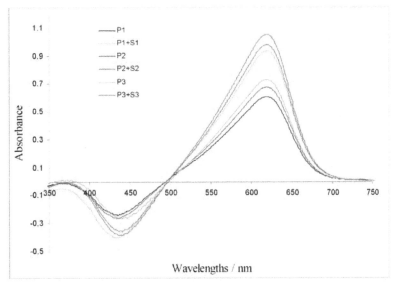

Figure 4. UV/Vis spectra of spiking experiments for recovery for BCG method (sample of Formulation 2 containing 20 μg mL^{-1} TMP + 10 μg mL^{-1} of standard solution TMP)

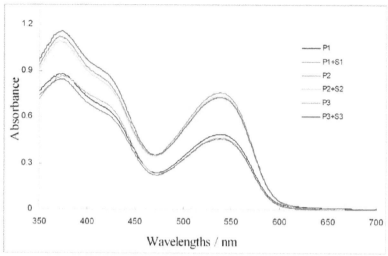

Figure 5. UV/Vis spectra of spiking experiments for recovery for DNFB method (sample of Formulation 2 containing 60 μg mL^{-1} TMP + 30 μg mL^{-1} of standard solution TMP)

adding 10 μg mL^{-1} of TMP standard solution to the different formulation sample extracts containing the analyte at level of 20 μg mL^{-1} and 60 μg mL^{-1} for the BCG and DNFB method, respectively. Afterwards, the samples were analyzed by the optimized BCG and DNFB methods. The results from the recovery testing for investigated formulations for both methods were within the range 97.57–100.56 %, and 97.53–103.13 % respectively (Table 2). On Fig. 4 and Fig. 5 examples of spectra of samples with TMP spiked with standard solutions with concentrations mentioned above are presented.

Precision of the BCG and DNFB method

The precision of the BCG and DNFB method was determined for all formulations tested on two different days, estimating the intra - and inter-day variations. The results from the precision experiments are presented in Tables 3 and 4. The within-day precision for the BCG method for investigated formulations ranged between 0.46 and 3.76 %. Regarding the DNFB method, in average,

we obtained higher precision, with estimated values between 0.40 and 1.35 %.

The between-day precision for the BCG method was estimated to be in the range 1.74 to 3.20%; while for the DNFB method, it was between 1.08 and 1.93 % (Table 4).

Fig's. 6 and 7 are examples of the overlapped spectra, from six measurements with the BCG and DNFB method, respectively obtained for Formulation 2.

To compare the BCG and DNFB method performances, in terms of closeness of the determined TMP content in investigated formulations and precision, we performed *t*-test and *F*-test, respectively. The obtained statistical values for significance are presented in Table 5. According to the data obtained, significant difference was observed when both methods were applied on Formulation 2. For other formulations tested, the statistical tests revealed that both methods are equally precise and accurate.

Table 3. Within-day precision for BCG and DNFB method

Samples	BCG method			DNFB method		
	γ(TMP)*/ μg mL^{-1}±SD	RSD*/%	% of DV[†]	γ(TMP)*/ μg mL^{-1}±SD	RSD*/%	% of DV[†]
Formulation 1	20.07±0.48	2.39	100.37	59.23±0.24	0.40	98.71
Formulation 2	19.20±0.72	3.76	96.02	60.72±0.70	1.15	101.21
Formulation 3	18.91±0.09	0.46	94.57	54.45±0.74	1.35	90.76
Formulation 4	19.17±0.56	2.94	95.85	59.12±0.55	0.93	98.53

* average values ± standard deviation of three replicates
[†] DV-Declared Value (by the producer)

Table 4. Between-day precision for BCG and DNFB method

Samples	BCG method			DNFB method			Horwitz criterion
	γ(TMP)*/ μg mL^{-1}±SD	RSD[†]/ %	% of DV[‡]	γ(TMP)*/ μg mL^{-1}±SD	RSD[†]/ %	% of DV[‡]	
Formulation 1	20.07±0.40	2.01	100.33	59.26±0.64	1.08	98.77	RSD< 4.19 %
Formulation 2	18.95±0.56	2.98	94.75	60.88±0.69	1.13	101.46	RSD< 4.19 %
Formulation 3	18.57±0.32	1.74	92.86	54.29±0.86	1.58	90.48	RSD< 5.40 %
Formulation 4	19.49±0.62	3.20	97.44	58.86±1.13	1.93	98.09	RSD< 5.40 %

* average values ± standard deviation of six replicates
[†] relative standard deviation
[‡] DV-Declared Value (by the producer)

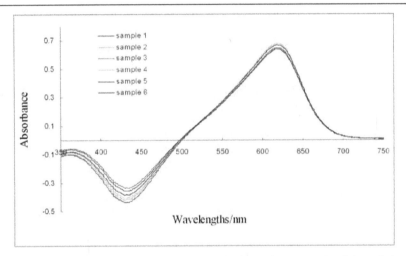

Figure 6. UV/Vis spectra from precision experiments for BCG method (Sample of Formulation 2 containing 20 μg mL^{-1})

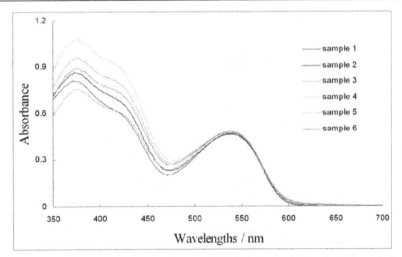

Figure 7. UV/Vis spectra from precision experiments for DNFB method (Sample of Formulation 2 containing 60 μg mL^{-1})

Table 5. Statistical evaluation of the performances of BCG and DNFB method

Samples	BCG method		DNFB method		Statistics ($p<0.05$)	
	γ(TMP)* (mg/tablet, mg/g powder)	RSD[†] /%	γ(TMP)* (mg/tablet, mg/g powder)	RSD[†] /%	t-test value[‡]	F-test value[§]
Formulation 1	80.26±1.62	2.01	78.99±0.85	1.08	1.56	3.62
Formulation 2	75.80±2.26	2.98	81.15±0.92	1.13	5.08	6.01
Formulation 3	18.57±0.32	1.74	18.08±0.29	1.58	2.44	1.27
Formulation 4	19.49±0.62	3.20	19.60±0.38	1.93	2.01	2.73

* determined average TMP content ± standard deviation in formulations, from six replicates

[†] relative standard deviation

[‡] t-test between the average values obtained for both methods (t_{crit}=2.57)

[§] F-test between the precision obtained for both methods (F_{crit}=5.05)

DISCUSSION

Method optimization for trimethoprim

The application of ultraviolet (UV) spectroscopy for determination of TMP in presence of some sulfonamide has often proved difficult due to the overlapping of their UV absorption spectra. Charge transfer complexation reactions have been widely applied in quality control of important chemical compounds of pharmaceutical interest in human and veterinary medicine, as well (5, 8, 15). For the methods we proposed, there were insufficient validation or applicability data on various real formulation forms (5, 15).

Bromcresol green method

It is based on the reaction where BCG is most probably acting as an acceptor of the π electrons from TMP (5). The optimal experimental conditions were chosen determining the recovery values of TMP at different conditions. Regarding the sonification time, the experiments reveled that for human formulations 30 min duration enables satisfactory recovery of TMP, while for veterinary formulations the optimal time was 45 min. During the optimization if was noticed that the reaction of TMP with BCG is more completed in basic media. Therefore, 20-25 µL of 0.1 mol/L NaOH solution was added for adjustment of the pH value of the media. Unlike our experiments, in the previously published report by El-Ansary (5), the influence of pH value on adduct formation was not taken into consideration; i.e. no pH adjustment was performed. As a first choice of solvents for TMP extraction from formulations were pure methanol and ethanol, considered as more environment friendly reagents. The recovery value of 106.49 % and 117.61 %, for methanol and ethanol, respectively, indicated that some of interfering substances are co-extracted, thus increasing the UV-Vis signal of the samples.

By modifying the methanol with 10 % solution of N,N-dimethylacetamide, we obtained recovery values between 95 and 105 % (Table 2) which is acceptable according to the ICH requirements (20). This was due to the fact that TMP is more soluble in N,N-dimethylacetamide (22) unlike pure ethanol and methanol. Second reason is that adding of N,N-dimethylacetamide increases the alkalinity of the solvent (methanol), which is necessary for the TMP extraction, especially in the presence of sulfonamides, for which the extraction is favorable in acidic environment. However, the use of pure N,N-dimethylacetamide is neither ecologically nor economically justified. Thus, by methanol modification adding 10% N,N-dimethylacetamide the conditions for better extraction of TMP are obtained in terms of obtaining better solubility of TMP in weakly basic environment, and is also ecologically and economically acceptable. Accordingly, in comparison to the previously published method for TMP determination with BCG (5), our method was improved in terms of excluding the use of environment non-friendly organic solvents such as chloroform, methylene chloride and chlorobenzene. The obtained spectra from TMP calibration solutions measured in wavelength range 350–750 nm, and concentration range 1–35 µg mL^{-1} (Fig. 2), confirmed that this solvent system was the best choice for carrying out further experiments.

2,4-Dinitro-1-fluorobenzene method

This method for determination of TMP applying UV-Vis spectroscopy is based on nucleophylic substitution on the free primary amino group in the TMP molecule (15). The rosy red colored complex formed exhibits two absorption bands at around 380 nm, and between 500 and 600 nm. The first one is a doublet of two overlapped peaks, while the second one is well-shaped symmetrical band (Fig. 3). Therefore, the choice of acetone as extraction solvent was logical because it absorbs at wavelengths lower than 300 nm. The heating of the solution is a crucial factor for completing the substitution reaction, i.e. complex formation. According to the previously published DNFB method (15), the solutions should be heated at 60°C for 40 minutes. Applying this temperature, after approximately 20 min we observed total acetone evaporation. Therefore, in our further experiments we heated the solutions at 50 °C for 45 min, obtaining solutions with pale pink color. By further heating at 60 °C for 10 min the solutions color became more intensive, resulting in well-defined absorption peak around 540 nm (Fig. 3). Al-Sabha and Hamody (15) concluded that the optimal pH value for complex formation is 7.4. Accordingly, we did not make any pH adjustment of the media before performing the substitution reaction.

Validation of the BCG and DNFB method
Linearity and sensitivity

The range for both methods was selected on the basis of TMP content in the formulations. Additionally, we had to have in mind the fact that for fulfilling the Lambert-Beers law the UV-Vis signal of the maximal concentration should be around one absorbance unit. On this basis, we decided that the linear dynamic range is going to be 1–35 µg mL^{-1} and 20–90 µg mL^{-1} for BCG and DNFB method, respectively (Table 2). Regarding the BCG method, the linearity was obtained measuring the signals from five repetitive measurements of each standard, at 618 nm. Thus, the method revealed good linearity (R^2=0.9976) for the range mentioned above. In comparison to the previously published method for BCG (5), where the linearity was determined within the range 2.9–20.3 µg mL^{-1}, we expanded the linearity range on our modified method. Applying the DNFB method within the range defined, the regression coefficient obtained was 0.9981; calculated from the absorbances at 538 nm, from five repetitive measurements for each standard concentration. The previously published method for DNFB (15) demonstrated the linearity within the range 10–75 µg mL^{-1}. For both methods we proposed, the linearity obtained was better than 0.99, fulfilling the requirements from the reference document (20). Even though the method sensitivity for determination of analytes that are present in the samples in sufficiently high amounts is not a critical parameter, yet we have determined the LOD and LOQ values. The BCG and DNFB method sensitivity parameters calculated from the calibration curve standard deviation (21), revealed values (Table 2) comparable to ones obtained by other authors (8). Thus, Adegoke et al. (8) obtained

values of 2.69 and 8.96 µg mL^{-1} for LOD and LOQ, respectively. On the other hand when applying the derivative spectrophotometric method for TMP determination, Zimmer et al. (10), estimated the LOD value to be 0.11 µg mL^{-1}.

Method accuracy

Comparing the recovery results for both methods one may conclude that they are equally accurate, except for Formulation 2 where the DNFB method revealed significantly higher recovery rate. This could be attributed to interferences due to greater acetone extractability for some of the unknown formulation excipients. The values obtained for the recoveries are in the range 97.57–100.91 % and 97.53–103.13 % for the BCG and DNFB method, respectively. The recovery values obtained indicate that the methods are fulfilling the method accuracy acceptable limits (95–105 %) according to the reference document requirements (20). Therefore, one may conclude that the modified and optimized methods are sufficiently accurate for performing quality control of medicinal products, regarding TMP determination. In reference to the BCG method, the previously published study (5) has not reported validation data regarding the recovery estimation. However, the recovery values obtained for the DNFB method within this study are comparable with those obtained applying colorimetric UV-Vis spectroscopic methods. Thus, Al-Sabha and Hamody (15) have obtained recovery values within the range 100.43±1.07 %. Recently, Adegoke et al. (8) have reported spectophotometric determination of TMP following charge-transfer complexation with chloranilic acid, whereas the recovery estimated was form 99.97 to 102.57 %. In another investigation, Shamsa and Amani (3) have proposed a diazotization procedure for TMP spectrophotometric determination in the visible spectra. The recovery values they have obtained are somewhat higher (104–105.5%) when compared with the results obtained within our study. In general, our proposed methods are satisfactorily accurate regarding the reference document (20) and comparable to ones reported by other authors.

Method precision

The precision of the BCG and DNFB method was determined for all formulations tested on two different days, estimating the intra- and inter-day variations (Table 3). Within-day precision for the BCG method determined from three repetitive measurements were estimated to be from 0.46 (Formulation 3) to 3.76 % (Formulation 2). Regarding the DNFB method, the precision ranged from 0.40 % (Formulation 1) to 1.35 %

(Formulation 3). The between-day accuracy of the BCG method, in terms of relative standard deviation (Table 4) ranged from 1.74 % (Formulation 3) to 3.20 % (Formulation 4). For the DNFB method, we obtained between-day precision values ranged from 1.08 (Formulation 1) to 1.93 % (Formulation 4). In general, the DNFB method pronounced higher precision with standard error variations between 1 and 2 %. All between-day precision data estimated (Table 4) are in accordance with Horwitz criteria for maximal acceptable precision, calculated from the proposed formula, based on analyte content in analyzed samples (23). The precision values obtained for the DNFB method are very similar to ones determined with the same method by Al-Sabha et al. (15), being in average around 1 %. In comparison, the precision values obtained for other complexation methods for TMP determination were within the range 1.3–1.7 % (8), and 1.3–2.2 % (3). However, applying spectrophotometric method with metol and potassium hexacyanoferrate(III), Ayad et al. (24) revealed significantly lower precision data for TMP, ranged from 0.274–0.748 %.

Statistical analysis for evaluation of the method applicability

Previously, by evaluating the recovery and relative standard deviation, we have presented the study on method linearity, sensitivity, accuracy, and precision (Tables 2, 3, and 4). The method applicability was tested through determination of TMP in four investigated formulations, and the corresponding results for both methods were tested for significance (Table 5). Statistical analysis was performed using F-ratio test and Student's t-test ($P<0.05$). The statistical analysis results indicated that regarding the formulation 1, 3 and 4 (Table 1), there was no difference in the accuracy and precision between both methods applied. The difference was observed for Formulation 2, whereas BCG and DNFB method exhibited significantly different average content of TMP in the formulation, as well as significantly different precision (Table 5). The TMP content on Formulation 1 and Formulation 2 is equal (80 mg/tablet); however such difference was not observed for Formulation 1. We assume that it could be a result of the probable interference of the unknown matrix from the tablet on the TMP– BCG reaction.

Clearly recognized advantages of the optimized and validated methods for determination of TMP are simplicity, high precision, and high accuracy. When compared to the previously reported BCG and DNFB methods, our study has made improvements towards enlarging of the method ranges, as well as avoiding of environmental non-friendly toxic solvents. Future investigations could be focused on interferences study using placebo as blank for the recovery and precision experiments.

CONCLUSION

Improvement and validation of two visible spectrophotometric methods applying BCG and DNFB as reagents for TMP determination in investigated formulations were successfully carried out. The near 100 % recoveries and low relative standard deviation values obtained, point to the suitability of the both modified and validated methods for determination of TMP in various potentiated sulfonamide formulations intended for use in human and veterinary medicine. This study could contribute towards improvement of the quality control of TMP in potentiated sulfonamides intended for use in veterinary medicine, applying simple, effective, precise and low cost testing methods.

REFERENCES

1. Fresta, M., Furneri, P.M., Mezzasalma, E., Nicolosi, V.M., Pugeisi, G. (1996). Correlation of trimethoprim and brodimoprim physicochemical and lipid membrane interaction properties with their accumulation in human neutrophils, Antimicrob. Agents Chemother. 40(12): 2865 - 2873. PMid:9124856 PMCid:PMC163637

2. Saha, N., Kar, S.K., (1977). Metal complexes of pyrimidine-derived ligands - I: Nickel (II) complexes of 2-hydrazino-4,6-dimethyl pyrimidine, J. Inorg. Nucl. Chem. 39, 195-200. http://dx.doi.org/10.1016/0022-1902(77)80465-X

3. Shamsa, F., Amani, L. (2006). Determination of sulfamethoxazole and trimethoprim in pharmaceuticals by visible and UV spectrometry, Iran. J. Pharm. Res. 1, 31-36.

4. Reisberg, B., Herzog, J., Weinstein, L. (1967). In vitro antibacterial activity of trimethoprim alone and in combination with sulfonamides. Antimicrob. Agents Chemother., 424-426.

5. El-Ansary, A.L., Issa, Y.M., Selim, W. (1999). Spectrophotometric determination of trimethoprim in pure form and in pharmaceutical preparations using Bromthymol blue, Bromocresol green and Alizarin red S. Anal. Lett. 32(5): 655-969. http://dx.doi.org/10.1080/00032719908542869

6. Gemperline, P.J., Cho, J. H., Baker, B., Batchelor, B., Walker, D.S. (1997). Determination of multicomponent dissolution profiles of pharmaceutical products by in situ fiber-optic UV measurements. Anal. Chim. Acta. 345, 155-159. http://dx.doi.org/10.1016/S0003-2670(97)00095-0

7. Ni, Y., Q. Zj., Kokot, S. (2006). Simultaneous ultraviolet-spectrophotometric determination of sulfonamides by multivariate calibration approaches. Chemometr. Intell. Lab. 82, 241-247. http://dx.doi.org/10.1016/j.chemolab.2005.07.006

8. Adekoge, O.A., Babalola, C.P., Kotila, O.A., Obuebhor, O. (2014). Simultaneous spectrophotometric determination of trimethoprim and sulphamethoxazole following charge-transfer complexation with chloranilic acid. Arabian Journal of Chemistry, in press

9. Othman S. (1989). Multicomponent derivative spectroscopic analysis of sulfamethoxazole and trimethoprim. Int. J. Pharm. 63, 173-176. http://dx.doi.org/10.1016/0378-5173(90)90168-4

10. Zimmer, Ł., Czarnecki, W. (2010). Derivative spectrophotometric method for simultaneous determination of sulfadimidine and trimethoprim. Annales Universitatis Mariae Curie-Skłodowska, Lublin - Polonia, Sectio DDD, 23(1-3): 27-36.

11. Medina, J.R., Miranda, M., Hurtado, M., Dominguez-Ramirez, A. M., Ruiz-Segura, J.C. (2013). Simultaneous determination of trimethoprim and sulfamethoxazole in immediate-release oral dosage forms by first-order derivative spectroscopy: Application to dissolution studies. Int. J. Pharm. Pharm. Sci. 5 (Suppl.4), 505-510.

12. Rezaee, A., Nejad, Q.B., Kebriaeezadeh, A. (2000). Simultaneous analysis of thrimethoprim and sulphamethoxazole drug combinations in dosage forms by High Performance Liquid Chromatography. Iran. Biomed. J. 4 (2&3): 75-78.

13. Akay, C., Özkan, S.A. (2002). Simultaneous LC determination of thrimethoprim and sulfamethoxazole in pharmaceutical formulations. J. Pharm. Biomed. Anal. 30, 1207-1213. http://dx.doi.org/10.1016/S0731-7085(02)00460-0

14. Lemus Gallego, J.M., Perez Arroyo, J. (2002). Simultaneous determination of dexamethazone and trimethoprim by liquid chromatography. J. Pharm. Biomed. Anal. 30, 1255-1261. http://dx.doi.org/10.1016/S0731-7085(02)00468-5

15. Al-Sabha, T.N., Hamody, I.A. (2011). Spectrophotometric determination of trimethoprim using 2,4-dinitro-1-fluorobenzene reagent. J. Edu. & Sci. 24(2): 1-12.

16. Chati, S., Wadookar, S.G., Kasture, A.V. (1979). Nonaqueous titrimetric method for timethoprim determination in combination. Indian J. Pahrm. Sci. 41(6): 231.

17. Carapuca, H.M., Cabral, D.J., Rocha, L.S. (2005). Adsorptive stripping voltammetry of trimethoprim: mechanistic studies and application to the fast determination in pharmaceutical suspensions. J. Pharm. Biomed. Anal. 38(2): 364-369. http://dx.doi.org/10.1016/j.jpba.2005.01.005 PMid:15925233

18. Chatten, L.G., Stanley-Pons, B., McLeod, P. (1982). Electrochemical determination of trimethoprim. Analyst 107, 1026-103. http://dx.doi.org/10.1039/an9820701026 PMid:7149266

19. British Pharmacopoeia 2009, Volume I & II, p. 6201-6207.

20. ICH Harmonized tripartite guideline. Validation of analytical procedures: Text and methodology. Q2 (R1). (2005). International conference on harmonization of technical requirements for registration of pharmaceuticals for human use.

21. Miler, J.C., Miler, J.N. (1994). Statistics for analytical chemistry. 3rd Edition, Ellis Horwood Ltd. Chichester, West Sussex PMid:7819605

22. Profiles of drug substances, excipients and related methodology. In: Klaus Florey (Ed.), Analytical profiles of drug substances. Volume 7. (pp. 459). 1978, San Diego, California: Academic Press, USA.

23. Horwitz, W. (1982). Evaluation of analytical methods used for regulation of foods and drugs, Anal. Chem. 54 (1): 67A-76A. http://dx.doi.org/10.1021/ac00238a765

24. Ayad, M.R.R., Huda, M.A., Halah H. (2012). Spectrophotometric determination of trimethoprim in pure form and pharmaceutical formulations with metol and potassium hexacyanoferrate (III). Tikrit Journal of Pharmaceutical Sciences 8(2): 209-220.

13

FACTORS AFFECTING FIN DAMAGE OF
FARMED RAINBOW TROUT

Aleksandar Cvetkovikj[1], Miroslav Radeski[1], Dijana Blazhekovikj-Dimovska[2],
Vasil Kostov[3], Vangjel Stevanovski[2]

[1]*Veterinary Institute, Faculty of Veterinary Medicine, Ss. Cyril and Methodius University
in Skopje, Lazar Pop-Trajkov 5-7, 1000 Skopje, Republic of Macedonia*
[2]*Fishery Department, Faculty of Biotechnical Sciences, St. Kliment Ohridski University
in Bitola, Partizanska bb, 7000 Bitola, Republic of Macedonia*
[3]*Fishery Department, Institute of Animal Science, Ss. Cyril and Methodius University
in Skopje, Bul. Ilinden 92-a, 1000 Skopje, Republic of Macedonia*

ABSTRACT

The aims of this study were to determine the influence of the factors affecting fin damage under different rainbow trout production systems and to compare the findings with the known experimental reports. The study was based on a questionnaire that included information about the main factors i.e. oxygen level in exit water, water temperature, stocking density, daily feed ration, number of meals and grading frequency on seven rainbow trout farms. Standard multiple regression analysis, based on a previously published fin damage dataset, was used to assess the relationship between the level of fin damage per fin and the factors. Daily feed ration received the strongest weight in the model for the caudal, anal and both pectoral fins, whereas number of meals received the strongest weight in the model for both pelvic fins. Grading frequency received the strongest weight only in the dorsal fin model. Lower levels of daily feed ration and number of meals combined with higher water temperature increased the level of fin damage, whereas stocking density had no effect. The results conform to the experimental research on fin damage in rainbow trout. The research model contributes to the overall assessment of fish welfare and the regression analysis used in this study could be used on rainbow trout farms to evaluate the effect of the main factors on the level of fin damage.

Key words: rainbow trout, factor, fin condition, fish welfare

INTRODUCTION

Fin damage is considered important for both economic and welfare reasons and continuous to be a significant problem in rainbow trout (*Oncorhynchus mykiss*) farms (1). The fin damage phenomenon has been studied for many decades, because fish with damaged fins are usually declared as less valuable by the consumers and the fishing public (2). Fin

Corresponding author: Dr. Aleksandar Cvetkovikj, DVM, MSc, PhD
E-mail address: acvetkovic@fvm.ukim.edu.mk
Present address: Veterinary Institute, Faculty of Veterinary Medicine
Ss. Cyril and Methodius University in Skopje
Lazar Pop-Trajkov 5-7, 1000 Skopje
Republic of Macedonia

damage is considered as an operational welfare indicator that is increasingly gaining attention (3, 4) and represents one of the key welfare outcomes (5). The ubiquitous presence of fin damage results with a growing interest in understanding it's the etiology and the factors that increase or reduce fin damage in farmed rainbow trout (1).

There is a significant body of experimental research which identified that the main factors affecting fin damage are feeding practices, water quality, stocking density and routine handling, not excluding the bacterial infections (3, 6, 7, 8, 9). However, despite the experimental approach, there are few research reports that determine the important factors having effect on fin damage and fish welfare under different commercial production systems (5, 10). Nevertheless, there are also differences between species. For example, the most frequently damaged fin in Atlantic salmon (*Salmo salar*) and rainbow trout is the dorsal fin, whereas in brown trout (*Salmo trutta*) it is the caudal fin (10, 11).

Table 1. Farming practices on the surveyed rainbow trout farms

Farm	Water temperature (°C)		Stocking density (kg/m³)		Daily feed ration (% of body weight)		Number of meals per day		Grading on every X days
	Min.	Max.	<30g	>100g	<30g	>100g	<30g	>100g	
1	1	18	30	37	4	1.3	4	2	45
2	2	16	35	40	6	2	6	2	20
3	10	18	20	45	8	4	5	2	20
4	4	12	20	65	6	2	4	2	20
5	10	12	30	45	8	2	5	2	15
6	5	10	20	40	7	2	7	2	30
7	11	11	30	40	8	2	4	2	30

Farmed rainbow trout generally experience varying degrees of fin damage, and the farms in Republic of Macedonia are no exception. We have previously proposed that some factor or group of factors influence the degree of damage (10) and these factors should be identified in order to apply management practices that can minimize the level of fin damage.

The aims of this study were to determine the influence of the main factors on the level of fin damage in different commercial rainbow trout farms and to compare the (on farm) findings with the experimentally determined effects on the level of fin damage.

MATERIAL AND METHODS

We did a questionnaire survey with the farm owner or the responsible technologist on the seven rainbow trout farms described by Cvetkovikj et al. (10). The questionnaire was designed to include information about water quality [oxygen level in exit water (DO) and water temperature (WT)], stocking density (SD), feeding practices [daily feed ration (DF) and number of meals (NM)] and routine handling [grading frequency (GR)] per fish category (Table 1).

Table 2. Level of the fin damage and significance of the results between the different fish farms [adapted from Cvetkovikj et al. (10)]. Values represent mean ± SE

	Farm 1	Farm 2	Farm 3	Farm 4	Farm 5	Farm 6	Farm 7	p
Dorsal < 30g	3.63 ±0.06	2.53 ±0.13	3.02 ±0.15	2.30 ±0.11	1.50 ±0.09	2.35 ±0.12	2.13 ±0.15	p < .001
Dorsal > 100g	4.27 ±0.06	3.23 ±0.12	4.07 ±0.09	2.77 ±0.12	2.10 ±0.09	2.72 ±0.13	3.32 ±0.15	p < .001
Caudal < 30g	1.43 ±0.06	1.30 ±0.06	1.37 ±0.06	1.33 ±0.06	1.03 ±0.02	1.13 ±0.04	1.07 ±0.03	p < .001
Caudal > 100g	2.95 ±0.3	1.73 ±0.07	2.07 ±0.07	1.85 ±0.10	1.73 ±0.09	1.73 ±0.08	2.28 ±0.11	p < .001
Anal < 30g	1.73 ±0.07	1.67 ±0.09	1.52 ±0.09	1.47 ±0.06	1.10 ±0.04	1.73 ±0.08	1.33 ±0.06	p < .001
Anal > 100g	3.60 ±0.10	1.85 ±0.08	2.37 ±0.09	2.07 ±0.11	1.80 ±0.10	2.03 ±0.09	2.40 ±0.11	p< .001
Pectoral left < 30g	2.10 ±0.13	2.02 ±0.12	1.78 ±0.09	1.82 ±0.09	2.10 ±0.08	2.03 ±0.09	1.73 ±0.17	p > .05
Pectoral left > 100g	4.10 ±0.13	2.70 ±0.11	2.57 ±0.08	2.43 ±0.13	3.07 ±0.14	2.43 ±0.06	3.08 ±0.18	p < .001
Pectoral right < 30 g	2.07 ±0.14	2.03 ±0.12	1.80 ±0.10	1.83 ±0.10	2.07 ±0.07	2.02 ±0.09	1.70 ±0.12	p > .05
Pectoral right > 100 g	4.12 ±0.13	2.67 ±0.09	2.53 ±0.08	2.47 ±0.14	3.10 ±0.10	2.40 ±0.08	3.05 ±0.17	p < .001
Pelvic left < 30 g	1.58 ±0.11	1.75 ±0.09	2.18 ±0.14	1.50 ±0.09	1.33 ±0.06	1.30 ±0.06	1.47 ±0.09	p < .001
Pelvic left > 100 g	3.07 ±0.10	1.93 ±0.11	3.03 ±0.06	2.13 ±0.12	1.87 ±0.07	1.90 ±0.09	2.47 ±0.12	p < .001
Pelvic right < 30 g	1.57 ±0.10	1.77 ±0.11	2.20 ±0.14	1.53 ±0.09	1.43 ±0.08	1.33 ±0.07	1.43 ±0.09	p < .001
Pelvic right > 100 g	3.05 ±0.10	1.97 ±0.10	3.07 ±0.13	2.15 ±0.12	1.97 ±0.08	1.93 ±0.09	2.43 ±0.11	p < .001

Table 3. Pearson's correlations of the damaged fins and the predictors (n=840)

	WT	SD	DF	NM	GR
dorsal fin	.072	.147	-.348	-.302	.365
caudal fin	-.026*	.320	-.518	-.474	.254
anal fin	-.069	.258	-.472	-.373	.356
left pelvic fin	.110	.266	-.335	-.375	.118
right pelvic fin	.097	.259	-.320	-.359	.085
left pectoral fin	.072	.262	-.449	-.376	.192
right pectoral fin	.078	.273	-.463	-.385	.190

*Non-significant correlation

The DO did not significantly differ between the farms (all farms had DO between 6.5 and 6.7 mg/L) so we excluded it from further analysis. All farms used extruded fish feed and were manually feeding and grading the fish. This survey was conducted in parallel with the second scoring of the fins during the summer in 2012 (10).

To assess the relationship between the dependent variable (damaged dorsal, left and right pectoral, left and right pelvic, anal and caudal fin) and the predictor variables (WT, SD, DF, NM and GR), we performed standard multiple regression analysis [IBM SPSS Statistics 22 (©IBM, Armonk, NY, USA)] using the same fin damage dataset (Table 2) from our previous research (10).

As fin damage represents a continuous process (3, 12), we merged the fin damage data per fin from the two different categories (< 30g and > 100g) and performed the analysis separately for every fin. The results were considered statistically significant at p < .05

In addition, the results from Table 2 were used for a meta-analysis. First the mean and errors of means were used to calculate a t-value (the difference of the mean value from zero), the t-value was converted into r-values (13) and finally those r-values used for calculating effect sizes for each fin listed in Table 2. For that purpose we used the statistical package MetaWin (14).

RESULTS

The correlations of the predictor variables and the damaged fins are shown in Table 3. All correlations except between the caudal fin and WT were statistically significant. The regression coefficients of the predictors, together with their correlations with the damaged fins and their squared semi-partial correlations are shown in Tables 4, 5, 6, 7, 8, 9 and 10.

The prediction model for the dorsal fin was statistically significant, $F(5, 834) = 48.812$, $p < .001$, and accounted for approximately 22% of the variance of dorsal fin damage ($R^2 = .226$, Adjusted $R^2 = .222$). Dorsal fin damage was predicted by higher levels of GR (Beta = .315, p < .001) and WT (Beta = .114, p < .001) and lower levels of DF (Beta = -.178, p = .008) and NM (Beta = -.154, p = .010) (Table 4). Stocking density was not a significant predictor in this model (p = .469). Grading frequency received the strongest weight in the model. For every additional point on the GR measure, we would predict an increment of .039 points (3.90 %) on the dorsal fin damage measure (B = .039). On the other hand, for every additional point on the NM measure, we would predict a decrement of .108 points (10.80 %) on the dorsal fin damage measure (B = -.108) (Table 4).

Table 4. Standard regression of the dorsal fin and the predictors

	Model	Unstandardized Coefficients		Standardized Coefficients			Correlations		
		B	Std. Error	Beta	t	Sig.	Pearson	Partial	Sr²
1	(Constant)	2.461	.358		6.873	.000			
	WT	.026	.007	.114	3.623	.000	.072	.124	.012
	SD	-.004	.005	-.037	-.724	.469	.147	-.025	.000
	DF	-.083	.031	-.178	-2.650	.008	-.348	-.091	.006
	NM	-.108	.042	-.154	-2.580	.010	-.302	-.089	.006
	GR	.039	.005	.315	8.672	.000	.365	.288	.069

Note: R^2=.226. Adjusted R2 = .222. Sr² is the squared semi-partial correlation

Table 5. Standard regression of the caudal fin and the predictors

Model		Unstandardized Coefficients		Standardized Coefficients	t	Sig.	Correlations		
		B	Std. Error	Beta			Pearson	Partial	Sr²
1	(Constant)	2.234	.229		9.744	.000			
	WT	.002	.005	.012	.417	.677	-.026	.014	.000
	SD	-.003	.003	-.046	-.963	.336	.320	-.033	.000
	DF	-.103	.020	-.330	-5.165	.000	-.518	-.176	.022
	NM	-.104	.027	-.221	-3.883	.000	-.474	-.133	.012
	GR	.013	.003	.150	4.337	.000	.254	.149	.015

Note: $R^2 = .299$. Adjusted $R^2 = .294$. Sr² is the squared semi-partial correlation

The prediction model for the caudal fin was statistically significant, $F(5, 834) = 71.023$, $p < .001$, and accounted for approximately 30% of the variance of caudal fin damage ($R^2 = .299$, Adjusted $R^2 = .294$). Caudal fin damage was predicted by lower levels of DF (Beta = -.330, $p < .001$) and NM (Beta = -.221, $p < .001$) and higher levels of GR (Beta = .150, $p < .001$) (Table 5). Water temperature ($p = .677$) and SD ($p = .336$) were not significant predictors in this model. Daily feed ration received the strongest weight in the model. For every additional point on the DF measure, we would predict a decrement of .103 points (10.30 %) on the caudal fin damage measure (B = -.103). On the other hand, for every additional point on the GR measure, we would predict an increment of .013 points (1.30 %) on the caudal fin damage measure (B = .013) (Table 5).

The prediction model for the anal fin was statistically significant, $F(5, 834) = 66.287$,

this model. Daily feed ration received the strongest weight in the model. For every additional point on the DF measure, we would predict a decrement of .122 points (12.20 %) on the anal fin damage measure (B = -.122). On the other hand, for every additional point on the GR measure, we would predict an increment of .025 points (2.50 %) on the anal fin damage measure (B = .025) (Table 6).

The prediction model for the left pelvic fin was statistically significant, $F(5, 834) = 32.254$, $p < .001$, and accounted for approximately 16% of the variance of left pelvic fin damage ($R^2 = .162$, Adjusted $R^2 = .157$). Left pelvic fin damage was predicted by lower levels of NM (Beta = -.298, $p < .001$) and higher levels of WT (Beta = .114, $p = .001$) and GR (Beta = .106, $p = .005$) (Table 7). Daily feed ration ($p = .583$) and SD ($p = .375$) were not significant predictors in this model. Number of meals received the strongest weight in the model.

Table 6. Standard regression of the anal fin and the predictors

Model		Unstandardized Coefficients		Standardized Coefficients	t	Sig.	Correlations		
		B	Std. Error	Beta			Pearson	Partial	Sr²
1	(Constant)	1.897	.259		7.321	.000			
	WT	-.002	.005	-.010	-.319	.750	-.069	-.011	.000
	SD	.001	.004	.012	.238	.812	.258	.008	.000
	DF	-.122	.023	-.351	-5.431	.000	-.472	-.185	.025
	NM	-.029	.030	-.055	-.963	.336	-.373	-.033	.000
	GR	.025	.003	.265	7.593	.000	.356	.254	.049

Note: $R^2 = .284$. Adjusted $R^2 = .280$. Sr² is the squared semi-partial correlation

$p < .001$, and accounted for approximately 28% of the variance of anal fin damage ($R^2 = .284$, Adjusted $R^2 = .280$). Anal fin damage was predicted by lower levels of DF (Beta = -.351, $p < .001$) and higher levels of GR (Beta = .265, $p < .001$) (Table 6). Stocking density ($p = .812$), WT ($p = .750$) and NM ($p = .336$) were not significant predictors in

For every additional point on the NM measure, we would predict a decrement of .164 points (16.40 %) on the left pelvic fin damage measure (B = -.164). On the other hand, for every additional point on the WT measure, we would predict an increment of .020 points (2.00 %) on the left pelvic fin damage measure (B = .020) (Table 7).

Table 7. Standard regression of the left pelvic fin and the predictors

	Model	Unstandardized Coefficients		Standardized Coefficients	t	Sig.	Correlations		
		B	Std. Error	Beta			Pearson	Partial	Sr²
1	(Constant)	2.003	.293		6.836	.000			
	WT	.020	.006	.114	3.482	.001	.110	.120	.012
	SD	.004	.004	.047	.887	.375	.266	.031	.000
	DF	-.014	.025	-.038	-.549	.583	-.335	-.019	.000
	NM	-.164	.034	-.298	-4.796	.000	-.375	-.164	.023
	GR	.010	.004	.106	2.806	.005	.118	.097	.007

Note: $R^2 = .162$. Adjusted $R^2 = .157$. Sr² is the squared semi-partial correlation

The prediction model for the right pelvic fin was statistically significant, $F (5, 834) = 27.820$, $p < .001$, and accounted for approximately 16% of the variance of right pelvic fin damage ($R^2 = .143$, Adjusted $R^2 = .138$). Right pelvic fin damage was predicted by lower levels of NM (Beta = -.281, $p < .001$) and higher levels of WT (Beta = .100, $p = .003$) (Table 8). Stocking density ($p = .526$), DF

hand, for every additional point on the WT measure, we would predict an increment of .018 points (1.80 %) on the right pelvic fin damage measure (B = .018) (Table 8).

The prediction model for the left pectoral fin was statistically significant, $F (5, 834) = 48.912$, $p < .001$, and accounted for approximately 22% of the variance of left pectoral fin damage ($R^2 = .227$,

Table 8. Standard regression of the right pelvic fin and the predictors

	Model	Unstandardized Coefficients		Standardized Coefficients	t	Sig.	Correlations		
		B	Std. Error	Beta			Pearson	Partial	Sr²
1	(Constant)	2.186	.306		7.141	.000			
	WT	.018	.006	.100	3.019	.003	.097	.104	.009
	SD	.003	.004	.034	.635	.526	.259	.022	.000
	DF	-.021	.027	-.056	-.788	.431	-.320	-.027	.000
	NM	-.159	.036	-.281	-4.465	.000	-.359	-.153	.020
	GR	.007	.004	.067	1.749	.081	.085	.060	.003

Note: $R^2 = .143$. Adjusted $R^2 = .138$. Sr² is the squared semi-partial correlation

($p = .431$) and GR ($p = .081$) were not significant predictors in this model. Number of meals received the strongest weight in the model. For every additional point on the NM measure, we would predict a decrement of .159 points (15.90 %) on the right pelvic fin damage measure (B = -.159). On the other

Adjusted $R^2 = .222$). Left pectoral fin damage was predicted by lower levels of DF (Beta = -.489, $p < .001$) and higher levels of WT (Beta = .125, $p < .001$) (Table 9). Number of meals ($p = .754$), SD ($p = .099$) and GR ($p = .066$) were not significant predictors in this model. Daily feed

Table 9. Standard regression of the left pectoral fin and the predictors

	Model	Unstandardized Coefficients		Standardized Coefficients	t	Sig.	Correlations		
		B	Std. Error	Beta			Pearson	Partial	Sr²
1	(Constant)	3.229	.337		9.586	.000			
	WT	.027	.007	.125	3.993	.000	.072	.137	.014
	SD	-.008	.005	-.083	-1.650	.099	.262	-.057	.002
	DF	-.213	.029	-.489	-7.282	.000	-.449	-.245	.049
	NM	-.012	.039	-.019	-.314	.754	-.376	-.011	.000
	GR	.008	.004	.067	1.843	.066	.192	.064	.003

Note: $R^2 = .227$. Adjusted $R^2 = .222$. Sr² is the squared semi-partial correlation

ration received the strongest weight in the model. For every additional point on the DF measure, we would predict a decrement of .213 points (21.30 %) on the left pectoral fin damage measure (B = -.213). On the other hand, for every additional point on the WT measure, we would predict an increment of .027 points (2.70 %) on the left pectoral fin damage measure (B = .027) (Table 9).

The prediction model for the right pectoral fin was statistically significant, F (5, 834) = 52.680, $p < .001$, and accounted for approximately 24% of the variance of right pectoral fin damage ($R^2 = .240$, Adjusted $R^2 = .235$). Right pectoral fin damage

was predicted by lower levels of DF (Beta = -.517, $p < .001$) and higher levels of WT (Beta = .134, $p < .001$) (Table 10). Number of meals (p = .961), SD (p = .101) and GR (p = .096) were not significant predictors in this model. Daily feed ration received the strongest weight in the model. For every additional point on the DF measure, we would predict a decrement of .221 points (22.10 %) on the right pectoral fin damage measure (B = -.221). On the other hand, for every additional point on the WT measure, we would predict an increment of .028 points (2.80 %) on the right pectoral fin damage measure (B = .028) (Table 10).

Table 10. Standard regression of the right pectoral fin and the predictors

	Model	Unstandardized Coefficients		Standardized Coefficients			Correlations		
		B	Std. Error	Beta	t	Sig.	Pearson	Partial	Sr²
1	(Constant)	3.220	.326		9.870	.000			
	WT	.028	.006	.134	4.304	.000	.078	.147	.016
	SD	-.008	.005	-.082	-1.641	.101	.273	-.057	.002
	DF	-.221	.028	-.517	-7.776	.000	-.463	-.260	.055
	NM	-.002	.038	-.003	-.049	.961	-.385	-.002	.000
	GR	.007	.004	.060	1.666	.096	.190	.058	.002

Note: R² = .240. Adjusted R² = .235. Sr² is the squared semi-partial correlation

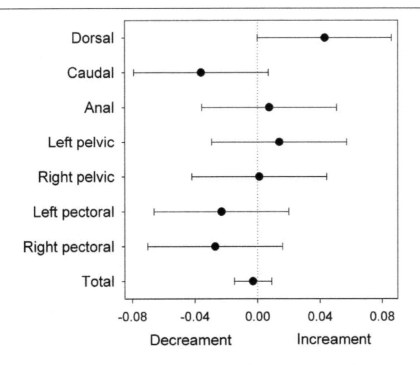

Figure 1a. Meta-analysis of the damaged fins. The dots in the figure show the mean effect sizes and the horizontal bars the range of 95% confidence interval. Thus, if the bar crosses the vertical dotted line (effect size=0) the mean is not significantly different from zero

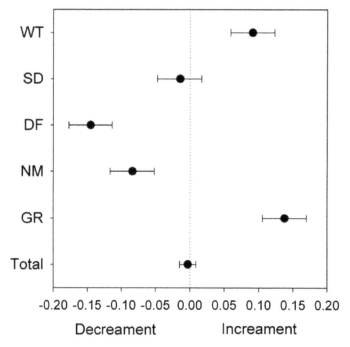

Figure 1b. Meta-analysis of the predictor variables. The dots in the figure show the mean effect sizes and the horizontal bars the range of 95% confidence interval. Thus, if the bar crosses the vertical dotted line (effect size=0) the mean is not significantly different from zero

The unique variance explained by each of the predictors indexed by the squared semi-partial correlations (Table 4 - Table 10) was low for every fin (GR accounts uniquely for about 7% of the variance of dorsal fin damage; DF accounts uniquely for about 2% of the variance of caudal fin damage; GR accounts uniquely for about 5% of the variance of anal fin damage; NM accounts uniquely for about 2% of the variance of the left and the right pelvic fin damage and DF accounts uniquely for about 5% of the variance of the left and the right pectoral fin damage, given the other variables in the model).

The meta-analysis based on the data in Table 2 revealed that there were no differences in fin damage among fins. Within the range of the variables studied, only the dorsal fin showed significant increment (Fig 1a). Increased DF and NM resulted in a decrement of fin damage. Decreased WT and fewer grading occasion also resulted in a decrement of fin damage (Fig 1b). Stocking density had no effect on the degree of fin damage.

DISCUSSION

This study shows that the feeding practices (DF and NM) have the most significant effect on the level of fin damage in different commercial rainbow trout farms. If the effects on all fins were combined,

DF tended to be more important than NM (Fig. 1b), but the variables had different effects on different fins. Daily feed ration received the strongest weight in the model for the caudal, anal and both pectoral fins, whereas NM received the strongest weight in the model for both pelvic fins. Dorsal, caudal, anal, left pectoral and right pectoral fin damage were predicted by lower levels of DF. Lower levels of NM predicted the damage of the pelvic fins, and, the same as DF, predicted the damage of the dorsal and the caudal fin.

Fish aggregate in small area during feeding and this is the time when the incidence of fin damage is highest (3, 6, 15). Our findings agree with previous research that lower feed rations increase erosion of the dorsal and caudal fins of rainbow and brown trout (16, 17) and that feed restriction causes fin damage (erosion) in small steelhead trout and Atlantic salmon (15, 18). The lower feeding ration strengthens the social hierarchy among the fish and worsens the fin condition. When feeding rainbow trout to satiety from self-feeders, reducing the daily number of meals from 3 to 1 significantly reduces the recovery from historical dorsal fin erosion (19). However, when rainbow trout receive a fixed satiation ration, increasing the daily number of meals from 1 to 3 increases the damage of the left pectoral fin (7). Fish should have the opportunity to feed without undue competition (5) and the contemporary feeding strategies promote self-feeding or on-demand feeding regimes than fixed feeding regimes (19, 20, 21, 22, 23, 24). These regimes provide feed access during longer period of time and result with lower presence of damaged fins thus improving the welfare of the fish. In the feeding strategy design, it must be taken into account that the feeding regime affects the welfare of fish by increasing the risk of aggression that results with fin damage (25).

Although extensively referred to, it cannot be assumed that the level of fin damage is proportional to higher rearing densities (3). The regression analysis showed that SD was not a significant predictor in every examined fin model (Table 4 - Table 10). Fin damage is historically linked to SD (3) and the main approach was that higher densities will increase the level of fin damage (26-31). In our study, SD was the only factor that did not have an effect on the level of fin damage. This finding conforms to other research that there is no relationship between SD and the level of fin damage (3, 6, 7, 9, 32). The normal recommended SD for rainbow trout is 2 - 80 kg/m^3 (26). According to the welfare standards for farmed rainbow trout (5), the maximum SD for first feeding and on-growing tanks, raceways and ponds must not exceed 60 kg/m^3. Except Farm 4 (Table 1), all surveyed farms practiced lower SD that conforms to the welfare standards (5). Rasmussen et al. (7) found that in rainbow trout reared at high temperatures, the anal fin was in better condition at low densities, but the dorsal fin condition was better in high densities. They concluded that density had only a minor impact on fin condition, and suggest that young rainbow trout can be reared at relatively high densities (up to 120 kg/m^3) without significant impairment of their welfare. On the other hand, Bosakowski and Wagner (33) by using stepwise multiple linear regression suggested that fin erosion was correlated with higher fish densities. The differences between their and our findings may be a result of the different methodological approach and combination of farm variables. Macintyre (34) found that SD was associated with fin damage only on the rainbow trout farms that were breeding fish for restocking purposes, with an increase in SD associated with deteriorating fin condition. This finding did not exist for fish farmed for human consumption. His findings support the hypothesis that the SD effect on fin damage is mediated through behavioral interactions, so, before recommending the SD on a specific site, other factors must be considered, such as water quality and flow, feeding strategies, size of the fish and available space (5, 7).

Water temperature plays a role in the process of fin damage and affects the rate of healing and regeneration, but there is no common trend and the effects differ between species (32, 35). If the effect on all fins were combined, increased WT resulted in higher degrees of fin damage (Fig 1b), *nota bene*: within the temperature ranges included in this study. Higher levels of WT predicted the damage of the dorsal, pelvic and pectoral fins but WT was not a significant predictor in the models for the caudal and the anal fin. Higher WT promotes higher feeding activity and faster metabolism (15), therefore WT is in close relation to other factors such as DF and NM. The welfare standards for rainbow trout recommend WT between 1°C and 16°C, depending on the fish category (5). Except Farms 1 and 3, the other farms had WT in the recommended range. Our findings agree with the research of Winfree et al. (15) that juvenile rainbow trout reared at 10°C have less damaged fins than the same trout category reared at 15°C. In contrast, Atlantic salmon had increased fin erosion as WT decreased (36) and the level of fin damage in Bonneville cutthroat trout (*Oncorhynchus clarki*) was not clearly related to WT (37).

There is little information about the role of handling in fin damage (3). Routine handling affects the level of fin damage as fish come into physical contact with surfaces (nets, grading equipment, vaccination tables) and with other fish during crowding within the rearing units prior to vaccination, grading and processing (3, 30, 38). In our study, GR received the strongest weight in the model only for the dorsal fin, but higher levels of GR predicted the damage of the dorsal, caudal, anal and left pelvic fin. Contrary, GR was not significant predictor in the model for the right pelvic and both pectoral fins. If the effects on all fins were combined, increased GR values returned increased values for fin damage. Grading frequency was the most important variable, although not significantly different from WT (Fig. 1b). To our knowledge, there is no published data that specifically examines the influence of grading on the level of fin damage. According to the welfare standards for rainbow trout (5), grading must be performed when absolutely necessary and all equipment used during handling must be designed to avoid physical damage and stress to the fish. Grading can temporarily increase the aggressive behavior due to the disordered hierarchy (39, 40). However, it reduces the individual differences in the size of fish and positively affects welfare reducing the dominant hierarchical placement and the aggressive behavior (38).

CONCLUSION

In summary, our results support the experimental research on fin damage in rainbow trout and show that the feeding practices (lower levels of DF and NM) combined with the higher WT have the most dominant and proportional effect on the level of fin damage. The results also show that the standard multiple regression analysis predicts the level of fin damage inline as previously published experiments. This leads to the conclusion that the research model and the statistical analysis used in this study could be used on rainbow trout farms to evaluate the effect of the main factors on the level of fin damage, resulting with contribution to the assessment of fish welfare. Nevertheless, this study only explained less than 30% of the variance in fin damage, which suggests that further research has to statistically identify the effects of other factors (e.g. pH, alkalinity, ammonium concentration, water current, light regime, rearing unit surface, absence/presence of tank cover, etc.) on fin damage. This will lead to development of a management plan and modification of the husbandry practices that will result with low level of fin damage (according to the welfare standards for rainbow trout (5), the acceptable level is minimal damage i.e. score 1) and improved fish welfare.

REFERENCES

1. Hoyle, I., Oidtmann, B., Ellis, T., Turnbull, J., North, B., Nikolaidis, J., Knowles, T.G. (2007). A validated macroscopic key to assess fin damage in farmed rainbow trout (Oncorhynchus mykiss). Aquaculture 270, 142–148.
http://dx.doi.org/10.1016/j.aquaculture.2007.03.037

2. Kindschi, G.A., Barrows, F.T. (2009). Effects and interaction of phenotype and rearing density on growth and fin erosion in rainbow trout. N Am J Aquacult 71 (1): 79–86.
http://dx.doi.org/10.1577/A07-063.1

3. Ellis, T., Oidtmann, B., St-Hilaire, S., Turnbull, J., North, B., MacIntyre, C., Nikolaidis, J., Hoyle, I., Kestin, S., Knowles, T. (2008). Fin erosion in farmed fish. In: Branson, E. (Ed.), Fish Welfare (pp. 121–149). Blackwell, Oxford.
http://dx.doi.org/10.1002/9780470697610.ch9
PMid:17929165

4. Ellis, T., Hoyle, I., Oidtmann, B., Turnbull, J., Jacklin T.E., Knowles, T. (2009). Further development of the "Fin Index" method for quantifying fin erosion in rainbow trout. Aquaculture 289, 283–288.
http://dx.doi.org/10.1016/j.aquaculture.2009.01.022

5. Royal Society for the Prevention of Cruelty to Animals (2014). RSPCA welfare standards for farmed rainbow trout. RSPCA, West Sussex. Available at http://www.freedomfood.co.uk/media/51298/RSPCA-welfare-standards-for-farmed-rainbow-trout-web-.pdf

6. Latremouille, D.N. (2003). Fin erosion in aquaculture and natural environments. Rev Fish Sci 11 (4): 315–335.
http://dx.doi.org/10.1080/10641260390255745

7. Rasmussen, R.S., Larsen, F.H., Jensen, S. (2007). Fin condition and growth among rainbow trout reared at different sizes, densities and feeding frequencies in high temperature recirculated water. Aquacult Int 15, 97–107.
http://dx.doi.org/10.1007/s10499-006-9070-1

8. Person-Le Ruyet, J., Le Bayon, N. (2009). Effects of temperature, stocking density and farming conditions on fin damage in European sea bass (Dicentrarchus labrax). Aquat Living Resour 22, 349–62.
http://dx.doi.org/10.1051/alr/2009047

9. Klima, O., Kopp, R., Hadašová, L., Mareš, J. (2013). Fin condition of fish kept in aquacultural systems. Acta Univ Agric Silvic Mendelianae Brun 61 (6): 1907-1916.
http://dx.doi.org/10.11118/actaun201361061907

10. Cvetkovikj, A., Radeski, M., Blazhekovikj-Dimovska, D., Kostov, V., Stevanovski, V. (2013). Fin damage of farmed rainbow trout in the Republic of Macedonia. Mac Vet Rev 36 (2): 73-83.

11. Petersson, E., Karlsson, L., Ragnarsson, B., Bryntesson, M., Berglund, A., Stridsman, S., Jonsson, S. (2013). Fin erosion and injuries in relation to adult recapture rates in cultured smolts of Atlantic salmon and brown trout. Can J Fish Aquat Sci 70 (6): 915-921.
http://dx.doi.org/10.1139/cjfas-2012-0247

12. Barrows, F.T., Lellis, W.A. (1999). The effect of dietary protein and lipid source on dorsal fin erosion in rainbow trout, Oncorhynchus mykiss. Aquaculture 180, 167–175.
http://dx.doi.org/10.1016/S0044-8486(99)00188-X

13. Rosenthal, R. (1994). Parametric measures of effect size. In Cooper, H. and Hedges, L.V. (Eds.), The Handbook of research synthesis. (pp. 231-244). Russell Sage Foundation, New York.
PMid:8005375

14. Rosenberg, M.S., Adams, D.C., Gurevitch, J. (2012). MetaWin 2.1, Release 5.10.

15. Winfree, R.A., Kindschi, G.A., Shaw, H.T. (1998). Elevated water temperature, crowding, and food deprivation accelerate fin erosion in juvenile steelhead. Prog Fish Cult 60, 192–199.
http://dx.doi.org/10.1577/1548-8640(1998)060<0192:EWTCAF>2.0.CO;2

16. Moutou, K.A., McCarthy, I.D., Houlihan, D.F. (1998). The effect of ration level and social rank on the development of fin damage in juvenile rainbow trout. J Fish Biol 52, 756-770.
http://dx.doi.org/10.1111/j.1095-8649.1998.tb00818.x

17. Bergman, E., Piccolo, J., Greenberg, L. (2013). Raising brown trout (Salmo trutta) with less food - effects on smolt development and fin damage. Aquacult Res 44 (6): 1002-1006.
http://dx.doi.org/10.1111/j.1365-2109.2011.03086.x

18. Canon Jones, H.A., Hansen, L.A., Noble, C., Damsgard, B., Broom, D.M., Pearce, G.P. (2010). Social network analysis of behavioural interactions influencing fin damage development in Atlantic salmon (Salmo salar) during feed-restriction. Appl Anim Behav Sci 127, 139–351. http://dx.doi.org/10.1016/j.applanim.2010.09.004

19. Noble, C., Mizusawa, K., Suzuki, K., Tabata, M. (2007). The effect of differing self-feeding regimes on the growth, behaviour and fin damage of rainbow trout held in groups. Aquaculture 264, 214–222. http://dx.doi.org/10.1016/j.aquaculture.2006.12.028

20. Noble, C., Kadri, S., Mitchell, D.F., Huntingford, F.A. (2007). Influence of feeding regime on intraspecific competition, fin damage and growth in 1+ Atlantic salmon parr (Salmo salar L.) held in freshwater production cages. Aquacult Res 38, 1137–1143. http://dx.doi.org/10.1111/j.1365-2109.2007.01777.x

21. Noble, C., Kadri, S., Mitchell, D.F., Huntingford, F.A. (2008). Growth, production and fin damage in cage-held 0+ Atlantic salmon pre-smolts (Salmo salar L.) fed either a) on-demand, or b) to a fixed satiation–restriction regime: data from a commercial farm. Aquaculture 275, 163–168. http://dx.doi.org/10.1016/j.aquaculture.2007.12.028

22. Suzuki, K., Mizusawa, K., Noble, C., Tabata, M. (2008). The growth, feed conversion ratio and fin damage of rainbow trout Oncorhynchus mykiss under self-feeding and hand feeding regimes. Fisheries Sci 74, 941–943. http://dx.doi.org/10.1111/j.1444-2906.2008.01610.x

23. Wagner, E. J., Routledge, M. D., Intelmann, S. S. (1996). Assessment of demand feeder spacing on hatchery performance, fin condition, and size variation of rainbow trout Oncorhynchus mykiss. J World Aquacult Soc 27 (1), 130–136. http://dx.doi.org/10.1111/j.1749-7345.1996.tb00604.x

24. Attia, J., Millot, S., Di-Poi, C., Begout M., Noble, C., Sanchez-Vazquez, F. J., Terova, G., Saroglia M., Damsgard, B. (2012). Demand feeding and welfare in farmed fish. Fish Physiol Biochem 38 (1), 107–118. http://dx.doi.org/10.1007/s10695-011-9538-4 PMid:21728053

25. Lopez-Olmeda, J.F., Noble, C., Sanchez-Vazquez, F. J. (2012). Does feeding time affect fish welfare? Fish Physiol Biochem 38 (1), 143-52. http://dx.doi.org/10.1007/s10695-011-9523-y PMid:21671025

26. Ellis, T., North, B., Scott, A.P., Bromage, N.R., Porter, M., Gadd, D. (2002). The relationships between stocking density and welfare in farmed rainbow trout. J Fish Biol 61, 493–531. http://dx.doi.org/10.1111/j.1095-8649.2002.tb00893.x

27. Turnbull, J., Bell, A., Adams, C., Bron, J., Huntingford, F. (2005). Stocking density and welfare of cage farmed Atlantic salmon: application of multivariate analysis. Aquaculture 243, 121–132. http://dx.doi.org/10.1016/j.aquaculture.2004.09.022

28. North, B.P., Turnbull, J.F., Ellis, T., Porter, M.J., Migaud, H., Bron, J., Bromage, N.R. (2006). The impact of stocking density on the welfare of rainbow trout (Oncorhynchus mykiss). Aquaculture 255, 466–479. http://dx.doi.org/10.1016/j.aquaculture.2006.01.004

29. Adams, C.E., Turnbull, J.F., Bell, A., Bron, J.E., Huntingford, F.A. (2007). Multiple determinants of welfare in farmed fish: stocking density, disturbance and aggression in salmon. Can J Fish Aquat Sci 64, 336–344. http://dx.doi.org/10.1139/f07-018

30. Person-LeRuyet, J., Labbe, L., Bayon, N.L., Severe, A., Roux, A.L., Delliou, H.L., Quemener, L. (2008). Combined effects of water quality and stocking density on welfare and growth of rainbow trout (Oncorhynchus mykiss). Aquat Living Resour 21, 185–195. http://dx.doi.org/10.1051/alr:2008024

31. Canon Jones, H.A., Noble, C., Damsgard, B., Pearce, G.P. (2011). Social network analysis of the behavioural interactions that influence the development of fin damage in Atlantic salmon parr (Salmo salar) held at different stocking densities. Appl Anim Behav Sci 133, 117–126. http://dx.doi.org/10.1016/j.applanim.2011.05.005

32. Noble, C., Canon Jones, H.A., Damsgard, B., Flood, M.J., Midling, K.Ø., Roque, A., Sæther, B.S., Cottee, S.Y. (2012). Injuries and deformities in fish: their potential impacts upon aquacultural production and welfare. Fish Physiol Biochem 38 (1), 61-83. http://dx.doi.org/10.1007/s10695-011-9557-1 PMid:21918861

33. Bosakowski, T., Wagner, E.J. (1994). A survey of trout fin erosion, water quality, and rearing conditions at state fish hatcheries in Utah. J World Aquacult Soc, 25, 308–316. http://dx.doi.org/10.1111/j.1749-7345.1994.tb00196.x

34. Macintyre, C. (2008). Water quality and welfare assessment on United Kingdom trout farms. PhD thesis. Institute of Aquaculture, University of Stirling.

35. Turnbull, J.F., Richards, R.H., Robertson, D.A. (1996). Gross, histological and scanning electron microscopic appearance of dorsal fin rot in farmed Atlantic salmon, Salmo salar L., parr. J Fish Dis 19, 415–427. http://dx.doi.org/10.1046/j.1365-2761.1996.d01-93.x

36. Schneider, R., Nicholson, B.L. (1980). Bacteria associated with fin rot disease in hatchery reared Atlantic salmon (Salmo salar). Can J Fish Aquat Sci 37, 1505–1513. http://dx.doi.org/10.1139/f80-195

37. Wagner, E.J., Arndt, R., Routledge, M.D., Bradwisch, Q. (1998). Hatchery performance and fin erosion of Bonneville cutthroat trout, Oncorhynchus clarki, at two temperatures. J App Aquacult 8, 1–12. http://dx.doi.org/10.1300/J028v08n02_01

38. Farm Animal Welfare Council (1996). Report on the welfare of farmed fish. FAWC, Surbiton, Surrey.

39. Abbott, J.C., Dunbrack, R.L., Orr, C.D. (1985). The interaction of size and experience in dominance relationships of juvenile steelhead trout (Salmo gairdneri). Behaviour 92, 241-253.

40. Jobling, M., Wandsvik, A. (1983). Effect of social interactions on growth rates and conversion efficiency of Arctic charr, Salvelinus alpinus L. J Fish Biol 22, 577-584.
http://dx.doi.org/10.1111/j.1095-8649.1983.tb04217.x

14

INFLUENCE OF METABOLIC CAGE ON *WISTAR* RAT PHYSIOLOGICAL STATE

Judita Zymantiene, Rasa Zelvyte, Vaidas Oberauskas, Ugne Spancerniene

Department of Anatomy and Physiology, Veterinary Faculty of Lithuanian University of Health Sciences, Tilzes st. 18, LT 47181 Kaunas, Lithuania

ABSTRACT

The aim of this study was to investigate the influence of metabolic cage housing on the *Wistar* rat physiological state and to analyze the correlation between the minerals in blood and urine. Thirty male rats were used in the experiment. Fifteen rats (control group) were housed individually in standard polycarbonate cages and fifteen rats (experimental group) in metabolic cages (Techniplast, Italy) for two weeks. Body weight, respiration rate, water and food consumptions were recorded for each animal at the beginning of the experiment. The same parameters, as well as blood and urine parameters of control and experimental animals were recorded during the experiment after 72 h, 168 h and 336 h of housing in standard cages and metabolic cages. Urine collection was measured only in the experimental group. Rats weight decreased from 3.84 % to 18.59 % (P<0.05), respiration rate from 18.65 % to 24.59 % (P<0.05) when rats were housed in metabolic cages. Consumption of food and water by the rat depended on how long the animal was kept in metabolic cage. Glucose concentration increased on average by 15.37 %, WBC count decreased by 5.83 % in the blood of rats housed in metabolic cages compared to the animals housed in standard cages. We did not observe significant changes of triglycerides concentration, red blood cells count and total protein between all rats. The positive moderate correlation of rat housing in a metabolic cage was between K blood and K urine, P blood and P urine, Na blood and K blood, between Na urine and P urine and significant negative moderate correlation was determined between K urine and P urine. These present study findings indicate that metabolism cage housing significantly affects rat's physiological parameters and potentially may influence animal health and wellbeing.

Key words: metabolic cage, rat, blood, urine, physiological parameters

INTRODUCTION

Rodents are mostly used in scientific and experimental studies. Rats are one of the primary mammalian species used for the evaluation of acute and chronic toxicity, metabolism and bioavailability in preclinical evaluation of drugs and preregistration evaluation of chemicals (1, 2). Rats are used for metabolism study, pharmacokinetic study, toxicity testing, vaccine potency testing, model for induction of tumors and etc. (3).

Metabolic cages are used to gain information about metabolic function and how different factors affect animal's metabolism processes (2, 4). Metabolic cages are equipped with a unique system for the separated collection of faeces and urine. The cage is designed to avoid contamination of the urine and effectively separate urine and faeces into collection tubes outside of the cage (2). The grid floor is a necessity to allow urine and faeces to be collected (5, 6).

Design and finish results are such that the animal has a minimum of comfort and housing on grid floors is negative for animal welfare. Preference tests have shown that most rats prefer to sleep in solid bottom cages (7). Rodents housed in metabolic cages can not perform some of their natural behaviors such as nest-building, hiding, social interaction process (8). Social isolation affected the central nervous system of mice and single housed wild type mice showed an increase of stereotypic behaviors which strongly indicate a lack of possibilities to perform natural behaviors in the environment (9, 10). Moreover, social isolation, lack of nesting material, housing on grid floor and small cage area are environmental factors that may expose rodents

Corresponding author: Dr. Zymantiene Judita, PhD
E-mail address: Judita.Zymantiene@lsmuni.lt
Present address: Department Anatomy and Physiology, Lithuanian University of Health Sciences , Tilzes 18, Kaunas LT-47181

to stress (8). Conducted surveys revealed that grid floor can cause hypersensitivity and nerve injury in the feet of rats and lead to elevated corticosterone levels, increased blood pressure, heart rate and body temperature.

There are limited scientific investigations performed on the influence of a metabolic cage on animal welfare. Stress can be defined as factor that alters the internal environment of the body (11). The body has some major adaptations to stress in order to maintain homeostasis, prepare for physical activity, such as increased glucocorticoid and catecholamine secretion (12, 13). According to scientists observations it was measured that young male rats housed in metabolic cages had reduced weight gains and produced more amounts of faeces after three days of metabolism cage housing (4). There are various reasons how the type of cage influences weight of rodents. Single housed mice had significantly lower body weights and lower bone mineral content, compared to animals held in groups. Some researches noticed several physiological disruptions due to increased levels of circulating corticosterone in single housed rodents (14, 15). Many scientists conducted studies on social isolation and the release of sympathetic neurotransmitter substances in the brains of mice. Since the reproductive, cardiovascular, gastrointestinal and the immune system are regulated by the sympathetic nervous system any change in the central nervous system will have great impact on the animal's physiology (16). Attempts to keep rodents in metabolic cages have been carried out in all EU countries, but some researchers noticed only changes in animals behavior, others (2, 8, 10, 17) determined only changes of hormonal activity in blood or lower animals weight, but there is still insufficient knowledge about systematic data changes of physiological parameters.

The aim of this study was to investigate the influence of metabolic cage housing on *Wistar* rat physiological state and to analyze the correlation between minerals in blood and urine.

MATERIAL AND METHODS

24-weeks-old male *Wistar* rats weighing 289.05±1.55g (mean±SEM (standard error of the mean)) were used. The rats were kept under normal conditions: light-dark cycle of 12:12 hours, temperature maintained at 22 ± 2^oC and relative humidity was 55±5 %. Rats were given ad libitum access to high-quality feed of the same batch and water throughout the whole study in both groups. The commercial standard diet (PA-11700000-171)

for rodents contained crude protein 19.91 %, fat 12.05 %, crude fiber 2.79 % and 7.72 % cellulose in 1 kg of feed. All procedures were approved by the local Animal Ethical Committee (No. license G2-16).

A control group of fifteen rats were housed individually in standard polycarbonate cages (Techniplast, Italy), where minimum enclosure size was 800 cm^2, floor area per animal 350 cm^2 and minimum 18 cm height according to the Directive 2010/63 EU of the European Parliament and of the Council of 22 September 2010 on the protection of animals used for scientific purposes. Fifteen rats of the experimental group were transferred to and housed in individual metabolic cages (Techniplast, Italy) with stainless steel grid floor for two weeks.

Body weight, respiration rate, water and food consumptions were recorded for each animal in the beginning of the experiment. The same parameters as well as blood and urine parameters of control and experimental animals were recorded during the experiment after 72 h, 168 h, 336 h of housing in standard cages and metabolic cages. Urine collection was measured only in the experimental group. Rats were weighed using the scales KERN PCB000-1 (Germany, 2014). Daily urine was collected at 9 a.m. for analysis and calculation of diuresis intensity. Water and food consumption were calculated via 24 hours. Respiration rate was measured by calculation of breaths per minute. The rats were killed by an overdose of carbon dioxide in camber and blood samples were collected from *v. jugularis.*

Blood samples collected in heparinized tubes were used for determination of red blood cells (RBC) and white blood cells (WBC) count. RBC and WBC count were calculated using hemacytometer Neubauer chamber (Germany) under the microscope OLYMPUS CX 22LED (Germany).

Serum was separated taking blood in microtubes without anticoagulant, using rotation 4000 x g for 10 min by centrifuge (EBA-200, Germany). Serum levels of glucose (GL), triglycerides (TG) and total protein (T-Pro) were measured by analyzer SPOTCHEM EZ SP-4430 (Arkray Inc., Japan).

The concentrations of minerals as sodium (Na), potassium (K), phosphorus (P) in serum and urine after 336 h housing in metabolic cages were assayed using Cobas Integra 400 plus analyzer and commercial kits (Tegimenta Ltd Roche, Switzerland).

The statistical analysis of the results were carried out using the SPSS (licence No. 9900457; version 15, SPSS Inc., Chicago, IL). All data are presented as mean±SEM. The level of statistical significance was set at P<0.05. Correlation coefficient (r) was used for measuring the relationship between two variables. The correlation is considered weak at r = 0.50, moderate at r = 0.50 – 0.75 and strong at r = 0.80 – 1.00.

RESULTS

At the beginning of the experiment body weight, respiration rate, consumption of food and water of control and experimental rats were similar within the range of the physiological norms for rats (Table 1). Variation of some functional parameters of the rats during the study have been presented in Table 2. Duration of the housing of rats in the metabolic cage influenced the body weight and respiration rate. Rats weight decreased 3.84 % and 18.59 % (P<0.05) respectively when rats were housed 72 h and 168 hours in metabolic cages, compared to the housing of animals in standard cages. We did not determine changes in breathing when rats were housed 72 h in metabolic cages, but the respiration rate decreased from 18.65 to 24.59 % (P<0.05) when rats were housed from 168 to 336 hours in metabolic cages

compared to the rats housed in the standard cages. We established a tendency of increasing water consumption by average of 37.68 % (P<0.01) when rats were housed 168 h and 336 hours in metabolic cages, but there were no changes when rats were 72 hours in these cages. The intensity of diuresis increased from 6.19 % to 28.32 % after 168 h and 336 h of housing rats in metabolic cages compared to the diuresis of rats after 72 h of housing in metabolic cages.

In vivo study in rats has demonstrated that metabolic cages have influence on the GL concentration in blood (Table 3). Glucose level increased from 13.95 to 16.79 % in blood of rats housed in metabolic cages compared to the rats housed in standard cages. Our experiment results did not reveal any significant changes of TG concentration, RBC and total protein counts between all rats, but WBC decreased by average 5.83 % (from 5.00 to 6.33 %) (P<0.05) in the blood of rats housed in metabolic cages compared to the analogical parameters of housing rats in standard cages.

Table 1. Body weight, respiration rate, consumption of food and water of control and experimental rats at the beginning of the study

Parameter	Group	
	Control, n=15	Experimental, n=15
Body weight, g	288.5±1.8	289.6±1.3
Respiration rate, breaths/min	60.0±2.3	60.0±1.4
Consumption of water, via 24 h, ml	25.0±1.7	24.0±1.5
Consumption of food, via 24 h, g	39.7±2.1	41.2±1.9

Table 2. Variations of rats' body weight, respiration rate, consumption of food and water and intensity of dieresis

Parameter	Control group			Experimental group		
	after 72 h	after 168 h	after 336 h	after 72 h	after 168 h	after 336 h
Number, n	5	5	5	5	5	5
Body weight, g	288.7±1.4*	288.4±1.7*	289.3±2.3	277.6±2.2*	234.8±1.5*	252.1±2.0
Respiration rate, breaths/min	60.0±1.9	59.0±2.0*	61.0±1.8*	61.0±1.7	48.0±1.9*	46.0±2.0*
Consumption of water, via 24 h, ml	25.6±2.1	24.8±1.7**	26.3±1.4**	27.6±1.9	40.0±1.5**	30.0±1.8**
Consumption of food, via 24 h, g	37.2±2.3	40.1±1.9	39.2±2.3	25.9±2.3	25.0±1.8	23.9±1.5
For a 24–h intensity of diuresis, ml	-	-	-	11.3±2.0	14.5±2.2	12.0±2.6

P<0.05*; P<0.01**

Table 3. Changes in some hematological parameters of rats

Parameter	Control group			Experimental group		
	after 72 h	after 168 h	after 336 h	after 72 h	after 168 h	after 336 h
Number, n	5	5	5	5	5	5
RBC, $\times 10^{12}$/L	4.2±0.05	4.0±0.15	4.3±0.10	4.3±0.07	4.4±0.20	4.2±0.14
WBC, $\times 10^{9}$/L	8.1±0.40*	8.0±0.31*	7.9±0.10*	7.6±0.51*	7.6±0.42*	7.4±0.09*
T-Pro, g/L	56.3±0.84	55.6±0.36	55.7±1.00	54.6±0.91	54.8±0.88	54.6±0.80
GL, mmol/L	6.88±0.10*	7.00±0.23	6.79±0.33*	7.84±0.21*	7.38±0.17	7.93±0.41*
TG, mmol/L	1.62±0.08	1.65±0.10	1.63±0.15	1.62±0.11	1.72±0.07	1.76±0.04

P<0.05*

We found that when rats were housed 336 hours in metabolic cages there were changes in the main minerals in blood and urine and results are presented in Table 4. Correlation coefficient was used for measuring the relationship between the two variables. The positive moderate correlation was between K blood and K urine (r=0.7328; P<0.01), P blood and P urine (r=0.6932; P<0.01), Na blood and K blood (r=0.6151; P<0.01), Na urine and P urine (r=0.7373; P<0.01) and significant negative moderate correlation was determined between K urine and P urine.

Table 4. Correlations between blood and urine minerals of rats housed in the metabolic cages for 336 h

Parameter		r
Na blood	Na urine	0.0769
K blood	K urine	0.7328
P blood	P urine	0.6932
Na blood	K blood	0.6151
Na blood	P blood	-0.1116
K blood	P blood	0.2831
Na urine	K urine	-0.0083
Na urine	P urine	0.7373
K urine	P urine	-0.5867

We did not determine significant correlation between Na blood and Na urine; among Na blood and P blood, between P blood and K blood and among Na urine and K urine when rats were accommodated in a different cage system.

DISCUSSION

Modern housing technologies, physical environmental factors, research experiments, human interaction and intervention are parts of the stimuli presented to rats every day, influencing their physiology and contributing to their welfare. Human interaction, certain environmental conditions and routine procedures in the animal facility might induce stress responses and when the animal is unable to maintain its homeostasis in the presence of a particular stressor, the animal's wellbeing is threatened. When rats were housed in metabolic cages, the human interaction process increased because of daily urine collection and cage washing. The present study focused on the impact of the metabolic cage on the laboratory rat physiological state and correlation between minerals in blood and urine. When rodents are used in experiments with preclinical animal models they are kept in metabolic cages with specific floor construction and this fact can influence some functional parameters (18). Our results revealed that the long-term effect of housing of rats in a metabolic cages lead to changes in feeding, water consumption and some blood parameters compared to the housing of rats in standard cages. This may be associated with the specific construction of the cage floor that influences changes in the respiration rate of rats and this parameter decreased by 21.62 %. We established a tendency of increasing water consumption by 14.07 % and decreasing of food consumption by 39.04 % when rats were housed for 336 hours in metabolic cages. Scientists indicated that consumption of water and food depends on the bedding material volume (19), but in our experiment bedding was not provided. According to our analysis if the plate of the feeding area in the metabolic cage is not a very small grid construction, the rats are feeling better because they stand in a normal position. Some scientists identified that cage design and construction may influence temperature in the cage, which can affect the physiological state of the organism (20).

We determined that long-term housing of rats when this duration is applied in preclinical studies has negative effect on rats' functional parameters. After 7-14 days of rat's social isolation there was a significant decreased WBC count. Glucose concentration in blood, as one of the stress factors, depended on the duration of metabolic cage housing. We noticed that when rats were housed in metabolic cages from 168 to 336 hours, the glucose concentration increased by average of 15.37 % if compared to the housing of animals in standard cages. Several authors have shown that cage cleaning promotes an acute stress response in laboratory animals (10, 21). They reported that cage cleaning of adult male Sprague-Dawley rats, housed in groups of three, elevated serum concentrations of corticosterone and prolactin (15, 22, 23). We found that daily cleaning of metabolic cages and urine samples taking caused fear in rats. This effect showed that activation of the sympathetic nervous system has also been associated with routine housing procedures such as cage cleaning and significant increases in plasma noradrenalin and adrenalin (15, 24). Furthermore, we determined positive moderate correlation between K blood and K urine, P blood and P urine, Na blood and K blood, Na urine and P urine, but also significant negative moderate correlation was found between K urine and P urine.

Researchers should be careful with animal housing in metabolic cages when planning studies, because this modern cage caused potential discomfort due to floor construction, there is no place for rest and the animal does not have social communication.

CONCLUSION

Housing rodents in cages that exposes them to social isolation, or not natural grid floor construction, may cause physiological changes due to stress responses. But stress levesl depended on the duration of housing in a metabolic cage. Rats weight decreased from 3.84 to 18.59 % (P<0.05), respiration rate from 18.65 to 24.59 % (P<0.05) when rats were housed in a metabolic cage. Consumption of food and water of the rat depended on how long the animal was kept in a metabolic cage. Glucose concentration increased by 15.37 %,

WBC count decreased by 5.83 % in the blood of rats housed in metabolic cages compared to the animals housed in standard cages. We did not observe significant changes in triglycerides concentration, red blood cells count and total protein between all rats. The positive moderate correlation in rats housed in metabolic cages was between K blood and K urine, P blood and P urine, Na blood and K blood, between Na urine and P urine and significant negative moderate correlation was determined between K urine and P urine. These findings indicate that metabolism cage housing significantly affects rat's physiological parameters and potentially may influence the animal health and wellbeing.

REFERENCES

1. Gordon, C.J., Fogelson, L. (1994). Metabolic and thermoregulatory responses of the rat maintained in acrylic or wire-screen cages: implications for pharmacological studies. Physiology & Behavior 56(1): 73–79.
http://dx.doi.org/10.1016/0031-9384(94)90263-1

2. Kurien, B.T., Everds, N.E., Scofield, R.H. (2004). Experimental animal urine collection: a review Laboratory Animals Ltd. Laboratory Animals 38, 333–361.
http://dx.doi.org/10.1258/0023677041958945
PMid:15479549

3. EU (2010) Directive 2010/63 EU of the European Parliament and of the Council of 22 September 2010 on the protection of animals used for scientific purposes. Official Journal of the European Communities L276, pp. 33–79.

4. Eriksson, E., Royo, F.K, Lyberg Carlsson, H-E., Hau, J. (2004). Effect of metabolic cage housing on immunoglobulin A and corticosterone excretion in faeces and urine of young male rats. Experimental Physiology 89(4): 427–433.
http://dx.doi.org/10.1113/expphysiol.2004.027656
PMid:15131075

5. Heidbreder, C.A., Weiss, I.C., Domeney, A.M., Pryce, C., Homberg, J., Hedou, G., Feldon, J. Moran, M.C., Nelson, P. (2000). Behavioral, neurochemical and endocrinological characterization of the early social isolation syndrome. Neuroscience 100(4): 749–768.
http://dx.doi.org/10.1016/S0306-4522(00)00336-5

6. Krohn, T.C., Hansen, A.K., Dragsted, N. (2003). Telemetry as a method for measuring the impact of housing conditions on rat's welfare. Animal Welfare 12(1): 53–62.

7. Manser, C.E. Morris, T.H., Broom, D.M. (1995). An investigation into the effects of solid or grid cage flooring on the welfare of laboratory rats. Laboratory Animals 29(4): 353–363.
http://dx.doi.org/10.1258/002367795780740023
PMid:8558816

8. Cvek-Hopkins K. (2007). Effect of metabolic cage housing on rodent welfare. SLU Uppsala, 7–9.

9. Yamada, K., Ohki-Hamazaki, H., Wada, K. (2000). Differential effects of social isolation upon body weight, food consumption, and responsiveness to novel and social environment in bombesin receptor subtype-3 (BRS-3) deficient mice. Physiology & Behavior 68, 555–561.
http://dx.doi.org/10.1016/S0031-9384(99)00214-0

10. Balcombe, J.P., Barnard, N.D, Sandusky, C. (2004). Laboratory routines cause animal stress. Contemp Top Lab Anim Sci. 43, 42–51.
PMid:15669134

11. Sjaastad, Ø.V., Hove, K., Sand, O. (2003). Physiology of Domestic Animals (pp. 141, 224, 226–227, 241). First edition. Oslo: Scandinavian Veterinary Press.

12. Qiang, D., Salva, A., Sottas, C.M., Niu, E., Holmes, M., Hardy, M.P. (2004). Rapid glucocorticoid mediation of suppressed testosterone biosynthesis in male mice subjected to immobilization stress. Journal of Andrology 25(6): 973–981.

13. Hunt, C., Hambly, C. (2006). Faecal corticosterone concentrations indicate that separately housed male mice are not more stressed than group housed males. Physiology & Behavior 87, 519–526.
http://dx.doi.org/10.1016/j.physbeh.2005.11.013
PMid:16442135

14. Nagy, T.R., Krzywanski, D., Li, J., Meleth, S., Desmond, R. (2002). Effect of group vs. single housing on phenotypic variance in C57BL/6J mice. Obesity Research 10, 412–415.
http://dx.doi.org/10.1038/oby.2002.57
PMid:12006642

15. Spangenberg, E.M.F., Augustsson, H., Dahlborn, K., Essén-Gustavsson, B., Cvek, K. (2005). Housing related activity in rats: effects on body weight, urinary corticosterone levels, muscle properties and performance. Laboratory Animals 39, 45–57.
http://dx.doi.org/10.1258/0023677052886457
PMid:15703124

16. D'Arbe, M., Einstein, R., Lavidis, N.A. (2002). Stressful animal housing conditions and their potential effect on sympathetic neurotransmission in mice. The American Journal of Physiology. Regulatory, Intergrative and Comparative Physiology 282, 1422–1428.
http://dx.doi.org/10.1152/ajpregu.00805.2000
PMid:11959685

17. Gil, M.C., Aguirre, J.A., Lemoine, A.P., Segura, E.T., Barontini, M.I. (1999). Influence of age on stress responses to metabolic cage housing in rats. Cellular and Molecular Neurobiologi 19(5): 625–633.
http://dx.doi.org/10.1023/A:1006984402291
PMid:10384260

18. Ollson, I.A.S., Westlund, K. (2007).The effect of social factors on behavior and welfare of laboratory rodents and non-human primates. Appl. Anim. Behav. Sci. 103, 229–254.
http://dx.doi.org/10.1016/j.applanim.2006.05.022

19. Freymann J., Tsai, P.P., Stelzer, H., Hackbarth, H. (2015). The amount of cage bedding preferred by female BALB/c and C57BL/6 mice. Lab animal Europe 15 (2): 13–19.

20. Hirsjärvi, P., Väliaho, T. (1995). Gentled and nonhandled Wistar rats in a mildly novel open-field situation. Scandinavian Journal of Laboratory Animal Science 22 (3): 265–269.

21. Van Loo, P.L.P., Kruitwagen, C.L.J.J., Van Zutphen, L.F.M., Koolhaas, J.M., Baumans, V. (2000). Modulation of aggression in male mice: influence of cage cleaning regime and scent marks. Anim Welf. 9, 281–295.

22. Armario, A., Montero, J.L., Balasch, J. (1986). Sensitivity of corticosterone and some metabolic variables to graded levels of low intensity stresses in adult male rats. Physiol Behav. 37, 559–561.
http://dx.doi.org/10.1016/0031-9384(86)90285-4

23. Castelhano-Carlos, M.J., Baumans, V. (2009). The impact of light, noise, cage cleaning and in-house transport on welfare and stress of laboratory rats. Laboratory Animals 43, 311–327.
http://dx.doi.org/10.1258/la.2009.0080098
PMid:19505937

24. De Boer, S.F., Koopmans, S.J., Slangen, J.L., Van der Gugten, J. (1990). Plasma catecholamine, corticosterone and glucose responses to repeated stress in rats. Effect of interstressor interval length. Physiol Behav 47, 1117–1124.
http://dx.doi.org/10.1016/0031-9384(90)90361-7

15

MICROBIOLOGICAL PROPERTIES AND CHEMICAL COMPOSITION OF MACEDONIAN TRADITIONAL WHITE BRINED CHEESE

Mojsova Sandra, Jankuloski Dean, Sekulovski Pavle, Angelovski Ljupco, Ratkova Marija, Prodanov Mirko

Food institute, Faculty of veterinary medicine
University of "Ss. Cyril and Methodius" in Skopje

ABSTRACT

The purpose of this study was to asses the chemical and microbial characteristics of 10 artisanal cheeses made from raw ewe's milk without addition of starters, during maturation. Microbial populations were numerous and diverse with Lactic acid bacteria and *Enterobaceriaceae* as a predominant groups of microorganisms. Pathogenic bacteria were not detected. The pH of the cheeses was within the range of 4.04 – 5.05, the moisture content within 46.97 – 51.58%, total protein from 18 – 21.37%, fat content from 26 - 30% and NaCl from 4.38 – 5.43%.

Key words: traditional, ewe's milk cheese, pathogen bacteria, lactic acid bacteria

INTRODUCTION

Dairy products made from locally produced raw milk are still a very important part of daily diet. The characteristics of these products are different from one to another region depending on the local indigenous microflora, which in turns reflects the climate conditions of the area.

Macedonian white cheese is a brined cheese variety with a soft or semihard texture. The main flavor characteristic is the salty acid taste. The cheese is rindless, white coloured and close textured. It is generally made from cow's milk, ewe's milk and less from goat milk, prepared in cubes and ripened for 3 months. Traditionally, this type of cheese have been manufactured by local farmers on a small scale for decades using raw milk and traditional techniques passed down from generation to generation using only basic equipment. Commercial starter cultures are not used in the production and instead, the cheese maker relies on the lactic acid bacteria (LAB) naturally present in the raw unpasteurized milk as adventitious contaminants.

Cheese is chemically, microbiologically and enzymatically a complex and dynamic system. This makes the process of cheese ripening highly complex. One of the characteristics of white-brined cheeses is their high salt content, and this probably accords with the fact that they are traditionally manufactured in countries with hot climates. it is important to note that the composition of different white brined cheeses varies within a broad interval due to the differences in the composition of raw milk, processing parameters and ripening conditions (22).

Bacterial biodiversity arising from the raw milk and environmental contamination (from farm and production practices) constitute the principal source of the microorganisms which are necessary for the development of the typical features (taste, flavor, consistency). The microbial diversity originating from environmental exposure during cheese manufacture and maturation and the initial natural

Corresponding author: Mojsova Sandra , MSc

e-mail address: kostova.sandra@fvm.ukim.edu.mk
Present address: Food institute, Faculty of Veterinary medicine-Skopje,
"Ss. Cyril and Methodius" University,
Lazar Pop- Trajkov 5-7, 1000 Skopje, R. Macedonia

diversity of the microbiota present in the raw milk all play a role in fermentation processes and are important in the final development of traditional dairy products (1).

Microbiological quality of white-brined cheeses can be influenced by numerous factors, including the quality of the milk, the use of pasteurization or thermization, various technological parameters and the level and type(s) of microbial contamination that occur throughout the manufacture and storage of the cheese. White-brined cheeses are matured for long periods in brine, and thus the dominant microflora make a significant contribution to the maturation process and, to a degree, regulate the quality of the final product (2).

When cheese is produced following traditional procedures from raw milk, the environmental microflora plays a fundamental role in fermentation and is one of the most important parameters affecting the cheese quality. In addition, the biodiversity of bacteria involved in cheese production can be considered a fundamental factor for the maintenance of the typical features of traditional cheese products. Recent investigations have shown that the indigenous microflora of raw milk influence the biochemical characteristics and flavor of cheeses (3).

No information is available on this cheese microflora and its evolution during ripening. The objective of this study was to obtain the initial insight into the biodiversity of the microbial community associated with this cheese during the ripening. The main purpose was to investigate the dynamics of the microflora and to characterize the dominant groups of LAB during the maturation process and pathogen bacteria as a main risk factor in making cheese in a traditional way.

MATERIAL AND METHODS

Collection of samples and sample preparation
Five samples of white brined ewe's milk cheese in the beginning of the ripening (second week) and five samples in the end of the ripening (after 3 months) made by traditional method were collected aseptically from local producers from five different regions of the country. Samples were brought to the laboratory under refrigerated conditions (4-6°C), and analyzed within 24h.

Microbial population counting and chemical analyses
All of the analysed parameters according to the tested matrix and reference methods (12-19) used are given in Table 1.

Table 1. Overview of the parameters and methods used in the study

No.	Parameter	Matrix	Reference method
1.	*Enterobacteriaceae*	Cheese	ISO 21528-2:2004
2.	*Listeria monocytogenes*	Cheese	ISO 11290-1:1996
3.	*Escherichia coli*	Cheese	ISO 16649-3:2005
4.	*Staphylococcus aureus*	Cheese	ISO 6888-1:1999
5.	Yeasts and moulds	Cheese	ISO 21527-2
7.	pH	Cheese	pH meter Sartorius
8.	Protein content	Cheese	ISO 8968:1 2001
9.	*Fat content*	Cheese	ISO 16266:2006
10.	Moisture content	Cheese	Mitrovic, 1954
11.	Sodium chloride content	Cheese	Titrimetric method

Lactobacilli were grown on Rogosa agar (RA, Sigma Aldrich) after 5 days at 30°C incubated anaerobically (Gas-Pack anaerobic system, Biomerieux, France). Gram positive, catalase negative cocci on M17 agar, after incubation at 30°C for 48h. Cycloheximide was added (100 mg⁻¹) to prevent the growth of yeasts in M17 agar (Sigma Aldrich). Enterococci were grown on kanamycin esculine azide agar (KAA, Fluka) at 37°C 24h. Presumptive leuconostoc on De Man, Rogosa,

Sharpe (MRS agar, Sigma Aldrich) with 30 μg/ml $^{-1}$ vancomycin.

After the incubation period, the plates containing between 10 and 300 colonies were selected for enumeration. The number of colonies grown on each medium was expressed as log cfu/g^{-1}. The cells from Rogosa and M17 agar were Gram-stained and the catalase activity was determined. All determinations were conducted two times.

RESULTS AND DISCUSSION

In our research ten cheese samples from five different regions have been analyzed. Five were tested at the second week of the ripening (day 10) and five in the end of ripening after three months (day 90). The changes of different microbial groups investigated during the maturation period are shown in the Fig. 1 and Fig. 2.

The chemical composition of all of the cheeses was generally within the range typical for white brined cheese. Macedonian white brined cheese may be characterized as a soft (50 - 60 %) moisture, high fat cheese (25-30%), protein (12–21%) high salt (3–5%) content and the final pH range of 4.20 – 5.05. Decreases in total solid content of brined cheeses throughout ripening generally originate from water soluble proteins and peptides passed from cheese matrix to brine. Increase in salt content during ripening could be attributed to the higher water content because salt penetrates the cheese matrix in water (6).

Table 2. Chemical composition of Macedonian white brined cheese

sample	day	pH	Moisture %	Protein%	Fat%	NaCl%
A	10	6.69	62.01	12.43	25.00	4.09
	90	5.05	50.00	18.21	30.00	4.60
B	10	6.38	59.03	12.41	26.50	3.51
	90	4.04	51.58	19.02	28.00	5.43
C	10	6.20	55.96	14.00	26.00	3.15
	90	4.45	47.83	20.01	27.50	4.38
D	10	6.23	56.10	14.40	26.00	4.09
	90	4.20	46.97	21.37	28.00	5.20
E	10	6.40	55.24	14.45	25.50	4.00
	90	4.25	47.52	21.50	27.00	5.10

The parameters for proteins, moisture content and pH are similar with the parameters determined in Teleme cheese and Feta cheese (20, 21). The salt content of our brined cheese appears to be same as it was found in Feta cheese 3.5-5.0 (21). pH values in the end of the ripening were found to be from 4.04 - 5.05. Tayar (23) stated that, in white cheeses produced in three different plants with traditional methods pH was found to be between 4.38-5.94. The fat content, the pH, moisture and the salt content were found to be the same as in Sjenicki cheese. The protein content had slightly lower levels than it was in found in our study (24). According to the obtained chemical results we can conclude that Macedonian white brined cheese does not greatly differ from the brined cheeses in the region.

In the beginning of the ripening high level of contamination with *Enterobacteriaceae* from 7.24 log cfu/g and *E. coli* 8.69 log cfu/g occurred because of the use of raw milk and artisanal rennet as well as high moisture and low salt content. All above factors mentioned could promote the growth of these bacteria. Furthermore during the maturation process the number of *Enterobacteriaceae* was reduced to 3.07 and 1.77 log cfu/g and in some cheese samples they were not present at all. *E. coli* was not detected in the mature cheese. Similar results were obtained in Feta cheese where number of *E. coli* at day 4 reached 5.3 log cfu/g, after significantly declined and in the end of ripening were not detected. Coagulase positive staphylococci were present at day 10 in some cheese samples within the range from 2.0 – 4.77 log cfu/g but at day 90 they were not detected in none of the samples (11). In addition, even though staphylococci tolerate salt, their growth is not favored by the cheese environment, because of the combined inhibitory effect of the pH and NaCl concentration (5). Listeria was not detected in the cheese samples.

Yeasts and moulds counts, which are environmental contamination indicators were within the interval from 3.64 – 4.99 log cfu/g at day 10 and moulds were detected only in one sample. In the mature cheese at day 90 the population of yeasts have increased and was between 4.30 – 7.00 log cfu/g. Yeast counts in this artisanal cheeses were higher than those reported by other authors

who have studied the microbiology of artisanal cheeses made from raw milk without addition of starter cultures (11). The high number of yeasts found in this study may account for the typical organoleptic characteristics of our traditional cheese since recent investigations have shown that some lipolytic and proteolytic enzymes produced by those microorganisms contribute to the development of aroma and flavor compounds (4). At day 90 moulds were found in three samples and could be probably due to contamination.

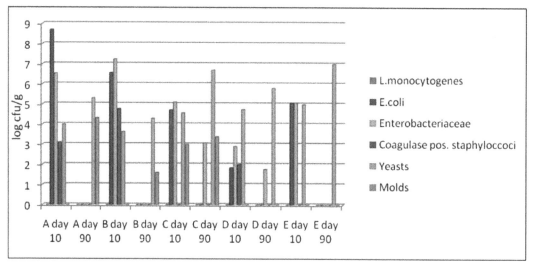

Figure 1. Log counts of microbial groups during cheese ripening

Lactic acid bacteria (LAB) constituted the predominant bacterial group during the ripening process with a population higher than 7 log cfu/g. Among LAB, lactococci were found at day 10 in higher numbers (5.44 – 7.94 log cfu/g) when compared with leuconostoc (4.11 – 6.58 log cfu/g) and lactobacilli from 5.17 in sample A to 6.9 log cfu/g in sample B (Fig. 2). These results indicate that lactococci constitute the predominant bacterial group in the beginning of the ripening period. At the end of the ripening lactobacilli were the most common group and their number was within the range 5.35 – 7.43 log cfu/g. The decline in lactococci is probably due to the inhibitory action of the low pH and high salt in moisture values in the maturing cheese (7). The presumptive leuconostoc at day 10 was found within the range from 4.11 – 6.50 log cfu/g. The obtained results are slightly higher than the one reported by Manolopoulou (11). At the end

of the ripening process at day 90, leuconostoc was detected in only one cheese sample. These groups of microorganisms may influence the ripening process through the production of lactic acid, the decrease in the oxidation – reduction potential and their proteolytic and lipolytic activities (10).

Enterococci were found also in high numbers at day 10 (from log 2.6 – 6.03 cfu/g). This results were similar with the results obtained in the Turkish white cheese (9) where the mean log was 5.34 cfu/g. At day 90 they rapidly decreased in two cheese samples to 2.69 log cfu/g in cheese B, and to 1.9 log cfu/g in cheese E. In cheese A, C and D enterococci were not detected. The presence of a high number of enterococci could be due to poor hygienic practices during the manufacturing process and the resistance of enteroccoci to unfavorable conditions (8). Enterococci may influence the ripening process due to their caseinolytic and lypolitic activity.

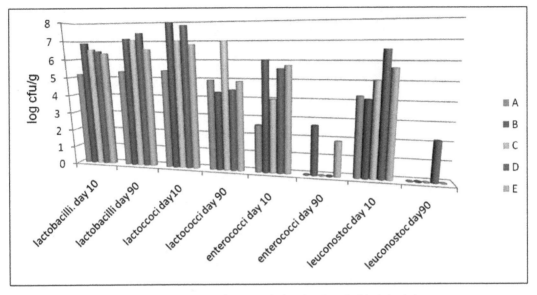

Figure 2. Log counts of the lactic acid bacteria groups during ripening of white brined cheese

Table 3. Microbiological criteria for food safety given in Official Gazette No.78/2008

Parameter	Acceptable limits
Listeria monocytogenes	Absence in 25 g
Escherichia coli	100 cfu/g
Coagulase-positive staphylococci	100 cfu/g

From the obtained microbiological results, Macedonian artisanal cheese could be considered as safe from a hygienic point of view and would be categorized as acceptable according to the Book of Rules for microbiological criteria in food (Official Gazette 78/2008).

It can be concluded that this study provides a new approach to ripening of white brined cheese, which is the most consumed cheese in Macedonia.

Further knowledge of the natural microbial communities present in this artisanal cheese may help to prevent loss of microbial diversity associated with local and regional traditions.

REFERENCES

1. Garabal JI. (2007), Biodiversity and the survival of autochthonous fermented products, Int Microbiol, 10, 1-3.

2. Bintsis, T., Papademas P. (2002). Microbiological quality of white brined cheeses: a review. International Journal of dairy Technology, 55 (3) : 113–120.

3. Demarigny, Y., Beuvier, E., Buchin, S., Pochet, S. and Grappin, R. (1997) Influence of raw milk microflora on the characteristics of Swiss-type cheeses. II. Biochemical and sensory characteristics. Lait 77, 151-167.

4. Marino M, Maifreni M and Rondinini G. (2003) Microbiological characterization of artisanal Montasio cheese: analysis of its indigenous lactic acid bacteria.FEMS Microbiology Letters 229 133-140.

5. Litopoulou-Tzanetaki, E., (1977) Staphylococci and micrococci in Kefalotyri cheese. Milchwissenshaft 32, 211-214

6. Hayaloglu, A.A.: (2003) Influence of the strains of Lactococcus used as a starter on the characteristics and ripening properties of Turkish white cheese. PhD Dissertation. Cukurova University, Adana, Turkey 2003.

7. Vafopoulou-Mastrogianaki A, Litopoulou-Tzanetaki E and Tzanetakis N (1990) Effect of Pediococcus pentosaceus on ripening changes of Feta cheese. Microbiologie-Alimnetis-Nutrition 8 53-62.

8. Moreno M R, Sarantinopoulos P, Tsakalidou E and De-Vuyst L (2006) The role and application of *Enterococci* in food and health. International Journal of Food Microbiology 106 1-24.

9. Oner Z, Karahan A G and Aloglu H (2006) Changes in the microbiological and chemical characteristics of an artisanal Turkish white cheese during ripening. Food Science and Technology 39 449-454.

10. Steele, J.L., (1995) Contribution of lactic acid bacteria to cheese ripening. In: Malin, E.L., Gibbs, M., Skinner, F.A. (Eds.), Chemistry of structure – Function Relationship in cheese. Academic Press, London, UK, pp. 65-79.

11. Manolopoulou E, Sarantinopoulos P, Zoidou E, Aktypis A, Moschopoulou E, Kandarakis IG, Anifantakis EM (2003). Evaluation of microbial population during traditional Feta cheese manufacture and ripening. Int. J. Food Microbiol., 82: 153-161.

12. ISO 11290-1:1996Microbiology of food and animal feeding stuffs -- Horizontal method for the detection and enumeration of Listeria monocytogenes -- Part 1: Detection method

13. ISO 21528-2:2004 Microbiology of food and animal feeding stuffs -- Horizontal methods for the detection and enumeration of Enterobacteriaceae -- Part 2: Colony-count method

14. ISO 16649-2:2001 Microbiology of food and animal feeding stuffs. Horizontal method for the enumeration of β-glucuronidase-positive Escherichia coli. Colony-count technique at 44°C using 5-bromo-4-chloro-3-indolyl-β-D-glucuronide

15. ISO 6888-1:1999 Microbiology of food and animal feeding stuffs -- Horizontal method for the enumeration of coagulase-positive staphylococci (Staphylococcus aureus and other species) -- Part 1: Technique using Baird-Parker agar medium

16. ISO 21527-2:2008 Microbiology of food and animal feeding stuffs -- Horizontal method for the enumeration of yeasts and moulds -- Part 2: Colony count technique in products with water activity less than or equal to 0,95

17. Mitrovic M., (1954), Prirucnik laboratoriskih (hemiskih) metoda za ispitivanje zivotnih namirnica, Medicinska knjiga, Beograd-Zagreb.

18. ISO 8968-1:2001 (IDF 20-1: 2001)Milk -- Determination of nitrogen content -- Part 1: Kjeldahl method

19. Litopoulou-Tzanetaki E., Tzanetakis N., Vafopoulou-Mastrojiannaki A., (1993) Effect of type of lactic starter on microbiological, chemical and sensory characteristics of Feta cheese. Food Microb., 1031–34.

20. Alichanidis, E., Polychroniadou, A., Tzanetakis, N. & Vafopoulou, A. (1981) Teleme cheese from deep-frozen curd. Journal of Dairy Science, 64, 732–739.

21. Abd El-Salam M.H., Alichanidis E., (2004) Cheese varieties ripened in brine (3rd ed.). In: P.F. Fox, P.L.H. McSweeney, T.M. Cogan, T.P. Guinee, Editors, Cheese: chemistry, physics and microbiology Vol. 2, Elsevier, Amsterdam, pp. 227-249.

22. Hayaloglu, A.A., Guven, M., Fox, P.F. (2002): Microbiological, biochemical and technological properties of Turkish White cheese, "Beyaz Peynir". International Dairy Journal 12, 635-648.

23. Tayar, M., (1995). Beyaz peynirlerin olgunlaşma süresince kimyasal ve mikrobiyolojik özelliklerindeki değişmeler. Gıda. 20 (2) 97-101.

24. Macej, O., Jovanovic, S., Barac, M.(2004): Biotehnologija u stocarstvu, vol. 20(1-2), 109-117.

16

INVESTIGATIONS ON PREVALENCE AND ANTIMICROBIAL RESISTANCE OF ENTEROHAEMORRHAGIC *ESCHERICHIA COLI* (EHEC) AMONG DAIRY FARMS IN THE NORTH PART OF THE REPUBLIC OF BULGARIA

Valentina Urumova, Mihni Lyutzkanov, Vladimir Petrov

Department of Veterinary Microbiology, Infectious and Parasitic Diseases
Faculty of Veterinary Medicine, Trakia University, 6000 Stara Zagora, Bulgaria

ABSTRACT

Over a 2-year period, from January 2011 to May 2013, a total of 1094 faecal swab samples were collected from cattle at different age at 4 farms in North Bulgaria: Okorsh, Slavyanovo (Popovo municipality), Dobri dol and Trem. Out of them, 36 coli strains (3.3%) positive in the *E. coli* O:157 antiserum agglutination test and identified by the BBL CRYSTAL identification system as belonging to the *E. coli* O:157 serotype were isolated. The distribution of isolates was as followed: 5 (0.5%) *E. coli* O:157 strains at the Okorsh dairy cattle farm, 7 (0.6%) *E. coli* isolates at the Slavyanovo dairy farm, 16 (1.5%) isolates at the Dobri dol farm and 8 (0.7%) isolates at the Trem farm. Colibacteria exhibited 100% sensitivity to oxyimino-cephalosporins, gentamicin and enrofloxacin, and were resistant to ampicillin (19.4%) and tetracycline (41.6%). From the 15 strains resistant to tetracycline, 11 were isolated from the cows at Dobri dol, while the other 4 originated from the other three farms. The 7 ampicillin-resistant *E. coli* isolates were detected only at the Dobri dol cattle farm.

Key words: EHEC, cattle, antibiotic resistance

INTRODUCTION

In 1982, the identification of a new intestinal pathogen, *E. coli* O157: H7, involved in the etiology of two disease outbreaks related to haemorrhagic colitis in humans, was reported (1). During the next decade, this intestinal bacterium was outlined as a pathogen of public health importance in a number of countries in North America and Europe. Soon after that, researchers described other coli serotypes of similar pathogenicity and the entire group was termed as enterohaemorrhagic *E. coli* (EHEC). *E. coli* O157:H7 is the most commonly investigated member of this group. The haemolytic uraemic syndrome was first described in 1955

Corresponding author: Assoc. Prof. Valentina Urumova, PhD
E-mail address: valentina_62@ abv.bg
Present address: Department of Veterinary Microbiology,
Infectious and Parasitic Diseases
Faculty of Veterinary Medicine, Trakia University
6000 Stara Zagora, Bulgaria

in Switzerland (2). Coli strains involved in the etiology of haemorrhagic uremic syndrome were also classified in the EHEC group. Levin et al. (3) determine the *E. coli* O157:H7 and *E. coli* O26:H11 serotypes as enterohaemorrhagic coli bacteria. Tzipori et al. (4) proposed also to include O4:NM, O45:H2, O111:NM, and O145:NM serotypes to this group.

The term enterohaemorrhagic *E. coli* bacteria applies to strains, which, similar to *E. coli* O157:H7 produce one or more *Shiga-like toxins*, as well as possess a 60-MDa plasmid linked to pathogenicity and are able to form A/E type lesions in the intestinal mucosa. Like the enteropathogenic *E. coli* bacteria (EPEC), the members of the EHEC group initially adhere to intestinal mucosal surface in local areas, then adhere more deeply and destroy the intestinal microvilli. The initial adherence of EHEC is mediated by the 60-MDa plasmid while the subsequent adherence to the mucosa is a chromosome-determined event.

Another feature of EHEC virulence is the production of *Shiga-like* toxin similar to that produced by *Shigella dysenteriae* type 1. Konowalchuk detected shiga-producing *E. coli* as early as in 1977, before the elucidation of the role of toxins in bacterial virulence. He introduced the term verotoxins due to the cytotoxicity of strains when they are cultivated in *Vero* cells.

Both types of shiga-toxic factors, Shiga-like toxin I and Shiga-like toxin II, killing both Vero and HeLa cells, induce fluid accumulation in ligated rabbit intestinal loops, and are lethal for mice and rabbits (5, 6, 7, 8, 9, 10). Both toxic factors differ antigenically as well as with respect to their biological effect. The second shiga-like toxin is less toxic for Vero cells but at the same time, is more toxic for mice and causes hemorrhagic colitis in rabbits. Genes, determining the production of both toxins are located in bacteriophages, which allows obtaining the toxins from *E. coli* O157:H7 by transfer of bacteriophages. The genes responsible for the production of shiga-like toxin type I are similar to those encoding shiga-toxin production in *Shigella*, while the homology for shiga-like toxin type II is 58%. It is believed that the shiga-like toxin produced by *E. coli* causing the pig oedema disease is a variant of shiga-like toxin type II which implies the existence of different cell receptors.

Dairy cattle are one of the main *E. coli* O157:H7 reservoirs (11, 12). Therefore, bovine foodstuffs are considered as important risk factor for human disease outbreaks. Animals are asymptomatic vectors for many representatives of the EHEC groups, and some *E. coli* strains other than EHEC could induce disease in young animals. For instance, the members of the O153 group cause a disease, similar to the human HUS in rabbits. The distal part of the rectum of so-called calves "super shedders" of *E. coli* O157:H7 is heavily colonized for a long period of time. A similar colonisation by *E. coli* O157:H7 could be observed in sheep. Animals, which are not natural reservoirs of this serotype could serve as secondary natural reservoirs. Apart from the consumption of contaminated foods, humans could be infected through contaminated water, direct contact with animals, with faecal masses and contaminated soils. The direct man to man transmission could occur during an epidemic. Human infections were described in connection with consumption of non-pasteurised goat milk, dry pork sausages, and after direct contact with horses, poultry and rabbits. It is assumed that the infectious doses for men could be less than 100 bacterial cells, even about 10 cells. Contaminated vegetables (spinach, lettuce, radishes) as well as non-pasteurised fruit juices could also pose a risk for infection to men. Data for contamination by herbs, e.g. parsley are reported. Drosophila melanogaster could spread the bacteria and in cases of impaired integrity of tissues, for instance in apples, the pathogens could develop.

It is acknowledged that *E. coli* O157:H7 could survive for 9 months in veal at -20 °C. They exhibit a certain tolerance to acid environments, which could explain their persistence for weeks in mayonnaise, acid sauces, apple juice, and fresh cheeses at fringe temperatures. These bacteria are also resistance to drying. Cases of disease in humans are described also after swimming in pools and lakes (13).

With respect to the other EHEC serotypes, there are a lot of unexplained facts about their epidemiological status. For example, the main natural reservoirs of EHEC O26 are cattle, sheep, pigs, goats, rabbits and poultry. They are isolated from both healthy and diarrhoeic animals. Disease outbreaks in humans have been reported after consumption of beef products and non-pasteurised cow milk, as well as after direct contact with animals and drinking water contaminated with faeces.

EHEC O103 strains are isolated from calves, sheep, goats, as well as healthy and diseased humans (10). It could be claimed that EHEC O157: H- strains are rarely isolated from the feces of cattle and horses, although human outbreaks after consumption of sausage or close contact with infected cows and horses have been reported. This fact gave ground to believe that in such cases, humans could also serve as reservoir of infection (14).

The available data for the prevalence of VTEC in animals and food contamination rates in Europe originate from various sources, such as public health sector, veterinary and research labs. This complicates the analysis and necessitates coordination of programmes dealing with research on foods, official food control, monitoring programmes and research projects.

One of the first source of information with this regard was the European Community System for Monitoring and Collection of Information on Zoonoses, created by Council Directive 92/117/ECC. The directive includes the rules for sample collection, analysis and annual reporting associated with specific zoonoses, zoonotic agents in animals, foods and feeds in EC member states. In order to improve the information system, a new Zoonoses Directive 2003/99 was created, brought into force on 12 June 2004. At present, the system monitors 16 zoonoses, including VTEC.

Microbiological examinations associated to zoonotic agent monitoring could include the so-called sentinel studies, determining the trends in human morbidity rates, the so-called baseline prevalence in primary site of production and at a later stage, in the food chain, investigations on good production practices, determination of control measures' effect etc. The criteria of the EC Zoonoses Directive monitoring programmes include detection of the zoonotic agent in the animal population, in feeds, foods, the adverse effect in men, the economic impact for animals and human health, for the business related to feeds and foods production, epidemiological trends for animal populations, for men, feeds and foods.

Therefore, the investigation of VTEC O157 prevalence among animal populations and some foods of animal origin is a task of primary significance, which could consequently set the diagnostic strategy for investigation of the other factors. The purpose of the present study was to investigate for a two year period 2011-2013, the prevalence of *E. coli* O157 among cattle in some of the biggest farm in North Bulgaria, and to evaluate the sensitivity of isolates to some major classes of antibacterial drugs.

MATERIAL AND METHODS

Number of samples

For the period of the study, from January 2011 to May 2013, a total of 1094 faecal swab samples were obtained from cattle at different ages in four cattle farms in North Bulgaria – the villages Okorsh, Slavyanovo (municipality of Popovo), Dobri dol and Trem.

Samples were distributed as follows:

• Okorsh village – 300 swab samples (30 from heifers, 10 from dry cows, 10 from suckling calves, 50 from 6-month-old calves and 200 from cows);

• Slavyanovo village (municipality of Popovo) – 300 swab samples (30 from suckling calves, 100 from 6-month-old calves, 100 from heifers, and 70 from cows);

• Dobri dol village – 194 swab samples from calves 3 to 6 months of age;

• Trem – 300 swab samples (140 from calves 3 to 6 months of age; 70 from heifers and 90 from cows).

Nutrient media and microbiological consumables

The initial inoculation of swab samples was done on tryptic soy broth (Difco, USA) and McConkey agar with sorbitol (Difco, USA). For identification of sorbitol-negative coli bacteria on McConkey agar with sorbitol, indole motility medium (NCPID, Sofia) was used, as well as triple sugar iron agar medium (Merck, Germany), Simmons citrate agar

(NCPID, Sofia), the methyl rot and Voges–Proskauer tests, panels of BBL CRYSTAL (Becton Dickinson, USA) for identification of enterobacteria and non-fermenting bacteria. Isolates were serotyped by means of the agglutination test with *E.coli* O157 antiserum, Difco, USA, as per manufacturer's instructions.

The sensitivity of isolates to antimicrobial drugs was tested by disc-difusion method, on Muller-Hinton agar and antibiotic disks (Emapol, Poland). Antibiogrammes were done with the following disks: ampicillin 10 µg, cefotaxime 30 µg, ceftazidime 10 µg, gentamicin 10 µg, enrofloxacin 5 µg and tetracycline 30 µg. Antibiogrammes were prepared in compliance with the Performance standards for antimicrobial disk and dilution susceptibility tests for bacteria isolated from animals, approved standard-Third Edition, M31-A3, №6, Clinical and Laboratory Standards Institute, Wayne, PA. The MICs to ampicillin and tetracycline were determined by the E-test, Liofilchem, Italy. The reference *E. coli* ATTC 25922 strain was used for disk diffusion test control and MICs determination (18).

RESULTS

Profile of sorbitol-negative strains isolated from the 4 studied farms

Out of the 1094 examined faecal swab samples, 36 (3.3%) sorbitol-negative strains were isolated, which were positive in the agglutination test with *E. coli* O157 antiserum and were identified by the BBL CRYSTAL system as belonging to the *E. coli* O:157 serotype. The distribution of isolates was as followed:

• *In the Okorsh cattle farm* – 5 *E. coli* O: 157 isolates (0.5%, CL- 0.08%÷0.9%) – 2 from cows and 3 from heifers;

• *In the Slavyanovo farm* – 7 *E. coli* O:157 isolates (0.6%, CL- 0.5%÷0.7%) – 2 from calves 3 to 6 months of age and 5 from heifers;

• *In the Dobri dol farm* – 16 *E. coli* O:157 isolates (1.5%, CL- 1.2%÷1.8%) – all from calves 3 to 6 months of age

• *In the Trem farm* – 8 *E. coli* O:157 isolates (0.7%, CL- 0.6%÷0.8%) – 4 from calves 3 to 6 months of age and 4 from heifers

The structural profile of E. coli O:157 isolates from the four studied farms is presented in Table 1.

Table 1. Structural profile of cattle EHEC isolates

Age groups/studied animals	Number of samples/EHEC			
	Okorsh farm number of samples/EHEC	Slavyanovo farm number of samples/EHEC	Dobri dol farm number of samples/EHEC	Trem farm number of samples/EHEC
Suckling calves	10/0	30/0	-	-
Calves 3-6 mo. of age	50/0	100/2	194/16	140/4
Heifers	30/3	100/5	-	70/4
Cows	210/2	70/0	-	90/0
TOTAL number of samples/EHEC	300/5	300/7	194/16	300/8

Investigations on the sensitivity of cattle EHEC isolates to antimicrobial drugs

Table 2 presents the results about the sensitivity of studied EHEC isolates from cattle to 6 antimicrobial drugs. The interpretation was in two groups – sensitive and resistant. The isolates in the respective groups are given in percent and confidence limits. When selecting the antibiotic disks, we focused on beta-lactam antibiotics and 3rd generation cephalosporins with regard to the possibility for phenotyping isolates as producers of ESBL and AmpC enzymes, and we also included representatives of the different classes of antimicrobial drugs. The results were interpreted as per EUCAST recommendations (Epidemiological values).

The results from the disk diffusion test were presented through cumulative curves of ampicillin (Fig. 1) and tetracycline (Fig. 2) in resistant cattle EHEC isolates. The strains were 100% sensitive to the other tested antimicrobial drugs – oxyimino-cephalosporins, gentamicin and enrofloxacin. From the 15 isolates resistant to tetracycline, 11 originated from the Dobri dol farm and 4 – from the other three farms. All seven ampicillin-resistant EHEC strains were from the Dobri dol farm.

Table 2. Sensitivity of cattle EHEC isolates to antimicrobial drugs

Antibacterial drugs	Sensitive isolates (%)/CL	Resistant isolates (%)/CL
Ampicillin	80.6/66.3÷91.6	19.4/8.3÷33.6
Cefotaxime	100	-
Ceftazidime	100	-
Gentamicin	100	-
Tetracycline	58.3/42.1÷73.6	41.7/26.2÷57.9
Enrofloxacin	100	-

Legend: CL - Confidence limits

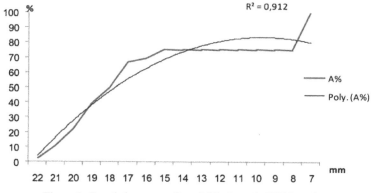

Figure 1. Cumulative curve of ampicillin in cattle EHEC strains

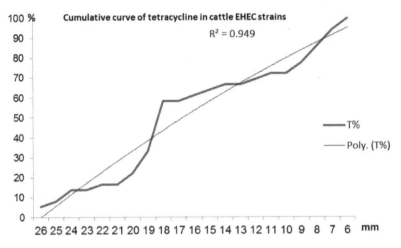

Figure 2. Cumulative curve of tetracycline in cattle EHEC strains

Figure 1 shows that the diameters of inhibition zones for ampicillin ranged between 22 mm and 6 mm. A bimodal pattern of behaviour was present. The inhibition zones beyond which 50% and 90% of strains were located, were 18 mm and 7 mm respectively.

Figure 2 depicts that inhibition zones of tetracycline ranged between 26 mm and 6 mm. The inhibition zones beyond which 50% and 90% of strains were located, were 19 mm and 7 mm respectively.

In connection with the resistance of EHEC isolates determined in the disk diffusion test to tetracycline (15 strains, 41.6%) and ampicillin (7 strains, 19.4%), the MICs of both antibiotics were determined. The data are presented in Table 3. Out of the 7 ampicillin-resistant strains, 5 had MIC of 16 µg/mL, one – of 32 µg/mL and one – of 64 µg/mL. Out of the 15 tetracycline isolates, 9 had MIC-of 16 µg/mL, 3 – of 32 µg/mL, 2 – of 64 µg/mL and 1 – of 128 µg/mL.

DISCUSSION

The aforementioned circumstances determined that a major part of *E. coli* O157 infections in humans are associated with consumption of contaminated animal foods after inadequate thermal processing and/or the consumption of contaminated water (19, 20, 21, 22, 23). Although the contamination at the farm level is believed to be minor (24), the risk for contamination of beef increases during transportation and the period of gathering of animals to slaughterhouses, and the end of the slaughter process. These facts are essential for investigations on the prevalence of EHEC in farm animals.

According to EFSA (15, 17) the prevalence of VTEC among the population of Europe is very low, 1.2 per 100,000. Nevertheless, EFSA declared the intestinal bacterial pathogens to be important zoonotic agents, usually affecting children and elderly people. According to Hussein and Bollinger (16) the worldwide prevalence of VTEC O157 in fecal swab samples ranged between 0.2 and 27.8% and for VTEC, other than O157 - from 2.1 to 70.1%.

Data from the international network Enter-net, founded by DG SANCO, European Commission in 2006 shows some differences in the data from EC countries with respect to VTEC infections. Regardless of the fact that more than 50% of EHEC infections in continental Europe are attributed to the O157 serotype, and that for countries like Belgium, France, Finland, Hungary, Netherlands, Sweden, Spain, O157 is the main serotype (data from Enter-net, 2005), in Denmark, Germany, Italy,

Table 3. MIC of ampicillin and tetracycline in cattle EHEC strains

Antimicrobial	MIC/ µg/mL													
Drugs	0.01	0.03	0.06	0.125	0.25	0.5	1	2	4	8	16	32	64	128	256
Ampicillin											5	1	1		
Tetracycline											9	3	2	1	

Norway and Luxemburg, other serotypes are more commonly reported. After the first epidemiological study on the prevalence of E. coli O157 among cattle, Montenegro et al. (25) affirmed that bovine population could be considered as the primary reservoir of VTEC. Other authors also suppose that cattle are the main reservoir of E. coli O157:H7, especially during the summer season (26, 27, 28, 29).

Low prevalence (0.28%) of E. coli O157 was established among cattle in the USA (29). In a 15-month survey on the prevalence of coli bacteria from the O157 serotype among the different categories of cattle at one farm, Mechie et al. (30) demonstrated a prevalence between 0% and 13.5% in dairy cows, between 0% and 68% in heifers and between 0% and 56.3% in calves. In our studies, we also observed EHEC in calves aged 3 to 6 months in three of the four studied farms (4.5%), and in heifers in three of farms (6%).

A critical analysis of data from 26 epidemiological surveys on the presence of E. coli O157:H7 among cattle in different regions of the world was performed (31). The data for North America showed that a prevalence for dairy cows of 7-8% and a high prevalence among feedlot calves –61%. In the same analysis however, other data from USA showed a low E. coli O157:H7 incidence in suckling calves (1.5%) and varying values in calves older than 8 months (1.8% to 5%). The prevalence among heifers was 2.3%, while in adult cows, it declined markedly up to 0.7%. In the opinion of the authors, data originating from Europe also evidenced a higher prevalence among younger animals. In adults, the incidence of E. coli O157:H7 was between 0 and 1%. We could hardly compare our data with those reported by Broseta et al. (31) 4.5% prevalence for calves 3-6 months, 6% for heifers and 0.5% for cows, as the information of the latter refers to a high number of farms, but it could be stated anyway that reported rates are comparable.

The investigations on the subject, carried out in different regions of the world (26, 28, 32, 33) also established higher prevalence of EHEC O157:H7 in calves aged 3 - 6 months. Hancock et al. (22) believe that heifers carried a significant amount of EHEC O157:H7 (CFU/g), compared to other categories of cattle. Ezawa et al. (34) outlined that the overall prevalence of EHEC O157:H7 among cattle in Japan (5-10%), but that heifers exhibited higher rates (32-46%). In Italy, a prevalence of 16% among cows was reported (35). According to Wray et al. (36), the shedding of EHEC in adult cows was shorter and no more than 2 weeks, whereas the shedding in weaned calves lasted for more than 58 days. Alali et al. (37) affirmed that in calves

experimentally infected with EHEC O157:H7, and calves fed milk replacer, an enhanced shedding of the pathogen occurred on the 6th and 10th day after the infection compared to calves fed milk. In England and Wales, Paiba et al. (38) reported EHEC O157:H7 prevalence rates at the farm level within a large range (from 1% to 51%,) with highest percentage among calves 2-6 months of age and lowest rates – among calves up to 2 months of age. In the Netherlands, the 2-year survey at the slaughterhouse level showed a 10% prevalence of EHEC serotype O157 in cows (39).

In comparison with the data of Johnsen et al. (40) evidencing a lower individual prevalence of E. coli O157:H7 – 0.19% and a correspondingly lower prevalence at the farm level (0.35%) in 15421 cattle in Norway, our data for the prevalence of coli bacteria from the O157 serotype in studied cattle at the farm level was higher, for Okorsh farm it was 1.6 %, for Slavyanovo -2.3%, Dobri dol -8.2% and for Trem- 2.6%.

The PhD thesis of Eriksson, Swedish University of Agricultural Sciences, Uppsala (41) has determined a prevalence of EHEC O157 in cattle at slaughterhouses for 2008-2009 of 3.3%, which agrees completely with our data for the two-year survey period, as well as with respect to the total number of examined faecal swab samples.

In the USA, it found out that 70% of EHEC O157 isolates from cattle were resistant to streptomycin, sulfamethoxazole and tetracycline (42). Furthermore, the authors included the resistance of ampicillin, kanamycin and ticarcillin in resistant phenotype profiles of coli bacteria. With respect to the sensitivity of E. coli isolates, the data from the present study are comparable to those of other authors (42, 43), except for the reported resistance to ceftazidime. In this study, the authors sought differences with respect to antimicrobial resistance of enterohaemorrhagic E. coli on the basis of the super-shedding ($\leq 10^4$ CFU) and low-shedding criteria. In the first group of isolates they determined resistance to ceftazidime, and for both groups the most common phenotype profiles included ampicillin, sulfamethoxazole, streptomycin and tetracycline, as well as the combination trimethoprim/sulfamethoxazole. Similar to the data from the present study, they did not observe resistance of enrofloxacin in studied coli strains. In Korea, You et al. (44) determined that cattle EHEC O157 were most frequently resistant to streptomycin, tetracycline, sulfamethoxazole, ampicillin, kanamycin, cefalotin, ticarcillin and sulfamethoxazole.

The resistance to beta-lactam antimicrobial drugs is essential for trends for the spread of coli bacteria producing beta-lactamases with broader spectrum of activity. In our study, in contrast to the aforementioned data, studied EHEC O157 strains showed no resistance to cephalosporins. In the USA, Fitzgerald et al. (45) reported that cattle EHEC 0157 isolates were resistant first to tetracyclines, and second, to spectinomycin, ampicillin and sulfonamides. They neither found out resistance to cephalosporins. Data about the sensitivity of cattle, pig and human EHEC 0157 isolates to antimicrobial drugs were published in South Africa (46). Cattle isolates demonstrated the highest percent of resistance to sulfamethoxazole (100%), tetracycline (100%), ampicillin (25%) and streptomycin (50%). The spread of resistance to tetracyclines, aminoglycosides, sulfonamides and lactam antibiotics in a number of intestinal bacteria occurs through integrons transfer by conjugation, facilitating the rapid dissemination among bacteria (47). Considering these events, another important aspect in studies on the prevalence of zoonotic agents among animal populations is the investigation of their resistance to antimicrobial drugs. Having in mind the public importance of this phenomenon, a number of regulations have been issued by the EC institutions for monitoring of resistance to various chemotherapeutic groups, which are essential for the out-hospital spread of resistance. Therefore, our study's emphasis was placed on the markers of resistance to oxyimino-cephalosporins due to the recent wide public discussion on the topic in European countries (48).

CONCLUSION

The prevalence of *E. coli* O157 between cattle in the four investigated farms in the North part of Bulgaria are low for cows 0.5%, in contrast with the prevalence of this serotype for heifers 6% and for calves 4.5%.

Taking into consideration the fact that the period and the scope of our survey were limited, the negative results with regard to the resistance of coli bacteria to 3rd generation cephalosporins could hardly be interpreted as optimistic. Moreover, there are data at a national level about the approval and use of cefquinome in dairy cattle farming and ceftiofur in pig farming, which are prerequisites for selective pressure and possibly at the background of the onset and spread of resistance to cephalosporins. At the Dobri dol farm, the resistance of ampicillin and tetracycline is a reliable proof for future trends, taking into account the mutation diversity with respect to beta lactamase enzymes.

REFERENCES

1. Riley, L.W., Remis, R.S., Helgerson, S. D. (1983). Hemorrhagic colitis associated with a rare Escherichia coli serotype. N. Engl. J. Med. 308, 681-685. PMid:6338386

2. Gasser, C., Gautier, E., Steck, A., Siebenmann, R.E., Oechslin, R. (1955). The haemolytic-uraemic syndrome. Schweiz. Med. Wschr. 85, 905 PMid:13274004

3. Levine, M. M., Xu, J., Kaper, J. B. (1987). A DNA probe to identify enterohemorrhagic Escherichia coli of O157:H7 and other serotypes that cause hemorrhagic colitis and haemolytic uremic syndrome. J. Infect. Dis. 156, 175-182. http://dx.doi.org/10.1093/infdis/156.1.175 PMid:3298451

4. Tzipori, S., Wachsmuth, I. K., Smithers, J. (1988). Studies in gnotobiotic piglets on non – O157:H7 Escherichia coli serotypes isolated from patients with hemorrhagic colitis. Gastroenterology 94, 590-597. PMid:3276573

5. Knutton, S., Baldwin, T., Williams, P. H. (1989). Actin accumulation at sites of bacterial adhesion to tissue culture cells: basis of a new diagnostic test for enteropathogenic and enterohemorrhagic Escherichia coli. Infect. Immunology 57, 1290-1298. PMid:2647635; PMCid:PMC313264

6. March, S. B., Ratnam, S. (1986). Sorbitol–MacConkey medium for detection of Escherichia coli O157:H7 associated with hemorrhagic colitis. J. Clin. Microbiol. 23, 869-872. PMid:3519658; PMCid:PMC268739

7. Walker, C. W., Upson, R., Warren, R. E. (1988). Hemorrhagic colitis: detection of verotoxin producing Escherichia coli O157:H7 in a clinical microbiology laboratory. J. Clin. Pathol. 41, 80-84. http://dx.doi.org/10.1136/jcp.41.1.80 PMid:2685050; PMCid:PMC501874

8. Chapman, P. A. (1989). Evaluation of commercial latex slide test for identifying Escherichia coli O157. J. Clin. Pathol. 42, 1109-1110. http://dx.doi.org/10.1136/jcp.42.10.1109 PMid:2685050; PMCid:PMC501874

9. Borczyk, A. A., Lior, H., Thomson, S. (1989). Sorbitol-negative Escherichia coli O157 other than H7. J. Infect. 18, 198-199. http://dx.doi.org/10.1016/S0163-4453(89)91486-2

10. Dorn, C. R., Scotland, S. M., Smith, H. (1989). Properties of Vero cytotoxin- producing Escherichia coli of human and animal origin belonging to serotypes other than O157:H7. Emidemiol. Infect. 103, 83-95. http://dx.doi.org/10.1017/S0950268800030387 PMid:2673828; PMCid:PMC2249490

11. Davis, M. A., Daniel, H. R., Haiqing, S. (2006). Comparison of cultures from rectoanal-junction mucosal swabs and feces for detection of Escherichia coli O157 in dairy heifers. Appl. Environ. Microbiol. 72(5): 3766-3770. http://dx.doi.org/10.1128/AEM.72.5.3766-3770.2006 PMid:16672532; PMCid:PMC1472398

12. Schouten, J.M., Graat, E.A., Frankena, K., Van Zijderveld, F., De Jong, M.C. (2009). Transmission and quantification of verocytotoxin-producing Escherichia coli O157 in dairy cattle and calves. Epidemiol. Infect. 137(1): 114-123. http://dx.doi.org/10.1017/S0950268808000320 PMid:18346284

13. Friedman, M. S., Roels, T., Koehler, J. E., Feldman, L., Bibb, W. F., Blake, P. (1999). Escherichia coli O157:H7 outbreak association with improperly chlorinated swimming pool. Clin. Infect. Dis. 29, 298-303. http://dx.doi.org/10.1086/520204 PMid:10476731

14. World Organisation for Animal Health (OIE). (2008). Manual of diagnostic tests and vaccines for terrestrial animals. Paris: OIE; Verocytotoxigenic Escherichia coli.

15. Europian Food Safety (EFSA). (2007). Monitoring of Verotoxigenic Escherichia coli (VTEC) and identification of human pathogenic VTEC types. Scientific Opinion of the Panel on Bilogical Hazards. EFSA J. 579, 1-61.

16. Hussein, H. S., Bollinger, L. M. (2005). Prevalence of Shiga toxin-producing E. coli in beef cattle. J.Food Prot. 68, 2224-2241. PMid:16245735

17. Europian Food Safety (EFSA) Scientific Report of EFSA (2009). Technical specifications for the monitoring and reporting of verotoxigenic Escherichia coli (VTEC) on animals and food (VTEC surveys on animals and food). EFSA J. 7 (11): D-RN-520.

18. CLSI. (2006). Performance standards for antimicrobial disk and dilution susceptibility tests for bacteria isolated from animals, approved standard-Third Edition, M31-A3, №6, Clinical and Laboratory Standards Institute, Wayne, PA.

19. Isaäcson, M., Canter, P.H., Effler, P., Arntzen, L., Bomans, P., Heenan, R. (1993). Haemorrhagic colitis epidemic in Africa. Lancet 341, 961. http://dx.doi.org/10.1016/0140-6736(93)91253-I

20. Paquet, C., Petea, W., Grimont, E., Collin, M., Guillod, M. (1993). Aetiology of haemorrhagic colitis epidemic in Africa. Lancet 342, 175. http://dx.doi.org/10.1016/0140-6736(93)91378-Y

21. Armstrong, G. L., Hollingsworth, J., Morris, J. R. (1996). Emerging foodborne pathogens Escherichia coli O157:H7as a model of entry of a new pathogen into the food supply of the developed world. Epidemiology Review 18, 29-51. http://dx.doi.org/10.1093/oxfordjournals.epirev.a017914 PMid:8877329

22. Müller, E. E., Ehlers, M. M., Grabow, W. O. K. (2001). The occurrence of E. coli O157:H7 in Southern African water sources intended for direct and indirect human consumption. Water Research 35, 3085-3088. http://dx.doi.org/10.1016/S0043-1354(00)00597-2

23. Olsen, S. J., Miller, G., Breuer, I., Kennedy, M., Higgins, C., Walford, J., Mckee, G., Fox, K., Bibb, W., Mead, P. (2002). A waterborne outbreak of Escherichia coli O157:H7 infections and haemolytic uraemic syndrome: implications for rural water systems. Emerging Infectious Diseases 8, 370-375. http://dx.doi.org/10.3201/eid0804.000218 PMid:11971769; PMCid:PMC2730238

24. Jordan, D. (1998). Pre-slaughter control of beef carcass contamination with Escherichia coli O157:H7: a risk assessment approach. PhD thesis, Univ. of Guelph, Guelph Canada, pp. 236.

25. Montenegro, M., Bülte, M., Trumpf, T., Aleksic, S., Reuter, G., Bulling, E., Helmuth, R. (1990). Detection and characterization of fecal verotoxin- producing Escherichia coli from healthy cattle. J Clinic. Microbiol. 28 (6): 1417-1421. PMid:2199502; PMCid:PMC267942

26. Wells, J. G., Shipman, L. D., Greene, K. D., Sowers, E. G., Green, J. H., Cameron, D. N., Downes, F. P., Martin, M. L., Griffin, P. M., Ostroff, S. M., Potter, M. E., Tauxe, R. V., Washsmuth, I. K. (1991). Isolation of Escherichia coli O157:H7 and other Shiga-like-toxin-producing E. coli from dairy cattle. J. Clin. Microbiol. 29, 985-989. PMid:2056066; PMCid:PMC269920

27. Chapman, P. A., Siddons, C. A., Malo, A. T. C., Harkin M. A. (1997). A one-year study of Escherichia coli O157 in cattle, sheep, pigs and poultry. Epidemiol. Infect. 119, 245-250. http://dx.doi.org/10.1017/S0950268897007826 PMid:9363024; PMCid:PMC2808847

28. Zhao, T., Doyle, M. P., Shere, J., Garber, L. (1995). Prevalence of enterohemorrhagic Escherichia coli O157:H7 in a survey of dairy herds. Appl. Envioron. Microbiol. 61, 1290-1293. PMid:7747951; PMCid:PMC167385

29. Hancock, D. D., Besser, T. E., Kinsel, M. L., Tarr, P. I., Rice, D. H., Paros, M. G. (1994). The prevalence of Escherichia coli O157:H7 in dairy and beef cattle in Washington State. Epidemiol. Infect. 113. 199-207. http://dx.doi.org/10.1017/S0950268800051633 PMid:7925659; PMCid:PMC2271540

30. Mechie, S. C., Chapman, P. A., Siddons, C. A. (1997). A fifteen month study of Escherichia coli O157:H7 in a dairy herd. Epidemiol. Infect. 118, 17-25. http://dx.doi.org/10.1017/S0950268896007194 PMid:9042031; PMCid:PMC2808768

31. Broseta, S. M., Bastian, S. N., Arné, P. D., Cerf, O., Sanaa M. (2001). Review of epidemiological surveys on the prevalence of contamination of healthy cattle with Escherichia coli sero group O157:H7. Int. J. Hyg. Environ. Health 203, 347-361.
http://dx.doi.org/10.1078/1438-4639-4410041
PMid:11434215

32. Cray, W. C., Moon, H.W. (1995). Experimental infection of calves and adult cattle with Escherichia coli O157:H7. Appl. Environ. Microbiol. 61, 1586-1590.
PMid:7747972; PMCid:PMC167413

33. Hancock, D. D., Besser, T. E., Rice, D. H., Herriot, D. E., Tazz, D. I. (1997). A longitudinal study of Escherichia coli O157 in fourteen cattle herds. Epidemiol. Infect. 118, 193-195.
http://dx.doi.org/10.1017/S0950268896007212
PMid:9129597; PMCid:PMC2808780

34. Ezawa, A., Gocho, F., Kawata, K., Takahashi, T., Kikushi, N. (2004). High prevalence of enterohemorrhagic Escherichia coli (EHEC) 0157 from cattle in selected region of Japan. J.Vet. Med. Sci. 66, 585-587.
http://dx.doi.org/10.1292/jvms.66.585
PMid:15187376

35. Bonardi, S., Maggi, E., Bottarelli, A., Pacciarini, M. L., Ansuini, A., Vellini, G., Morabito, S., Caprioli, A. (1999). Isolation of Verocytotoxin – producing Escherichia coli O157:H7 from cattle at slaughter in Italy. Vet. Microbiol. 67: 203-211.
http://dx.doi.org/10.1016/S0378-1135(99)00039-5

36. Wray, C., McLaren, I. M., Randall, L. D., Pearson, G. R. (2000). Natural and experimental infection of normal cattle with Escherichia coli O157:H7. Vet. Rec. 147: 65-68.
http://dx.doi.org/10.1136/vr.147.3.65
PMid:10958486

37. Alali, W. Q., Sargeant, J. M., Nagaraja, T. G., De Bey, B. M. (2004). Effect of antibiotics in milk replacer on fecal shedding of Escherichia coli O157:H7 in calves. J. Anim. Sci. 82, 2148- 2152.
PMid:15309963

38. Paiba, G. A., Willsmith, J. W., Evans, S. J. et al. (2003). Prevalence of fecal excretion of Verocytotoxigenic Escherichia coli 0157 in cattle in England and Wales. Vet. Rec. 153, 347- 353.
http://dx.doi.org/10.1136/vr.153.12.347
PMid:14533765

39. Heuvelink, A. E., Van Biggelaar, F. L., De Boer, E., Herbes, R. G., Melchers, W. J., Huis, I. T., Veld, J. H., Monnens, L. A. (1998). Isolation and characterization of verocytotoxin-producing Escherichia coli 0157 strains from Dutch cattle and sheep. J. Clin. Microbiol. 36, 878-882.
PMid:9542902; PMCid:PMC104654

40. Johnsen, G., Wasteson, Y., Heir, E., Berget, I. O., Herikstad, H. (2001). Escherichia coli O157:H7 in feces from cattle, sheep and pigs in southwest part of Norway during 1998 and 1999. Int. J. Food Microbiol. 65, 193-200.
http://dx.doi.org/10.1016/S0168-1605(00)00518-3

41. Eriksson, E. (2010). Verotoxinogenic Escherichia coli O157:H7 in Swedish cattle and pigs. Doctoral Thesis, Swedish University of Agricultural sciences, Upsala.

42. Meng, J., Zhaos, S., Doyle, M. P., Joseph, S. W. (1998). Antibiotic resistance of Escherichia coli 0157:H7 and 0157: NM isolated from animals, food and humans. J. Food Prot. 61(1): 1511-1514.
PMid:9829195

43. Stanford, K., Agopsowicz, C. A., McAllister, T. A. (2012). Genetic diversity and antimicrobial resistance among isolates of Escherichia coli 0157:H7 from feces and hides of super shedders and low-shedding pen –mates in two commercial beef feedlots. BMC Vet. Rec. 8, 178.
http://dx.doi.org/10.1186/1746-6148-8-178
PMid:23014060; PMCid:PMC3582550

44. You, I. Y., Moon, B. M., Oh, I. G., Back, B. K., Li, L. G. et al. (2006). Antimicrobial resistance of Escherichia coli 0157 from cattle in Korea. Int. J. Food Microbiol. 106 (1): 74-78.
http://dx.doi.org/10.1016/j.ijfoodmicro.2005.05.013
PMid:16300850

45. Fitzgerald, A. C., Edrington, T. S., Looper, M. L., Callaway, T. R. et al. (2003). Antimicrobial susceptibility and factors affecting the shedding of Escherichia coli 0157:H7 and Salmonella in dairy cattle. Letters in Applied Microbiology 37, 392-398.
PMid:14633110

46. Ateba, C. N., Bezuidenhout, C. C. (2008). Characterisation of Escherichia coli 0157 strains from humans, cattle and pigs in the North- West Province, South Africa. Int J Food Microbiol. 128 (2): 181-8.
http://dx.doi.org/10.1016/j.ijfoodmicro.2008.08.011
PMid:18848733

47. Zhao, S., White, D. C., Ayers, G. B., Friedman, S. et al. (2001). Identification and characterization of integrin-mediated antibiotic resistance among shiga-toxin-producing Escherichia coli isolates. Appl. Environ. Microbiol. 67, 1558- 1564.
http://dx.doi.org/10.1128/AEM.67.4.1558-1564.2001
PMid:11282605; PMCid:PMC92769

48. Efsa Panel on Biological Hazards (BIOHAZ). (2011). Scientific opinion on the public health risks of bacterial strains producing extended-spectrum β-lactamases and/or AmpC β-lactamases in food and food-producing animals. EFSA J. 9 (8): 2322.

17

FATAL SNAKE BITE IN A BROWN BEAR
(*Ursus arctos L.*)

Romel Velev[1], Toni Tankoski[2], Maja Tankoska[2]

*[1]Department of Pharmacology and Toxicology, Faculty of Veterinary Medicine - Skopje,
"Ss. Cyril and Methodius" University in Skopje, R. Macedonia
[2]Veterinary Practice Toni, Makedonski Prosvetiteli b.b., T.C. Ohrigjanka lok. 1,
6000 Ohrid, R. Macedonia*

ABSTRACT

Poisoning from snake venom in animals is an emergency which requires immediate attention or otherwise, the delayed and inadequate treatment leads to untoward consequences and death. The present paper describes a case of venomous snakebite in a brown bear cub (*Ursus arctos L.*) and its therapeutic management. The brown bear cub of which was found alone on the slopes of a mountain in the southwest part of the country was presented to the peripheral veterinary practice in Ohrid with a history of dullness, disorientation and excessive swelling around the left forepaw. It was diagnosed for snakebite based on the history and physical examination. The hematological parameters showed reduced values of hemoglobin, packed cell volume and increased total leukocyte count. The biochemical values showed elevated levels of alanine aminotransferase and creatinine. After immobilization of the animal, the treatment was conducted with fluids, corticosteroid and broad spectrum antibiotic with careful monitoring. Despite the treatment which was initiated immediately, it was only partially effective, and the animal died one hour after the beginning of its course. Poisonous snakes are common in the mountainous part of Macedonia and, just like humans, wild bears especially their cubs are susceptible to the deadly venom of some species. The severity of the reaction to snake venom and prognosis in animals depends on a number of factors: on the type and species of snake, on how much venom was injected, on the location of the bite, on the age, health and body weight of the animal and crucially, the time interval between the snakebite and the application of the treatment.

Key words: venomous snakebite, brown bear *(Ursus arctos L.)*, treatment

INTRODUCTION

Generally, snakes are harmless and play an important environmental role in the fragile ecosystems of the nation's wildlife areas. They usually use camouflage and methods like hissing and biting. Despite the fact that many of them are non-venomous, a few of them are venomous. In Macedonia there are three venomous species of snakes (1): *Vipera ammodytes L.* (Macedonian: poskok, kamenjarka); *Vipera berus L.* (Macedonian:

Corresponding author: Prof. Romel Velev, PhD
E-mail address: vromel@fvm.ukim.edu.mk
Present address: Ss. Cyril and Methodius University in Skopje
Faculty of Veterinary Medicine - Skopje
Department of Pharmacology and Toxicology
Lazar Pop-Trajkov 5-7 1000, Skopje, Macedonia

sharka, lutica, osojnica) and *Vipera ursinii L.* (Macedonian: ostroglava sharka, ostroglava osojnica, stepska lutica). Most accidental bites usually occur whenever a snake is encountered and does not have time or space to slip away. In Macedonia, most of the cases of snakebite in animals have been reported in dogs, goats and horses. Snakebites can be serious, especially in young animals that get bit multiple times. Poisonous snakes are common in the mountainous part of Macedonia and, just like humans, wild bears, especially their cubs, are susceptible to the deadly venom of some species.

The brown bear (*Ursus arctos L.*) is the largest of the carnivore species found in the Republic of Macedonia. They belong to the same nominal subspecies as the whole European brown bear population. Today, their population is restricted to the mountainous forest areas in the western, central and southern parts of the country. It occupies the slopes of Shara Mountain, Korab, Bistra, Stogovo, Karaorman, Jablanica, Plaknenski Planini, Galichica and Baba Mountain (2). The current population estimates vary between 160-200 brown bears (3). Both the restricted distribution and the decline of the population are a result of intensive hunting, destruction and fragmentation of the bear's habitat and other disturbances by humans.

Poisoning from snake venom in animals is an emergency which requires immediate attention or otherwise, the delayed and inadequate treatment leads to untoward consequences. The present paper describes a case of a venomous snakebite in a brown bear cub and its therapeutic management.

CASE HISTORY AND OBSERVATION

In the beginning of May, 2014, a male brown bear cub (2 - 3 months of age), weighing about 7-10 kg, was presented to the peripheral veterinary practice in the city of Ohrid with a history of dullness, disorientation, depression, and in a recumbent position (Fig.1 and Fig. 2). According to the onlookers, the teddy bear was found alone on the slopes of Slavej Planina near the Karaorman mountain in the southwest part of the country. Its left forepaw was swollen and bleeding in the front region (Fig. 4).

by an unidentified venomous snake. The clinical parameters like rectal temperature, capillary refill time (CRT), pulse and respiratory rate showed 36.0 °C (normal range: 37.0 – 37.5 °C), CRT > 2 sec., 50 heart beats per min. (normal range in adult bear: 40 – 50/min) and 20 respirations per min. (normal range: 15–30/min) (4). Further examination revealed almost white gums, weak pulse, presence of cold extremities, reduced reflexes, unfocused eyes which appear to glaze over and an apparent depressed "mental" state.

The blood samples were collected with and without ethylene diamine tetra acetic acid (EDTA) for hematological parameters like hemoglobin, packed cell volume and total leukocyte count estimation and biochemical parameters such as alanine aminotransferase and creatinin estimation. The hematological parameters revealed decreased hemoglobin concentration (12.6 g/dl) (normal range: 14.0 – 20.0 g/dl) and packed cell volume (35%) (Normal range: 42 – 63.0%) and increased total leukocyte count (18000/ml) (normal range: 7000 – 12000/ml) (5). The biochemical values showed elevated levels of alanine aminotransferase (62 IU/dl) (normal range: 10 – 49 IU/dl) and creatinine (2.2 mg/dl) (normal range: 0.5 – 2.0 mg/dl) (6).

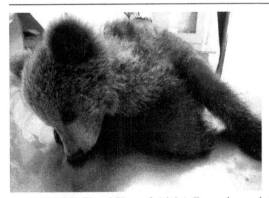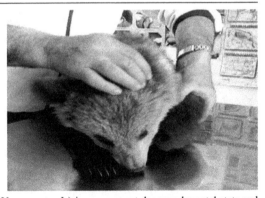

Figure 1 (left) and **Figure 2 (right).** Brown bear cub (*Ursus arctos L.*) in an apparent depressed mental state and in a recumbent position

DIAGNOSIS

The physical examination of the bear revealed a markedly discolored swollen area on the left forepaw. The hairs of the fur hide the typical fang marks of a snakebite. A marked increase in volume around the left forepaw, extending to the region of the shoulder and bleeding (dark bloody fluid which oozes from the wound) was also noticed (Fig. 3 and Fig. 4). Bleeding was also easily observed through the perforation left by the needles used for blood collection and drug administration.

Based on the history and physical examination of the bear, the case was suspected for snakebite

TREATMENT

The snakebite site was shaved, and the wound cleaned thoroughly with germicidal soap. Once immobilized, the animal received 300 mL Ringer's lactate solution (Lactated Ringers injection, Vioser) and 15 mL hetastarch 6% (Voluven 6%, Fresenius Kabi) intravenously, 10.0 mg dexamethazone (Colvasone 0.2%, Norbrook) also intravenously, and 250 mg procaine benzyl penicillin and 250 mg dihydrostreptomycin sulfate (Sustrepen, Genera) subcutaneously (14). Since the snake fangs can be contaminated with different types of bacteria, we administrated subcutaneously the combination

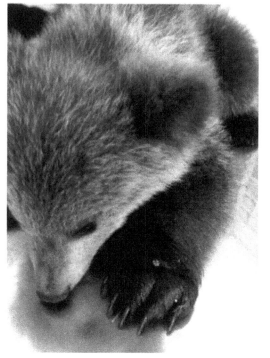

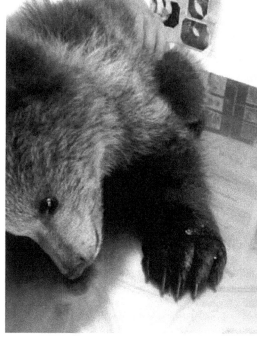

Figure 3. Increased size of the left forepaw

Figure 4. Dark bloody fluid which oozes from the wound

of procaine benzyl penicillin and 250 mg dihydrostreptomycin sulfate (Sustrepen, Genera) to expand the spectrum of antibiotics. Then the animal was kept under observation, but the clinical symptoms worsened. Despite the treatment which was initiated immediately, it was only partially effective, and the animal died one hour after the beginning of the course of the treatment. The bear was not treated with specific anti-snake venom. The private practice in Ohrid at that moment did not possess snake antivenin, which in Macedonia is permitted to be possessed and applied only by human medical institutions. It may be available only on an as-needed basis through a larger human hospital/outpatient emergency room. The clinical condition and the time required to supply snake antivenin did not permit for the animal to be treated specifically.

Necropsy of the animal was done the next day by an authorized veterinary inspector who conducted the postmortem protocol and confirmed a venomous snakebite of the brown bear cub. At necropsy, an area of hemorrhagic edema was found around the left front paw that reached the subcutaneous tissue. The liver presented congestion, mainly centrilobular. In the lung, there were areas of congestion. The other organs did not show significant alterations.

DISCUSSION

Snakebite presents as a minor mechanical trauma, allergy to venom (rare) and an evenomation syndrome. Three main clinical envenomation syndromes in snakebite should be identified: painful progressive swelling, progressive weakness and bleeding. Snake venoms are complex mixture of proteins and peptides, consisting of both enzymatic and non enzymatic compounds. The other components of snake venoms are glycoproteins, lipids, and biogenic amines, such as histamine, serotonin and neurotransmitters (catecholamines and acetylcholine) (7). Snakes venoms are often characterized as either hemotoxic (those that have hemorrhagic effects; traditionally associated with vipers from family Viperidae) or neurotoxic (those that produce paralysis and death by respiratory shock; traditionally associated with elapids from family Elapidae); many venoms, such as those from some rattlesnakes, show evidence of both types of effects (8, 9). While the term hemotoxic implies effects only to the circulatory system, hemotoxic venoms often cause tissue destruction in other body systems (9). Most of these tissue destructive properties are attributed to proteins and digestive enzymes such as phospholipase A2 which are commonly present in venom (9).

In our case, the cyanotic edema observed at the site of the bite may be attributed to enzyme hyaluronidase which acts as a spreading factor. Hyalurinadase cleaves internal glycoside bonds in certain acid mucopolysaccharides resulting in decreased viscosity of connective tissues, allowing other fractions of venom to penetrate the tissues (7). The increased size of the affected paw, is probably due to local inflammation. Snake venom has proteolytic activity, which is believed to be responsible for the inflammation (8). It is important to notice that although the bite was on the paw, the animal developed systemic problems and died. Haemotoxic effect of snake venom may interfere with many components of the haemostatic system (10). Moreover, the toxins such as the haemorrhagins cause spontaneous bleeding in the gingival sulci, nose, skin and gastrointestinal tract (11). However, bleeding tendencies were not noticed in our case. The decrease of hematocrit and hemoglobin levels in our case may be attributed to damage of the blood cells by the snake venom. The increased biochemical values like alanine aminotransferase and creatinine may be due to the hepatotoxic and nephrotoxic effect of snake venom (12).

Generally, the therapy for snakebite is comprised of, the first aid, antivenin, fluid therapy, anti-inflammatory agents and antibiotics. First aid measures which attempt to denature the venom (topical applications, electrotherapy, cryotherapy), remove the venom (incision and suction, excision) or retard its absorption (various types of tourniquet, cryotherapy) have not proved effective in controlled studies and can be potentially harmful. Therefore, syndromic management of snakebite without knowing the species of the snake is logical and effective.

Treatment for viper envenomation should be directed toward preventing or controlling shock, neutralizing venom, preventing or controlling coagulopathy, minimizing necrosis, and preventing secondary infection. Any animal presented within 24 hr of a snakebite showing signs of vipers envenomation requires intensive treatment, starting with IV crystalloids to combat hypotension. Hetastarch may be helpful to manage hypovolemia; however, colloids should be used with caution because of their potential to leak out of damaged vessels and pull fluids into tissue beds. Rapid-acting corticosteroids may be of benefit in the first 24 hr to help control shock, protect against tissue damage, and minimize the likelihood of allergic reactions to antivenin. However, prolonged use of corticosteroids is not recommended (13).

Antivenom is the only direct and specific means of neutralizing snake venom. Animals bitten by a viperine snake in Macedonia may be treated with antivenin, which may be available on an as-needed basis through larger human hospital emergency rooms. A polyvalent antivenin (Viekvin® equine-origin polyvalent $F(ab)^2$ fragment antivenin – Institute Torlak) against European vipers (*Vipera ammodytes* and *Vipera berus*) is available in Macedonia and should be used in all cases of substantial snake envenomation, if is not too late.

It is most effective if administered in the first 6 hr after the bite. The efficacy of antivenin is diminished if the bite occurred > 24 hr previously. Because of the cost, usually its use is generally reserved for small and young animals, animals that have received multiple bites, and/or animals that are showing signs of shock. In severe envenomations, multiple vials of antivenin may be required, although this is frequently cost-prohibitive in veterinary patients. In our case, clinical condition and the time required to supply snake antivenin has not permitted for the animal to be treated specifically.

Several potential pathogens, including *Pseudomonas aeruginosa*, *Clostridium spp*, *Corynebacterium spp*, and staphylococci have been isolated from the mouth of snakes. However, the incidence of wound infection after snake bites is low, and many clinicians use broad-spectrum antibiotics only when significant tissue necrosis is present (13).

CONCLUSION

This paper describes for the first time a case of venomous snakebite of a brown bear cub in Macedonia and provides details of the treatment of this endangered wild animal. Snakebite in animals, with envenomation, is a true emergency. Rapid examination and appropriate treatment are paramount. Intensive therapy should be instituted as soon as possible, because irreversible effects of venom begin immediately after envenomation. Unfortunately, the severity of the reaction to the snake venom and prognosis in animals depends on a number of factors: on the type and species of snake, on how much venom was injected, on the location of the bite, on the age, health and body weight of the animal and crucially the time interval between the snakebite and the application of treatment. Mortality is generally higher from bites to the thorax or abdomen than from bites to the extremities. However, this may relate to the size and vulnerability of the victim. In our case, it is important to notice that although the bite was on the paw, the animal developed systemic problems and died because it was found, delivered and treated too late. Animals bitten by a viperine snake may be treated with antivenin, but the problem is that they are available only on an as-needed basis through larger human hospital emergency rooms. The provided case report should be used as a baseline reference for venomous snakebite treatment in the species, especially in scenarios where individual animals are of significant value to conservation efforts.

REFERENCES

1. List of snakes in the Republic of Macedonia: http:// en.wikipedia.org /wiki/ List_of_snakes_in_ the_Republic_of_Macedonia

2. Stojanovski, L., Arsovska, S. (1996). Report on the Status of the brown bear (*Ursus arctos L. 1758*) in the Republic of Macedonia.

3. Melovski, L., Godes, C. (2002). Large carnivores in the "Republic of Macedonia" In Psaroudas, S. (Ed.), Protected areas in the Southern Balkans - Legislation, large carnivores, transborder areas. (pp. 81-93). Thessaloniki, Greece

4. Detailed physiology notes with literature reports for the Brown bear - Ursus arctos. http://wildpro.twycrosszoo.org/S/0MCarnivor/ursidae/ ursus/Ursus_arctos/10Ursus_arctosDetPhy.htm

5. Pearson, A.M., Halloran, D.W. (1972). Hematology of the brown bear (*Ursus arctos*) from southwestern Yukon Territory, Canada. Canadian Journal of Zoology 50(3): 279-286. http://dx.doi.org/10.1139/z72-038 PMid:5014061

6. Kuntze, A., Hundsdorf, P. (1985). Haematological and biochemical parameters of clinically intact and pathologically affected polar bears (*Thalarctos maritimus*) and brown bears (*Ursus arctos*). Verhandlungsbericht des 27. Internationalen Symposiums über die Erkrankungen der Zootiere (pp. 385–391). 9–13 June 1985, St Vincent/Torino, Akademie-Verlag Berlin

7. Klaassen, C.D. (2008). Properties and toxicities of animal venoms. In McGraw-Hill (Ed.), Toxicology 7th Ed. (pp 1093-1098). New Delhi

8. Jiminez-Porras, J.M. (1968). Pharmacology of peptides and proteins in snake venoms. Annual Review of Pharmacology 8, 299-318. http://dx.doi.org/10.1146/annurev.pa.08.040168.001503 PMid:4875394

9. Greene, H.W. (1997). Snakes: The evolution of mystery in nature. Berkeley, California: University of Berkeley Press

10. Wolff, F. A. D. (2006). Natural toxins. In: Clarke's analysis of drugs and poison. Pharmaceutical press, London, Electronic Version

11. Warrell D. A., Fenner, P. J. (1993). Venomous bites and stings. Br. Med. Bull, 49, 423–439.

12. O'Shea, M. (2005). Venomous snakes of the world. Princeton: Princeton University Press

13. Overview of Snakebite. Snakebite: Merck Veterinary Manual www. merckmanuals.com /vet/.../snakebite/overview _of_snakebite.html

14. Velev, R., Krleska – Veleva, N. (2013). Practical use of registered veterinary medicinal products in Macedonia in identifying the risk of developing of antimicrobial resistance. Mac Vet Rev., 36(1): 5 – 12.

18

THE DYNAMICS OF BIOCHEMICAL PARAMETERS IN BLOOD OF CLINICALLY HEALTHY HOLSTEIN COWS FROM DAY 5 BEFORE TO DAY 60 AFTER CALVING

Irena Celeska[1], Aleksandar Janevski[2], Igor Dzadzovski[2],
Igor Ulchar[1], Danijela Kirovski[3]

[1]Department of Pathophisiology, Faculty of Veterinary Medicine-Skopje,
Ss. Cyril and Methodius University in Skopje
[2]Department of Farm Animal Health, Faculty of Veterinary Medicine-Skopje,
University Ss. Cyril and Methodius University in Skopje
[3]Department of Physiology and Biochemistry, Faculty of Veterinary Medicine,
University of Belgrade

ABSTRACT

The peripartal period in Holstein dairy cows is critical, due to the transition from pregnancy to lactation. We have studied the dynamics of biochemical parameters from day 5 before to day 60 after calving. The study included 10 multiparous Holstein cows, examined at days -5, 5, 10, 30 and 60 relative to calving. Blood samples were taken from *vena jugularis*. Analyzed biochemical parameters were glucose, triglycerides, total cholesterol, total bilirubin, albumin, total protein, urea, NEFA and BHBA. Milk production and body condition score were also estimated. Obtained results showed that cows were exposed to mild to marked metabolic distress. Energy status was changed due to increased values of NEFA and BHBA and decreased value of glucose after calving. Protein concentrations were increased at day 10 after calving, despite the decrease of the level of albumin. Urea concentrations before and after calving were within physiological range indicating an optimal protein diet. Increased values of total bilirubin at day 5 after calving indicated liver increased activity. Lipid status presented by triglycerides and total cholesterol revealed no differences in blood concentrations. Milk production was highest at day 30 after calving. BCS were highest in dry cows, thereafter they declined and recovered at day 60 after calving.
In conclusion, biochemical parameters can be used as relevant indicators of metabolic distress in cows around calving with milk and BCS recording as aside parameters. Changes in some biochemical parameters indicate liver increased activity and metabolic stress, that could lead to decreased milk production, impaired reproductive performance and, finally, to illness.

Key words: Holstein cows, biochemical parameters, transition period

INTRODUCTION

Production diseases are metabolic disorders in animals with genetically determined high production capacities, based on disbalance between the animal's input (feed utilization) and output (animal's product,

Corresponding author: Dr. Irena Celeska, PhD
E-mail address: iceleska@fvm.ukim.edu.mk
Present address: Faculty of Veterinary Medicine – Skopje
Ss. Cyril and Methodius University in Skopje
Lazar Pop-Trajkov 5/7, 1000 Skopje, R. of Macedonia

e.g. milk). In dairy cows this disbalance is evident usually during the so-called "transition period" (3 weeks prior and 3 weeks after calving) (1), when very significant changes in the hormonal status occur, which leads to redirection of metabolic pathways, i.e. favoring of anabolic processes in the mammary gland (milk compounds production) vs. metabolic processes in other tissues. These high production performances also cause high nutrition demands, which exceed the animal's metabolic capacities (inadequate feed utilization), which usually leads to an aberrant physiological state known as negative energy balance (NEB) (2). Developing of NEB is closely related with specificities of the ruminant's metabolism. In ruminants, alimentary glucose is converted by ruminal microflora into short-chain volatile fatty acids, and only some of them are substrate for gluconeogenesis which occurs in liver, and is the main source of serum glucose in ruminants. This causes blood glucose in ruminants to have a relatively lower level compared with non-ruminants, and it ranges from 2.2 to 3.3 mmol/L (3). There are physiological variations in the glucose level in different phases of the production-reproduction cycle. In normal cows, at the end of the gestation the glucose level is within its physiological range for maintaining of the gluconeogenesis process (4). During the calving the glucose level rapidly increases, which is explained as a result of stress and hormonal status changes (5, 6). After calving, during the early lactation, the glucose level is significantly lower compared with the period before calving (7, 8), and this could be considered as introduction to NEB where synthesis of milk compounds in the mammary gland exceeds the gluconeogenesis capacities of liver, and leads to development of metabolic (production) diseases (8, 9). Increased utilization of glucose by the mammary gland vs. decreased glucoplastic compounds input and decreased gluconeogenesis cause development of hypoglycemia, which very often could be associated with a disorder of the lipid metabolism (7, 10). In cows with hepatic lipidosis gluconeogenesis is decreased, hepatic glycogen pools are depleted, which causes hypoglycemia (11, 12). All these changes in the glucose and lipid metabolisms are also related with hepatocyte morpho-functional integrity.

Animals typically response to NEB by mobilizing body fat reserves, as an attempt to maintain energy homeostasis, so non-esterified fatty acids (NEFAs) are mobilized from the adipose tissue and utilized by the liver, where they could be fully oxidized to CO_2, converted to ketone bodies, mainly in beta-hydroxybutyrate (BHBA), or re-esterified into triglycerides. Further, these triglycerides are delivered into the blood as very low density lipoproteins (VLDL), or stored as cytosolic lipid droplets (1). Like other ruminants, dairy cows' liver has very low capacities of VLDL synthesis and secretion (13), which makes these animals very susceptible to lipid metabolism disorders, manifested as hepatic lipidosis or fatty liver (retention of high levels of triglycerides in hepatocytes), or as ketosis (high concentration of ketone bodies in the blood) (14).

It could be summarized that metabolic disbalance which occurs during the transitional period in dairy cows is a real, but often encrypted problem, with significant implications for milk production, causing enormous economic losson one side, and on the other it can be a predisposition for many clinically manifested health problems, like milk fever, ketosis, retained fetal membranes, metritis (1), abomasum displacement (1, 15) and mastitis (16, 17). In looking at the multifactorial regulatory mechanisms in energy turnover in high-yielding dairy cows during the transition period, the aim of this survey was a monitoring of the metabolic profile during the transition period and detection of the intensity of morphological injury of the hepatocytes.

MATERIAL AND METHODS

The examination included 10 (n=10) Holstein cows, that were 3-6 years of age, with an average body weight 450-650 kg. All cows were kept at free stall system, managed and fed under the same conditions.

Blood samples were taken by puncturing of the jugular vein, -5, 5, 10, 30 and 60 days relative to calving. Blood samples were taken into sterile serological tubes and after the spontaneous coagulation, the serum was separated with *Sanyo Mistral 2500* centrifuge on 2500 rpm. The serum samples were stored on -18°C до -20°C till the analysis. Analyzed biochemical parameters included parameters that are related to carbohydrate and lipid metabolism (glucose, triglycerides, total cholesterol, non-esterified fatty acids - NEFA, and β-hydroxybutirate - BHBA), as well as parameters related to liver functional status (albumin, total protein, urea and total bilirubin).

The level of glucose was determined in the whole blood, immediately after sampling with commercial strips, using *Accu-Chek* (Roche, USA) glucometer.

Triglycerides, total cholesterol, albumin, total protein, urea and total bilirubin were determined by commercial kits, *Human* (Germany). NEFA and BHBA were analyzed by *Randox* (UK) commercial kits. According to the manufacturer's instructions, the methods were "end-point" and kinetic-enzymatic reaction on photometer *STAT FAX 3300* (Awareness Technology Inc, USA).

Body Condition Score was estimated according to Elanco Animal Health Bulletin AI 8478, at days -10, 10, 30 and 60 relative to calving.

Milk production was recorded by an automatic milking system, DeLaval, Sweden at days 10, 30, and 60 relative to calving.

RESULTS

Biochemical parameters presented in Tables 1 to 4, include the dynamics of biochemical parameters starting from day 5 before to day 60 after calving. Results for BCS and milk production are presented in Table 5.

Table 1. Biochemical parameters ($\bar{x}\pm$SD) related to energy status in a Holstein dairy cows (n=10)

	Days relative to calving - energy status				
	- 5	5	10	30	60
Glucose (mmol/L)	4,52±0,30[A]	3,66±0,32[B]	3,66±0,37[B]	3,62±0,32[B]	3,54±0,22[B]
BHBA (mmol/L)	0,81±0,27[AC]	1,29±0,37[BD]	1,03±0,43[ADF]	0,80±0,24[CEF]	0,66±0,21[C]
NEFA (mmol/L)	0,74±0,29[A]	1,08±0,51[A]	0,76±0,43[A]	0,35±0,19[B]	0,15±0,10[C]

[ABCD]- The different letter indicates the statistical difference between parameters within rows (p < 0.05)

Table 2. Biochemical parameters ($\bar{x}\pm$SD) related to the lipid status in Holstein dairy cows (n=10)

	Days relative to calving - lipid status				
	- 5	5	10	30	60
Triglycerides (mmol/L)	0,29±0,16[BCD]	0,33±0,18[BCD]	0,29±0,08[BC]	0,27±0,04[C]	0,18±0,047[D]
Total cholesterol (mmol/L)	2,11±0,33[A]	3,91±1,54[BC]	3,99±1,64[C]	5,23±1,40[DC]	6,35±0,87[E]

[ABCD]- The different letter indicates on the statistical difference between parameters within rows (p < 0.05)

Table 3. Biochemical parameters ($\bar{x}\pm$SD) related to the hepatic status in Holstein dairy cows (n=10)

	Days relative to calving - hepatic status				
	- 5	5	10	30	60
Total bilirubin (μmol/L)	4,58±0,43[A]	5,52±0,88[BC]	5,07±1,31[AC]	4,58±0,56[A]	4,54±0,72[A]

[ABCD]- The different letter indicates thestatistical difference between parameters within rows (p < 0.05)

Table 4. Biochemical parameters related to the protein status in Holstein dairy cows (n=10)

	Days relative to calving - protein status				
	- 5	5	10	30	60
Albumin (g/L)	43,09±5,60[A]	42,66±6,01[AC]	38,59±2,39[BC]	41,31±1,88[A]	42,80±1,67[A]
Total protein (g/L)	77,22±10,84[AC]	80,42±6,76[AC]	93,56±13,39[B]	75,28±11,66[AC]	70,25±8,96[C]
Urea (mmol/L)	4,78±1,83[A]	3,90±1,02[A]	4,09±2,06[A]	4,73±1,95[A]	4,89±1,74[A]

[ABCD]- The different letter indicates the statistical difference between parameters within rows (p < 0.05)

Table 5. BCS and milk production in Holstein dairy cows (n=10)

	Days relative to calving			
	-5	10	30	60
BCS	3.60±0.32[A]	2.36±0.45[B]	2.18±0.19[B]	2.61±0.81[B]
Daily milk production (L)	-	12.57±2.37[A]	14.85±2.11[A]	13.86±3.29[A]

[ABCD]- The different letter indicates the statistical difference between parameters within rows (p < 0.05)

DISCUSSION

Dairy cows with high genetic merit for milk production, during the peripartal period change the serum glucose level in different stages of the reproduction cycles (1, 11). We have studied the dynamics of biochemical parameters from day 5 before to day 60 after calving, in order to establish if a cow is capable to maintain those parameters within the physiological range, despite the challenges she is exposed to. Glucose serum concentrations depend on many factors, especially neuro-hormonal regulation and proper feeding management (3). Normoglycemia was observed in the examined cows during the antepartal period, indicating supply of energy precursors from alimentary recourses. Onset of lactation caused hypoglycemic condition due to enhanced utilization of glucose in galactogenesis. There was significant decrease of glucose serum concentrations combined with increased milk production. During the early lactation, the energy balance was switched in udder synthetic processes. NEFA are a "direct indicator" for lipomobilisation (18) and a very dynamic parameter. Subcutaneous and visceral fatty tissue broke down, releasing NEFA which are used in peripheral tissues as an energy source, or they become ingredients of the milk fat (4, 7). Besides the normal glucose status before calving, higher, compared to physiological, serum concentration of NEFA during the antepartal period revealed early lipolysis, as a result of adaptation to high energy demand for fetus growth and milk producing. (5, 9) Early stage lactation is characterized by intensive lipomobilisation for udder anabolism. (6, 14) Significant decrease of NEFA during 30 and 60 days postpartum means balanced metabolic requirements, form alimentary recourses and milk producing. Another parameter for energy status is BHBA, as an "indirect indicator" for negative energy balance. (17, 18) Obtained results for serum BHBA concentration during the antepartal period revealed intensive ketogenesis in hepatocytes, due to inappropriate oxidation of non-esterified fatty acids. BHBA follow the trend of NEFA serum concentration, so the highest values of BHBA were at days 5 and 10 after parturition, but on days 30 and 60 values return in referent ranges. Triglyceridemia indicates the capability of liver for synthesis apolipoprotein B-100, VLDL for elimination of triglycerides in the blood stream during the whole peripartal period, but diminished concentration was significant on day 60 after calving, when NEFA concentrations were very low. These results agree with some previously published results from other investigators (8, 10).

Hypocholesterinemia was maintained during the antepartal period, as a result of low "de novo" synthesis of cholesterol. During the postpartal period, serum cholesterol concentration significantly increased, thus 30 and 60 days after calving they reached the highest value. Also, the liver ability for synthesis of apolipoproteins for cholesterol transport was maintained and the highest significant cholesterol concentration was reached 30 and 60 days after calving. Total bilirubin as relevant indicator of liver impairment, (6) during the peripartal period showed an increased value at day 5 relative to calving, because the pathobiochemical processes of gluconeogenesis, glucogenolysis, phosphorilation, beta oxidation happened simultaneously in hepatocytes. Protein status through albumin and total protein concentrations showed changes at day 10 after calving. There were significant increases of protein concentrations at day 10 after calving, with a significant decrease of the level of albumin at the same time period, probably due to decreased synthesis in the liver and increased utilization in the udder.

CONCLUSION

Biochemical parameters can be used as reliable indicators of degree and duration of metabolic distress in Holstein cows. During the transition period, the lowest value of BCS is achieved at day 30 after calving due to prolonged lipolysis in those cows. Cows included in our study did not achieve their genetic merit for milk production. Although the examined cows were clinically healthy, changes in some biochemical parameters indicate liver increased activity and metabolic stress that could lead to decreased milk production, impaired reproductive performance and, finally, to illness.

REFERENCES

1. Drackley, J.K. (1999). ADSA Foundation Scholar Award. Biology of dairy cows during the transition period: the final frontier? J Dairy Sci. 82 (11): 2259-2273.
http://dx.doi.org/10.3168/jds.S0022-0302(99)75474-3

2. Wathes, D.C., Cheng, Z., Chowdhury, W., Fenwick, M.A., Fitzpatrick, R., Morris, D.G., Patton, J., Murphy, J. J. (2009). Negative energy balance alters global gene expression and immune responses in the uterus of postpartum dairy cows. Physiol Genomics. 39 (1): 1-13.
http://dx.doi.org/10.1152/physiolgenomics.00064.2009
PMid:19567787 PMCid:PMC2747344

3. Bell, A.W. Bauman D. E. (1997). Adaptations of glucose metabolism during pregnancy and lactation. Journal of Mammary Gland Biology and Neoplasia 2(3): 265-278.
http://dx.doi.org/10.1023/A:1026336505343
PMid:10882310

4. Yasothai, R. (2014). Importance of energy on reproduction in dairy cattle. International Journal of Science, Environment and Technology 6(3): 2020 – 2023.

5. Herdt, T.H. (1988). Fuel homeostasis in the ruminant. Vet. Clin. North. Am Food Anim Pract. 4: 213-231 PMid:3061608.

6. Kunz, P.L., Blum, J.W. (1985). Relationship energy balances and blood levels of hormones and metabolites in dairy cows during late pregnancy and early lactation. Z. Z. Tierphysiol. Tierernhrg. u. Futtermittelkde 54: 239-248.
http://dx.doi.org/10.1111/j.1439-0396.1985.tb01537.x

7. Mahapatra, R.K., Sahoo, A. (2006). Ketosis and fatty liver in dairy animals: preventive nutritional approaches. Clinical Nutrition of Livestock and Pets 23(3): 45-53.

8. García, A.M.B., Cardoso, F.C., Campos, R. Thedy, X.D., González H.D.F. (2011). Metabolic evaluation of dairy cows submitted to three different strategies to decrease the effects of negative energy balance in early postpartum. Pesq.Vet. Bras. 31(1): 11-17.
http://dx.doi.org/10.1590/s0100-736x2011001300003

9. Drackley, J.K., Overton, T.R., Douglas, G.N. (2001). Adaptations of glucose and long-chain fatty acid metabolism in liver of dairy cows during the periparturient period. Journal of Dairy Science. 84: 100-112.
http://dx.doi.org/10.3168/jds.S0022-0302(01)70204-4

10. Šamanc, H., Kirovski, D., Lakić, N., Celeska, I., Bojković-Kovačević, S., Sladojević, Ž., Ivanov I., (2014). A comparison of the concentrations of energy-balance-related variables in jugular and mammary vein blood of dairy cows with different milk yield. Acta Veterinaria Hungarica 62(1): 52-63.
http://dx.doi.org/10.1556/AVet.2013.055
PMid:24334081

11. Bobe, G., Young, J.W., Beitz, D.C. (2004). Invited review: pathology, etiology, prevention, and treatment of fatty liver in dairy cows. 87(10): 3105–3124.
http://dx.doi.org/10.3168/jds.s0022-0302(04)73446-3

12. Veenhuizen, J.J., Drackley, J.K., Richard, M.J., Sanderson, T.P., Miller, L.D., Joung, J.W. (1991). Metabolic changes in blood and liver during development and early treatment of experimental fatty liver and ketosis in cows. J. Dairy Sci. 74: 4238-4253.
http://dx.doi.org/10.3168/jds.s0022-0302(91)78619-0

13. Pullen, D.L., Liesman, J.S., Emery, R.S. (1990). A species comparison of liver slice synthesis and secretion of triacylglycerol from nonesterified fatty acids in media. J Anim Sci. 68 (5): 1395-1399.
PMid:2365651

14. McCabe, M., Waters, S., Morris, D., Kenny, D., Lynn, D., Creevey, C. (2012). RNA-seq analysis of differential gene expression in liver from lactating dairy cows divergent in negative energy balance. BMC Genomics 13: 193.
http://dx.doi.org/10.1186/1471-2164-13-193
PMid:22607119 PMCid:PMC3465249

15. Dezfouli, M.M., Eftekhari, Z., Sadeghian, S., Bahounar, A., Jeloudari, M. (2013). Evaluation of hematological and biochemical profiles in dairy cows with left displacement of the abomasum. Comp Clin Path. 22 (2): 175-179.
http://dx.doi.org/10.1007/s00580-011-1382-5
PMid:23483814 PMCid:PMC3590408

16. Mallard, B.A., Dekkers, J.C., Ireland, M.J., Leslie, K.E., Sharif, S., Vankampen, C.L., Wagter, L., Wilkie, B.N. (1998). Alteration in immune responsiveness during the periparturm period and its ramification on dairy cow and calf health. J. Dairy Sci. 81: 585-595.
http://dx.doi.org/10.3168/jds.S0022-0302(98)75612-7

17. Leslie, K.E., Duffield, T.F., Schukken, Y.H., LeBlanc, S.J. (2000). The influence of negative energy balance on udder health. National Mastitis Council Regional Meeting Proceedings, 25-33.

18. Van Saun, R.J. (2004). Metabolic profiling and health risk in transition cows. Proc Am Assoc Bov Pract. 37: 212-213.

19

CANINE ADIPOSE-DERIVED STEM CELL AGGREGATES AS A VIABLE SUBSTITUTE TO ACTUAL CANINE DERMAL PAPILLAE

Sohee Bae, Jina Kim, Li Li, Aeri Lee, Hyunjoo Lim, Junemoe Jeong,
Seung Hoon Lee, Oh-kyeong Kweon, Wan Hee Kim

Department of Veterinary Clinical Sciences, College of Veterinary Medicine and Research Institute for Veterinary Science, Seoul National University, 1 Gwanak-ro, Gwanak-gu, Seoul 151-742, Republic of Korea

ABSTRACT

Hair loss is a major dermatological disease in veterinary and human medicine. Active studies on hair regeneration with mesenchymal stem cells have been performed in an effort to solve the limitations of conservative treatments in human medicine. Our understanding of the canine hair follicle (HF), considering a useful model for the study of the human alopecia, is limited. This study was designed to broaden our understanding of canine dermal papilla (DP), and to reconstruct dermal papilla-like tissue (DPLT) using canine adipose-derived mesenchymal stem cells (AD-MSCs), as an alternative to actual DP. We cultured canine DPs, observed their culture patterns and compared their expression level of DP-related genes and proteins with those of DPLTs by performing RT-PCR analysis and Western blotting. Canine dermal papilla cells (DPCs) showed multilayer culture patterns with pseudo-papillae. Reconstruction of DPLTs was performed successfully. Not only were they morphologically similar to actual DPs, but we also observed similarities between DPCs and DPLTs in molecular characteristics. These findings suggested that DPLT was a viable substitute for DP. This study will not only be helpful for understanding the morphological and molecular characteristics of canine DPCs, but may also serve as a basis for understanding human hair follicle biology and potential therapeutic strategies for alopecia.

Key words: dog, dermal papillae, dermal papillae-like tissue, adipose-derived mesenchymal stem cells, hair regeneration

INTRODUCTION

Alopecia is a common dermatological disease in veterinary and human medicine. It may be caused by inflammation, infection, traumatic damage as a result of chemotherapy or radiotherapy, nutritional deficiencies, hormonal or autoimmune disease, or stress. Even though the classification of alopecia in humans is more complex, certain types of human alopecia can be found in canine hair loss (1-3).

The condition, especially in humans, may be mentally stressful to patients going through it due to its effect on their appearance, which is why many different treatment methods have been tried.

Out of these, auto hair transplantation has been the most effective. In addition, because of critical limitations due to cost, amount of hair and number of operations (4), studies on hair regeneration have been attempted using cultured hair follicle cells or mesenchymal stem cells (4-8).

Hair growth is a result of active epidermal and dermal interactions (6, 9-14). In general, the dermal component is thought of as an inducer and the epidermal component as a responder in the process of hair growth (15). Dermal papilla (DP) is a cluster of highly specialized fibroblasts located at the base of the hair follicle (HF). It is believed that DP not only determines the length, thickness and shape of the hair shaft (16), but also regulates hair follicle development and growth. For this reason, active research on DPs has been performed.

Hair regeneration has been attempted using tissue and cellular recombination of the epidermal and dermal component (15, 17). However, DP isolation is technically laborious and difficult, and cultured dermal papilla cells (DPCs) lose their hair inductive abilities after a few passages. To overcome these limitations, studies on the reconstruction of

Corresponding author: Prof. Wan Hee Kim, PhD
E-mail address: whkim@snu.ac.kr
Present address: Department of Veterinary Clinical Sciences, College of Veterinary Medicine and Research Institute for Veterinary Science, Seoul National University, 1 Gwanak-ro, Gwanak-gu, Seoul 151-742, Republic of Korea

dermal papilla-like tissues have been performed with human umbilical cord-derived mesenchymal stem cells (4, 5, 7).

This study represents the first reconstruction of DPLTs using canine adipose-derived mesenchymal stem cells (AD-MSCs); we compared them to actual canine DPCs in order to evaluate DPLTs as an alternative to actual DPs. We expect the findings of this study to broaden our understanding of the morphological and molecular characteristics of canine DPCs, and to represent a valuable source for the investigation of canine and human hair regeneration.

MATERIAL AND METHODS

Canine AD-MSC cultures

We used canine AD-MSCs that were supplied from Seung Hoon Lee (Department of Veterinary Clinical Sciences, College of Veterinary Medicine, Seoul National University); these AD-MSCs were previously characterized (18). The AD-MSCs were cultured in low-glucose Dulbecco's modified eagle medium (DMEM, Gibco®, Life Technologies, Grand Island, NY, USA) with 10% fetal bovine serum (FBS, Gibco®, Life Technologies, Grand Island, NY, USA), 100 units/mL penicillin and 100 mg/mL streptomycin at 37.0 °C, in a 5% CO_2 incubator.

Canine DP isolation and cell culturing

Full-thickness skin biopsies obtained from the flank region of healthy beagle dogs approximately 3 years old were immediately placed in phosphate-buffered saline (PBS). Under a dissecting microscope, the hair follicles were isolated using a No. 15 blade, watchmaker's forceps, and 23G needles. Isolated hair follicles were then transferred to a fresh medium-containing dish for further isolation. After the hair cycle stage was evaluated by the position of DP and tip of hair shaft, DPs in late anagen were isolated (19). Five DPs were placed together in a single well of a 12-well cell-culture cluster, which contained 1.2 mL of AmnioMAX™-C100 complete medium (AmnioMAX™, Invitrogen, Carlsbad, CA, USA) supplemented with 10% inactivated and steroid-free canine serum at 37 °C, in a 5% CO_2 incubator (6, 8, 20-22). The culture medium was replaced every third day. Primary cultured DPCs were harvested when confluent and then passaged on every tenth day. All procedures were approved by the Seoul National University's Institutional Animal Care and Use Committee (SNU-140729-5).

Reconstruction of DPLTs

Canine AD-MSCs were subjected to a monolayer culture in DMEM supplemented with 10% FBS, 100 units/mL penicillin and 100 mg/mL streptomycin, until the cells occupied approximately 80% of the culture dish. Next, the culture medium was replaced with dermal papilla-forming medium (DPFM) (23) that contained 10 ng/mL hydrocortisone, 5 mL Insulin-Transferrin-Selenium liquid media (ITS, Gibco®, Life Tecnologies, Grand Island, NY, USA), and 100 units/mL penicillin, 100 mg/mL streptomycin, and 20 ng/mL HGF (recombinant human HGF, Gibco®, Life Tecnologies, NY, USA). The medium was changed every third day for three weeks, after which the culture was treated with the StemPro® Accutase® Cell Dissociation Reagent (Accutase®, Gibco®, Life Technologies, Grand Island, NY, USA) at concentrations ranging from 20 to 40 µL/cm² to detach the cells from the culture dish (detach-attach step). Cell distribution was changed and cell aggregation was observed 24 h after treatment with Accutase; the aggregated cell mass became suspended in the medium five to seven days after the treatment. The suspended cell aggregates were then isolated from the culture by centrifugation at 500 rpm for 3 min. All procedures were performed based on those of previous studies (4, 23).

RT-PCR analysis

Total RNA from all three cell types (canine AD-MSCs, DPCs and DPLTs) was isolated using Hybrid-R™ with RiboEx® (GeneAll®, Seoul, Korea) according to the manufacturer's instructions. cDNA was then synthesized, using one microgram of the total RNA, with a PrimeScript™ RT-PCR Kit (Takara Bio Inc., Shiga, Japan) for RT-PCR processing according to the manufacturer's instructions. Cycling conditions included initial denaturation for 10 min at 94 °C, followed by thirty-five 15-s cycles at 95 °C and 60-s cycles at 60 °C. The products were then analyzed by electrophoresis on a 1.6% agarose gel and subsequently visualized by the Redsafe™ Nucleic Acid Staining Solution (iNtRON Biotechnology, Gyeonggi-do, Korea). We tested well-known hair-inductive markers of canine DPCs, such as alkaline phosphatase detection (ALP), Wnt inhibitory factor 1 (WIF1), laminin, vimentin, versican, and prominin-1 (1, 8, 13, 15, 24). Glyceraldehyde 3-phosphate de hydrogenase was used as the reference gene.

Western Blot

The cell and tissue extracts were prepared using the PRO-PREP™ protein extraction solution (iNtRON Biotechnology, Gyeonggi-do, Korea).

Protein samples were run on a 10% sodium dodecyl sulfate (SDS)-polyacrylamide gel, transferred onto a nitrocellulose membrane, and incubated with an anti-human versican (VCAN) antibody (R&D systems, Minneapolis, MN, USA), anti-laminin antibody (ab11575, Abcam, Cambridge, MA, USA), and anti-vimentin antibody (ab8069, Abcam, Cambridge, MA, USA). An anti-beta actin antibody was used (sc-47778, Santa Cruz Biotechnologiy, Paso Robles, CA, USA) as an internal control. Blots were then incubated with a peroxidase-conjugated secondary antibody and visualized using a Novex® ECL Chemiluminescent Substrate Reagent Kit (ECL, Novex®, Grand Island, Life Technologies, NY, USA).

Statistical Analysis

A student's *t*-test was used for comparing the size between the canine DPCs and DPLTs. A value of $p<0.05$ was considered to be statistically significant. The statistical analyses were performed using GraphPad Prism version 6.00 for Windows (GraphPad Software, La Jolla, CA, USA).

RESULTS

Morphological and cultural characteristics of actual canine DPs and DPCs

The DPs were teardrop-shaped (Fig. 1a). Their approximate sizes were measured and compared with those of DPLTs (Fig. 1b). The mean actual canine DP maximal width was 265.8 ± 11.50 μm. The first outgrowth of dermal papilla cells presented after five days, and the cells had a flattened, polygonal morphology (Fig. 1c) with multiple cytoplasmic processes. We also observed the aggregative growth pattern in the multi-layer culture with the formation of the pseudo-papillae (Fig. 1d) and cells formed multilayered conglomerates on day 8.

Reconstruction of the DPLTs

After the cell detach-attach process, cell aggregates were formed within five days. The mean DPLT size was 296 ± 12.43 μm, and there was no statistical difference when compared to actual DP size ($p = 0.1465$) (Fig. 1e). Various factors affected DPLT formation; of these, cell inoculation density was one of the most prominent factors. We tried DPLT formation with different cell inoculation densities, from 2.0×10^4 cells/cm^2 to 8.0×10^4 cells/cm^2. It was found that the optimal inoculation cell density was from 6.0×10^4 cells/cm^2 to 8.0×10^4 cells/cm^2 (data not shown). Cell migration only occurred in densities lower than 2.0×10^4 cells/cm^2. Even though significant aggregation was observed from a density of 4.0×10^4 cells/cm^2, in the optimal density, the number of DPLTs was higher and the sizes were more regular than those of DPLTs in a density of 4.0×10^4 cells/cm^2.

Evaluating DPLTs as an alternative to DPs

We performed RT-PCR and Western blotting to evaluate molecular similarities between DPLTs and DPs. Well-known hair-inductive markers, as previously mentioned, were assessed for evaluating the hair-inductive abilities of three groups on a genetic level. In addition, we assessed the quantitative protein expression level with laminin, vimentin and versican.

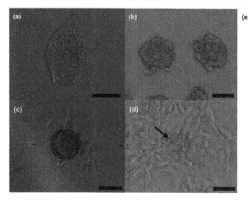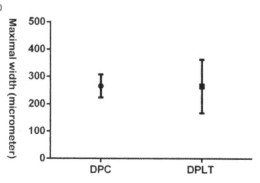

Figure 1. Dermal papilla (DP), cultured dermal papilla cells (DPCs) and dermal papilla-like tissues (DPLTs) (a). Isolated DP (200X) (b). Reconstructed DPLTs from canine AD-MSCs (100X) (c). Primary DPCs culture. The first outgrowth cell was seen on day 5 (100X) (d). Typical multilayered, aggregative DPC growth pattern and the formation of pseudopapaillae (arrow) (100X) (e). Comparison of DPs and DPLTs: There was no statistically significant difference in the maximal width between two groups

According to previous studies, ALP was used as an indicator for hair inductivity (6, 15), and versican was expressed in anagen hair follicles but absent in telogen hair follicles. This might support the idea that DP played an important role in anagen induction and maintenance (15, 24). WIF1, vimentin and laminin were related to signal transduction, cellular junction and cytoskeleton, and extracellular matrix and cell adhesion of DPs, respectively (12). In previous studies, WIF1 was considered to positively relate to *in vivo* murine hair-inductive capacity and was significantly over-represented in freshly isolated canine DPs (1, 6, 11, 13). Vimentin is known for the functions of promoting the proliferation of DPCs and increasing cell migration and growth factor expression and laminin plays an important role in promoting DP development and function during early hair morphogenesis (25).

RT-PCR analysis revealed that AD-MSCs, DPCs, and DPLTs expressed all markers as mentioned above (Fig. 2). In western blotting, all three groups showed similar versican expression level, which was reflected by their hair-inducing ability. However, we also observed that vimentin and laminin had a higher level of expression in DPCs and DPLTs compared to AD-MSCs (Fig. 3), which might mean that DPLTs have higher hair inductivity than AD-MSCs and the potential to be a viable substitute for actual DPs.

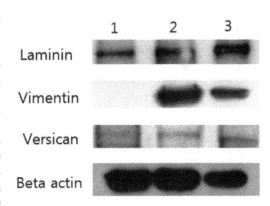

Figure 3. Western blot of reconstructed DPLTs. Lane 1, monolayer cultured canine AD-MSCs (third passage). Lane 2, third passage of cultured canine DPCs. Lane 3, DPLTs reconstructed from third passage canine AD-MSCs. Vimentin and laminin had a higher level of expression in DPC and DPLT than in AD-MSCs

DISCUSSION

Limited research has been done on canine hair follicles, and our understanding of hair follicles in veterinary and human medicine relies heavily on murine studies (14, 15, 26). Not only are canine primary anagen hair follicles morphologically analogous to human anagen hair follicles in terms of size and structure but dogs also develop most major human alopecia (2, 27). Therefore, canine hair follicles could be a helpful model for the investigation of human hair follicle biology.

There have been many trials and successes of regeneration of hair with epidermal and dermal components, both *in vitro* and *in vivo* (15). Yoo et al. (23) also observed hair regeneration on the scalps of mice through transplantation of epidermal and mesenchymal compartments. The difference was that they applied aggregates from human umbilical cord-derived mesenchymal stem cells as an alternative to the dermal components comparing to former studies.

DP plays an important role not only in regulating hair follicle development and growth, but also as a reservoir of mesenchymal stem cells. Driskell et al. (27) noted that DPC expansion and generation might be one way of strategically treating alopecia. However, cultured DPCs lose their trichogenic properties in vitro after few passages (15, 27, 28). Reconstructing DPLTs is one of the ways to overcome that limitation.

In this study, we found that the expression level of hair-inductive markers and proteins between

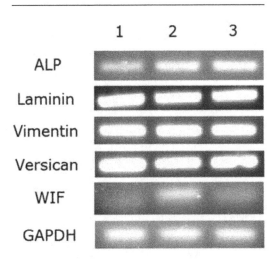

Figure 2. RT-PCR of reconstructed DPLTs. Lane 1, monolayer cultured canine AD-MSCs (third passage). Lane 2, third passage of cultured canine DPCs. Lane 3, DPLTs reconstructed from the third-passage canine AD-MSCs. Hair-inductive markers, ALP, WIF1, laminin, vimentin, versican, and prominin-1, were similarly expressed in all three groups

DPCs and DPLTs showed similar patterns, which suggested that cell aggregates reconstructed from AD-MSCs might be excellent substitutes for actual DPs. DPLTs may have the potential to be a key structure in a future treatment method of alopecia that does not respond to medical treatments, and in auto-transplantations. We may also consider a new trial to treat alopecia in veterinary medicine.

In previous study, it was demonstrated that AD-MSC, which had various cytokine-secreting properties and paracrine functions, showed an effect on hair growth by promoting the survival and proliferation of DPCs (29). In addition, Osada et al. (30) demonstrated that aggregates made from later passage DPCs (more than 10 passages) did induce new hair follicles unlike dissociated DPCs that lost their hair follicle-inducing ability at later passage (over passage 4). Considering the results of previous and present studies, we cautiously speculate that DPLTs would have a direct effect on hair re-growth as an alternative structure of DPs and show analogous behavior patterns *in vivo* or under epidermal-mesenchymal interactions (EMIs) compared to dissociated AD-MSCs.

In the culture of canine DPCs, they showed a typical growth pattern and morphology, as in previous studies (1, 21, 30). We hypothesized that early-passage canine DPCs cultured in AminioMAX had the same capacity for hair induction as canine DPs, based on previous studies (1, 21). We used third-passage DPCs and observed their aggregative culture patterns. In the DP microdissection procedures, we selected late-anagen-phase hair follicles based on morphological criteria; to make the procedures simple, we chose large hair follicles, which could explain why DP sizes were measured larger than expected.

In conclusion, in this study, we reconstructed canine DPLTs with AD-MSCs, which are a more easily accessible source than other mesenchymal stem cells and DPCs, and evaluated them as alternatives to canine DPs. We believe that DPLTs may form the basis of potential therapeutic applications. However, further investigations on DPLTs under active EMIs or *in vivo* should be performed.

ACKNOWLEDGMENTS

This research was supported by the Basic Science Research Program of the National Research Foundation of Korea (NRF), funded by the Ministry of Education, Science and Technology (2013-011357).

REFERENCES

1. Kobayashi, T., Fujisawa, A., Amagai, M., Iwasaki, T., Ohyama, M. (2011). Molecular biological and immunohistological characterization of canine dermal papilla cells and the evaluation of culture conditions. Vet Dermatol, 22(5): 414-422. http://dx.doi.org/10.1111/j.1365-3164.2011.00964.x PMid:21410799

2. Tobin, D., Gardner, S., Luther, P., Dunston, S., Lindsey, N., Olivry, T. (2003). A natural canine homologue of alopecia areata in humans. Br J Dermatol, 149(5): 938-950. http://dx.doi.org/10.1111/j.1365-2133.2003.05610.x PMid:14632797

3. Al-Refu, K. (2012). Stem cells and alopecia: a review of pathogenesis. Br J Dermatol, 167(3): 479-484. http://dx.doi.org/10.1111/j.1365-2133.2012.11018.x PMid:22533551

4. Yoo, BY., Shin, YH., Yoon, HH., Seo, YK., Song, KY., Park, JK. (2010). Optimization of the reconstruction of dermal papilla like tissues employing umbilical cord mesenchymal stem cells. Biotechnol Bioprocess Eng, 15(1): 182-190. http://dx.doi.org/10.1007/s12257-009-3050-z

5. Yoo, BY., Shin, YH., Yoon, HH., Seo, YK., Song, KY., Park, JK. (2010). Application of mesenchymal stem cells derived from bone marrow and umbilical cord in human hair multiplication. J Dermatol Sci, 60(2): 74-83. http://dx.doi.org/10.1016/j.jdermsci.2010.08.017 PMid:20956069

6. Mc Elwee, KJ., Kissling, S., Wenzel, E., Huth, A., Hoffmann, R. (2003). Cultured peribulbar dermal sheath cells can induce hair follicle development and contribute to the dermal sheath and dermal papilla. J Invest Dermatol, 121(6): 1267-1275. http://dx.doi.org/10.1111/j.1523-1747.2003.12568.x PMid:14675169

7. Yoo BY, Shin YH, Yoon HH, Kim YJ, Song KY, Hwang SJ, et al. (2007). Improved isolation of outer root sheath cells from human hair follicles and their proliferation behavior under serum-free condition. Biotechnol Bioprocess Eng;12(1):59. http://dx.doi.org/10.1007/BF02931804

8. Gledhill, K., Gardner, A., Jahoda, CA. (2013). Isolation and establishment of hair follicle dermal papilla cell cultures. Methods Mol Biol, 989, 285-292. http://dx.doi.org/10.1007/978-1-62703-330-5_22 PMid:23483403

9. Chuong, CM. (2007). Regenerative biology: new hair from healing wounds. Nature 447(7142): 265-266. http://dx.doi.org/10.1038/447265a PMid:17507966; PMCid:PMC4377231

10. Ito, M., Yang, Z., Andl, T., Cui, C., Kim, N., Millar, SE., et al. (2007). Wnt-dependent de novo hair follicle regeneration in adult mouse skin after wounding. Nature 447(7142): 316-320.
http://dx.doi.org/10.1038/nature05766
PMid:17507982

11. Kishimoto, J., Burgeson, RE., Morgan, BA. (2000). Wnt signaling maintains the hair-inducing activity of the dermal papilla. Genes Dev, 14(10): 1181-1185.
PMid:10817753; PMCid:PMC316619

12. Rendl, M., Lewis, L., Fuchs, E. (2005). Molecular dissection of mesenchymal–epithelial interactions in the hair follicle. PLoS Biol, 3(11):e331.
http://dx.doi.org/10.1371/journal.pbio.0030331
PMid:16162033; PMCid:PMC1216328

13. Rendl, M., Polak, L., Fuchs, E. (2008). BMP signaling in dermal papilla cells is required for their hair follicle-inductive properties. Genes Dev, 22(4): 543-557.
http://dx.doi.org/10.1101/gad.1614408
PMid:18281466; PMCid:PMC2238674

14. Schneider, MR., Schmidt-Ullrich, R., Paus, R. (2009). The hair follicle as a dynamic miniorgan. Curr Biol, 19(3): R132-142.
http://dx.doi.org/10.1016/j.cub.2008.12.005
PMid:19211055

15. Yang, CC., Cotsarelis, G. (2010). Review of hair follicle dermal cells. J Dermtol Sci, 57(1): 2-11.
http://dx.doi.org/10.1016/j.jdermsci.2009.11.005
PMid:20022473; PMCid:PMC2818774

16. Schlake, T. (2007). Determination of hair structure and shape. Semin Cell Dev Biol, 18(2): 267-273.
http://dx.doi.org/10.1016/j.semcdb.2007.01.005
PMid:17324597

17. Kim, H., Choi, K., Kweon, OK., Kim, WH. (2012). Enhanced wound healing effect of canine adipose-derived mesenchymal stem cells with low-level laser therapy in athymic mice. J Dermatol Sci, 68(3): 149-156.
http://dx.doi.org/10.1016/j.jdermsci.2012.09.013
PMid:23084629

18. Ryu, HH., Lim, JH., Byeon, YE. et al. (2009). Functional recovery and neural differentiation after transplantation of allogenic adipose-derived stem cells in a canine model of acute spinal cord injury. J Vet Sci, 10(4): 273-284.
http://dx.doi.org/10.4142/jvs.2009.10.4.273
PMid:19934591; PMCid:PMC2807262

19. Müntener, T., Doherr, MG., Guscetti, F., Suter, MM., Welle, MM. (2011). The canine hair cycle– a guide for the assessment of morphological and immunohistochemical criteria. Vet Dermatol, 22(5): 383-395.
http://dx.doi.org/10.1111/j.1365-3164.2011.00963.x
PMid:21401741

20. Warren, R., Chestnut, MH., Wong, TK., Otte, TE., Lammers, KM., Meili, ML. (1992). Improved method for the isolation and cultivation of human scalp dermal papilla cells. J Invest Dermatol, 98(5): 693-699.
http://dx.doi.org/10.1111/1523-1747.ep12499909
PMid:1569320

21. Bratka-Robia, CB., Mitteregger, G., Aichinger, A., Egerbacher, M., Helmreich, M., Bamberg, E. (2002). Primary cell culture and morphological characterization of canine dermal papilla cells and dermal fibroblasts. Vet Dermatol, 13(1): 1-6.
http://dx.doi.org/10.1046/j.0959-4493.2001.00276.x
PMid:11896964

22. Magerl, M., Kauser, S., Paus, R., Tobin, DJ. (2002). Simple and rapid method to isolate and culture follicular papillae from human scalp hair follicles. Exp Dermatol, 11(4): 381-385.
http://dx.doi.org/10.1034/j.1600-0625.2002.110414.x
PMid:12190949

23. Yoo, BY., Shin, YH., Yoon, HH., Kim, YJ., Seo, YK. (2009). Evaluation of human umbilical cord-derived mesenchymal stem cells on in vivo hair inducing activity. J Tissue Eng Regen Med, 6(1): 15-22.

24. Soma, T., Tajima, M., Kishimoto, J. (2005). Hair cycle-specific expression of versican in human hair follicles. J Dermatol Sci, 39(3): 147-154.
http://dx.doi.org/10.1016/j.jdermsci.2005.03.010
PMid:15871917

25. Kobayashi, T., Shimizu, A., Nishifuji, K., Amagai, M., Iwasaki, T., Ohyama, M. (2009). Canine hair-follicle keratinocytes enriched with bulge cells have the highly proliferative characteristic of stem cells. Vet Dermatol, 20(5-6): 338-346.
http://dx.doi.org/10.1111/j.1365-3164.2009.00815.x
PMid:20178470

26. Osada, A., Iwabuchi, T., Kishimoto, J., Hamazaki, TS., Okochi, H. (2007). Long-term culture of mouse vibrissal dermal papilla cells and de novo hair follicle induction. Tissue Eng, 13(5): 975-982.
http://dx.doi.org/10.1089/ten.2006.0304
PMid:17341162

27. Gao, J., DeRouen, MC., Chen, C-H., Nguyen, M., Nguyen, NT., Ido, H., et al. (2008). Laminin-511 is an epithelial message promoting dermal papilla development and function during early hair morphogenesis. Genes Dev, 22(15): 2111-2124.
http://dx.doi.org/10.1101/gad.1689908
PMid:18676816; PMCid:PMC2492752

28. Driskell, RR., Clavel, C., Rendl, M., Watt, FM. (2011). Hair follicle dermal papilla cells at a glance. J Cell Sci, 124(8): 1179-1182.
http://dx.doi.org/10.1242/jcs.082446
PMid:21444748; PMCid:PMC3115771

29. Ehama, R., Ishimatsu-Tsuji, Y., Iriyama, S., Ideta, R., Soma, T., Yano, K., et al. (2007). Hair follicle regeneration using grafted rodent and human cells. J Invest Dermatol, 127(9): 2106-2115. http://dx.doi.org/10.1038/sj.jid.5700823 PMid:17429436

30. Won, CH., Kwon, OS., Sung, MY. et al. (2010). Hair growth promoting effects of adipose tissue-derived stem cells. J Dermatol Sci, 57, 132-146. http://dx.doi.org/10.1016/j.jdermsci.2009.10.013 PMid:19963355

20

TICK POPULATION IN GOATS AND SHEEP IN ŠABAC

Ivan Pavlović[1], Snežana Ivanović[1], Aleksandar Dimitrić[2], Mensur Vegara[3],
Ana Vasić[4], Slavica Živković[5], Bojana Mijatović[5]

[1]*Scientific Veterinary Institute of Serbia, V. Toze 14, 11000 Belgrade, Serbia*
[2]*Agrimatco DOO, Narodnog Fronta 73/I, 21000 Novi Sad, Serbia*
[3]*Department of International Environment and Development Studies Norwegian
University of Life Science (NMBU) Campus As, Postboks 5003, No-1432 Aas, Norway*
[4]*Faculty of Veterinary Medicine, Belgrade University, Bul.Oslobođenja 18,
11000 Belgrade, Serbia*
[5]*Agricultural School PKB, Pančevački Put 39, 11000 Krnjača-Belgrade, Serbia*

ABSTRACT

During our examination performed in the period from 2010 to 2012, we collected ticks from 52 flocks of sheep and 38 goat flocks. Ticks infestation occured in 15.97% (214/1340) of sheep and 16.93% (107/632) of goats. The result showed the presence of *Ixodes ricinus, Rhipicephalus sanguineus, R. bursa, Dermacentor marginatus, D. pictus, Haemaphysalis punctata* and *Ha. inermis*. Additional to determination of tick species during the research, the sex ratio and the monthly influence of microclimate conditions (temperature, relative humidity and precipitation quantity) on the dynamics of populations of ticks were followed. Obtained results indicate the importance of the impact of climatic factors on the population dynamics of some species of ticks as well as the dynamics and abundance of different sexes within established species of ticks.

Key words: ecological factors, goat, sheep, ticks

INTRODUCTION

Ticks are obligate haematophagous ectoparasites which have multiple adverse effects on the host organism. A particular problem is that they spread diseases to humans, domestic and wild animals, which can be reservoirs, vectors and/or transient hosts for the tick-borne pathogens (5, 12, 14, 20, 23, 35, 36, 37, 41).

Most of the tick species of the family *Ixodidae* are egsophilic and during the search for the host they inhabit open habitats. During this development, ticks go through four life stages. These stages are egg, larvae (or seed tick), nymph, and adult (1, 5). *Ixodidae* ticks mainly belong to three host life cycle

Corresponding author: Dr. Ivan Pavlović, PhD
E-mail address: dripavlovic58@gmail.com
Present address: Scientific Veterinary Institute of Serbia,
V. Toze 14, 11000 Belgrade, Serbia

group of ticks, while during each developmental stage it feeds once on a separate host and will remain attached to the host for several days (8, 43).

An important feature of the life cycle of ticks is the diapause (10, 15). Throughout diapause, a tick goes into hibernation, during which the metabolism slows (49, 50). Diapause allows ticks to survive adverse conditions, such as extreme temperatures, drought and lack of food (19).

We have taken into account the epidemiological significance of ticks, because they carry many disease pathogens that belong to the group of natural focal infections, characterized by endemic and seasonal occurrence (27, 41). That was the starting point of our investigation of domestic animals tick fauna in certain areas of Serbia. In our paper we present the tick fauna of sheep and goats from the area of Šabac (Serbia) in the 2010-2012 period.

MATERIAL AND METHODS

Sheep and goat breeds play important role in the Šabac area. Usually, they are kept in small herds of 20 to 25 animals. From early spring to late autumn, they are kept on pastures and graze on any land that is not being cultivated. It is common that flocks of goats and sheep are found on the same pastures. During the winter, goats and sheep are kept in stables. During the course of our study, we collected ticks from 52 flocks of sheep and 38 goat flocks. Ticks were collected monthly during the period from the exit to the pasture to the retreat to the barn (March to October). All specimens were placed into glass specimen bottles which had a piece of hard paper inserted bearing the name of locality, name of host and date and hour of collection. The tick species and sex/gender were identified by morphometric characteristics (24, 25, 47).

The data obtained wase analyzed using Chi-square test (χ^2) to determinate if the tick species and the prevalence of infection with ticks depended on the host animal species. For all analyses, the confidence level was kept at 95%.

Our studies were carried out in the period from March 2010 to November 2012 in the municipality of Šabac, which is located at 44° 46' northern latitude and 19° 41' east longitude and is in the western part of Serbia. Morphologically, the municipality of Šabac has three natural zones. North of the town there is a vast plain area known as Mačva where lowland humus is the dominant soil type. The second morphological unit constitutes the western part of the territory of the municipality of Šabac, which is characterized by a hilly relief - the Pocerina area, where the plain area Mačva gradually turns into a hilly area down to the Cer Mountain, where the relief and forest caused degradation and evolution of lowland soils into brown forest soil. The third morphological unit covers the southeastern part and

pressure occurs in the coldest month of January, while the lowest in April. In this area winds blow from all quadrants. On windless periods as waste 1/3 the frequency of occurrence of winds. The mean air temperature in Šabac is around 11,7°C. Humidity is on average 78-92% in winter and 51-63% in summer. The annual precipitation is about 435 l/m2. Insolation increases from January to July and then decreases until December (official data by the Hydrometeorological Service of Serbia).

The climatic vegetation zones in this area correspond to the vegetation that is usually found on the territory of Serbia, such as forests of Hungarian oak (*Quercus confestim*), oak oak (*Quercus*) and beech (*Fagetum montanuum*), while in the underwater terrain we commonly encounter poplar (*Populus alba)* and white willow *(Salicerum alba)*. With regards to bushes and low trees the most common are: mandrel *(Prunus spinosa)*, hawthorn *(Scataegus monogyna)*, wild service tree *(Sorbus aria)* and maple *(Acer compestere)*. From the terrestrial plants, most common are: meadow fescue *(Festuca pratensis)*, meadow grass *(Poa pratensis)*, couch grass *(Agropyrum repens)*, couch grass without awns *(Bromus inermis)*, sheep fescue *(Festuca ovina)*, French ryegrass *(Arrhenatherum elatius)*, red clover *(Trifolium pratense)*, common vetch *(Vicia sativa)* and meadow pea *(Lathyrus sativa)* (21, 22).

RESULTS

During our examination we examined 1.340 sheep and 632 goats (Table 1).

Table 1. Number of examined sheep and goats in the period 2010-2012

host	Examined animals / years			Total
	2010.	2011.	2012.	
Sheep	502	486	352	1.340
Goats	215	246	171	632

it represents Posavina - the river valley along the right bank of the Sava River water intersected by former backwaters. There the most common type of soil is sandy black soil, which appears as a young Pedogenic creation and is most frequently found in the bottomlands of major rivers (2).

The municipality of Šabac has a continental climate. On the north side, Šabac is widely open to the Srem and therefore in terms of climate is strongly influenced by the Panonian continental climate. This climate is characterized by cold winters and warm, dry summers. The highest air

Tick infestation has occured in 15.97% (214/1340) of sheep and 16.93% (107/632) of goats. The results showed presence of *Ixodes ricinus, Rhipicephalus sanguineus, R. bursa, Dermacentor marginatus, D. pictus, Haemaphysalis punctata* and *Ha. inermis.* Their prevalence is presented in Table 2.

Relative abundance analysis revealed that the *I. ricinus* was absolutely dominant species in sheep, followed by *Rhipicephalus bursa, R. sanguineus, Haemaphysalis punctata, Dermacentor marginatus* and *D. pictus* and *Ha. inermis*. Similar fauna of ticks

Table 2. Percent of sheep and goats infected with ticks in the period 2010-2012

Tick species	Examined animals					
	sheep's			goats		
	total	infected	%	total	infected	%
Ixodes ricinus	1340	214	15.97	632	107	16.93
Rhipicephalus sanguineus	1340	112	8.35	632	34	0.53
Rhipicephalus bursa	1340	209	15.59	632	101	15.98
Dermacentor marginatus	1340	98	7.31	632	19	3.00
Dermacentor pictus	1340	87	6.49	632	7	1.10
Haemaphysalis punctata	1340	101	7.53	632	21	3.32
Haemaphysalis inermis	1340	4	0,29	632	2	0.31

was found in goats, since the herds of goats graze at the same pasture areas with herds of sheep.

The chi-square test showed there was a diference present between sheep and goats with regards to the prevalence and intensity of infection with *R. sanguineus, Ha. punctata, D. marginatus* and *D. pictus* (Fig. 1).

Ixodes ricinus reached maximum abundance in May, in which we also found the maximum occurrence of the species *Dermacentor pictus*. In June, the population peak is observed for the species *Rhipicephalus sanguineus* and *Rhipicephalus bursa*, which are the most common types both in July and August. In September, we saw an increase in the

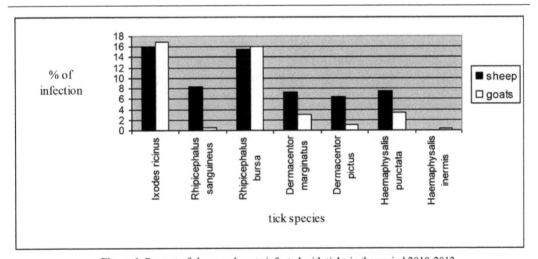

Figure 1. Percent of sheep and goats infected with ticks in the period 2010-2012

Population dynamics of the established species of ticks can be observed every year from March to October. No sampling took place from November to February, therefore their presence in nature cannot be confirmed. During the three years of examination, in the month of March the following types of ticks were found: *Ixodes ricinus, Rhipicephalus sanguineus, Dermacentor marginatus* and *Haemaphysalis punctata*. In April, we observed the occurrence of the following species: *Dermacentor pictus, Rhipicephalus bursa* and *Haemaphysalis inermis*. In April, species that reached maximum numbers were *Dermacentor marginatus, Haemaphysalis punctata* and *Haemaphysalis inermis*. Species

population of two species of ticks: *Ixodes ricinus* and *Dermacentor marginatus*, while in October we observed the emergence of the following species: *Haemaphysalis punctata* and *Ha. Inermis*, and *Rhipicephalus sanguineus* and *R. bursa*.

According to the Chi-square test for averages of the three year sampling periods, there is no significant difference between population dynamics of tick species infection with sheep and goats.

Overall, the female-male ratio during the course of our study was 61.02% : 38.98% in favor of females, with a higher percentage of females established in all three years of research. The ratio of males and females of the same species is

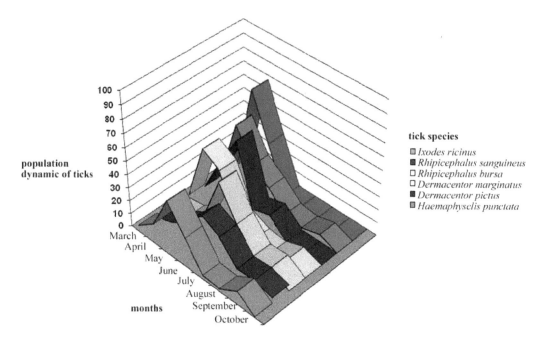

Figure 2. Population dynamics of the established species of ticks by months in the period 2010-2012

also interesting. Of the seven species established, a greater number of males than females (65.08% : 34.92%) occurred only in the species *Rhipicephalus bursa*, while for the other six species we established a larger number of females. For the two most commonly found species *Rhipicephalus sanguineus* and *Ixodes ricinus*, this ratio was 69.50%: 30.50% and 63.42%: 36.58%, respectively in favor of females.

DISCUSSION

Comparison of the obtained results with findings in other regions of Serbia indicated that there is a great similarity in the established tick species. Examination performed in the Belgrade area established *I. ricinus. R. sanguineus, D. pictus* and *D. marginatus* as the most abundant species (12, 31, 32, 40, 44).

Results obtained during the examination of the tick fauna of sheep and goats in the northeastern, eastern and western part of Serbia showed that *Ixodes ricinus* and *Dermacentor marginatus* are the dominant tick species in those areas (31, 34, 35, 44, 46). Examination performed in sheep in the Prizren district (Kosovo) during 1991 (39) pointed to the presence of the same tick species, including *Hy. savignyi, Ha. inermis, Boophilus calcaratus* and *Ornythonisus lachorenis*. The latest examination conducted during 2013 in the Kumanovo area

(Macedonia) established that most abudant in sheep were *Ixodes ricinus,* followed by *Dermacentor marginatus, Rhipicephalus sanguineus, R. bursa, Haemaphysalis punctata* and *D. pictus* (45). During all the examinations, *Ixodes ricinus* was the most abundant tick species insheep and goats. The found species of ticks are most common in sheep and goats in the regions of the Western Balkans, Mediterranean and Central Europe (14, 16, 25, 27, 28, 37, 38, 48).

Climate conditions have a great influence on the population dynamics of ticks. Population dynamics of ticks is related to the impact of climate factors like air temperature, relative humidity and rainfall (32, 49).

Our results confirmed the results of the studies carried out in northeast, eastern and south-eastern Serbia (29, 33, 34) which established that *I. ricinus* was by far the most abundant species with the largest number of specimens collected in the spring at a temperature of about 15°C, relative humidity of 76.00% and rainfall of 81.11 l/m^2. March marks the start of, the increase in the number of *Haemaphysalis* (*punctata* and *inermis*) species, whilesimilar results were obtained during examination in France (26), Romania (28) and in Macedonia (45). April is the month of greatest abundance of *D. marginatus, Haemaphysalis punctata* and *Ha. inermis* which reached their peak at a temperature of 9.01° C, relative humidity of 75.66% and rainfall of 35.80 and 36.06 mm/m^2.

This data is in correlation with the results of other examinations of the seasonal dynamics of ticks in Europe (3, 6, 9, 11, 17, 29, 37). Similar values were obtained during research in Serbia (12, 41), France (26), Italy (27, 38) and in a Berlin forest (11). The authors point out that the low temperature, high humidity and rainfall significantly affect the life cycle of ticks, particularly the *I. ricinus* species (20, 28, 46). Same results were obtained worldwide e.g. in coastal areas of New York (7) and in South Africa (18, 20). Both studied the temperature below which the activity of ticks is completely stopped and the temperature at which it expressed its full activity and found a significant relationship of tick activities and the degree of reduction of temperature for adult forms. This agrees with the data published about ticks in various part of Russia, Central Europe and the West Balkans (4, 12, 13, 14, 20, 21, 25, 26, 29, 31).

The female abundance of established tick species has been in correlation with previously established population dynamics. The females of *Ixodes ricinus* species were present from March to October, with a peak population in May and June. Females of two species of the genus *Rhipicephalus* (*sanguineus* and *bursa*) have been found most often in the summer months - June and July. Findings of the females of species *Dermacentor marginatus* and *Haemaphysalis punctata* were most common in April and May, while sporadic finding of females of *Dermacentor pictus* and *Haemaphysalis inermis* species was attached to the spring months. This population dynamics of female ticks is characteristic for this microclimate (3, 8, 9, 15).

Males of the species *Ixodes ricinus* were found from March to October, with the spring peak population in May and autumnal in September which corresponds to the values obtained in our earlier research (12, 17). Males of the species *Rhipicephalus sanguineus* were established from March to October, a species *Rhipicephalus bursa* from April to September with a population peak of both species in June, which also corresponds to values for this geographical area (28, 30, 32, 38). Males of the two species of the genus *Dermacentor* (*marginatus* and *pictus*) were usually found from April to June, while the males of *Haemaphysalis punctata* species were established from April to June. A small number of males of *Haemaphysalis inermis* was found only in April which corresponds to values of research in this area and in Central Europe and the Mediterranean basin (16, 20, 35, 42, 47).

CONCLUSION

Being the vectors and reservoirs for many endemic tickborne pathogens, the tick transmit diseases that cause health disturbance in domestic animals and humans in affected areas.

The occurence of tick born diseases in this species is usual during the exposure time period. The population dynamics and the climatic factors that influence the tick population need to be studied in order to predict the critical points and implement adequate protection measures in animals with the final goal of disease prevention and control.

ACKNOWLEDGEMENT

Paper is accomplished as a part of scientific and technological project BT 31053 of the Ministry of Education, Science and Technical Development of Republic of Serbia

REFERENCES

1. Anderson, J.F., Magnarelli, L.A. (2008). Biology of ticks. Infect Dis Clin North Am. 22 (2): 195-215. http://dx.doi.org/10.1016/j.idc.2007.12.006 PMid:18452797

2. Anonimus (2015). Geografski Atlas. Republički geodetski zavod. Beograd.

3. Babenko, L.V. (1974). Sutočnie kolebanija aktivnosti golodnih nimf Ixodes ricinus L. i Ixodes persulcatus P. SCH (Parazitiformes: Ixodidae). Med. Parazitol. Parazit. Bolezn. 42, 520-527.

4. Babenko, L.V., Arumova, E.A., Bush, M.A., Skadinsh, E.A. (1977). O sootonošenii polov v prirodnih populaciah imago Ixodes ricinus L. i Ixodes perculacatus P. SCH (Ixodidea, Ixodidae). Med. Parazitol. Parazit. Bolezn. 46, 294-301.

5. Belozerow, V.N. (1982). Diapausa and biological rhythms in ticks. In: F.D.Obenchain and R.Galun (Ed.), Physiology of ticks, 1st edition (pp.469-500). Oxford: Pergamon Press. http://dx.doi.org/10.1016/B978-0-08-024937-7.50018-4

6. Carrol, J.F., Kramer, M. (2003). Winter activity of Ixodes scapularis (Acari: Ixodidae) and the operation of deer-targeted tick control devices in Mryland. J.Med.Entomol. 40, 238-244. http://dx.doi.org/10.1603/0022-2585-40.2.238

7. Clark, D.D. (1995). Lower temperature limits for activity of several Ixodid ticks (Acari: Ixodidae): effects of body size and rate of temperature change. J.Med.Entomol. 32, 449 - 452. http://dx.doi.org/10.1093/jmedent/32.4.449 PMid:7650705

8. Černy, V., Daniel, M., Rosicky, B. (1974). Some features of developmental cycle of the tick Ixodes ricinus L. (Acarina, Ixodidae). Folia Parasitol. 21, 85-87.

9. Černy, V., Szymanski, S., Dusbabek. F., Daniel. M., Hozakova, E. (1982). Survival of unfed Dermacentor recitulatus adults under natural conditions. Wiadom. Parasitol. 28, 27-31.

10. Daniel, M. (1978). Microclimate as a determining element in the distribution of ticks and their developmental cycles. Folia Parasitol. 25, 91-94.

11. Dautel, H., Dippel, C., Kammer, D., Werkhausen, A., Kahl, O. (2008). Winter activity of Ixodes ricinus in a Berlin forest. Int. Med. Microbiol. 298, 50-54. http://dx.doi.org/10.1016/j.ijmm.2008.01.010

12. Dimitrić, A. (1999). Fauna i ekologija krprelja (Acari:Ixodidae) kao prenosioca metazoonoza. MSc thesis, Faculty of Veterinary Medicine University in Belgrade, Serbia

13. Duffy, D.C., Campbell, S.R. (1994). Ambient air temperature as a predictor of activity of adult Ixodes scapularis (Acari: Ixodidae). J. Med. Entomol. 31, 178-180. http://dx.doi.org/10.1093/jmedent/31.1.178 PMid:8158624

14. Dumitrache, M.O., Gherman, C.M., Cozma, V., Mircean, V., Györke, A., Sándor, A.D., Mihalca, A.D. (2012). Hard ticks (Ixodidae) in Romania: surveillance, host associations, and possible risks for tick-borne diseases. Parasitol.Res. 110, 2067-2070. http://dx.doi.org/10.1007/s00436-011-2703-y PMid:22033737

15. Dyk, V., Boučkova, L. (1968). Die Temperature -Feuchte-Relation in der Aktivitat des gemeinen Holzbocks. Angew Parasitol. 9, 83-87.

16. Estrada-Pe-a, A., Martinez Avilez, M., Mu-oz Reoyo, M.J. (2011). A population model to describe the distribution and sesonal dynamics of the ticks Hyalomma marginatus in the Mediterranean basin. Transbound. Emerg. Dis. 58, 213-223. http://dx.doi.org/10.1111/j.1865-1682.2010.01198.x PMid:21223534

17. Fourie, L.J., Horak, I.G., Mrais, L. (1988). The seasonal abundance of adult Ixodid ticks on Merino sheep in the Soulth-Western Orange Free State. J.S.A.V.A. 59,191-194.

18. Fourie, L.J., Horak, I.G. (1991). The seasonal activity of adult Ixodid ticks on Angora goats in the Soulth-Western Orange Free State. J.S.A.V.A. 62, 104-106.

19. Harlan, H.J., Foster, W.A. (1990). Micrometeorologic factors affecting field host-seeking activity of adult Dermacentor variabilis (Acari : Ixodidae). J. Med. Entomol. 27, 471-479. http://dx.doi.org/10.1093/jmedent/27.4.471 PMid:2388223

20. Hornok, S. (2009). Allochronic seasonal peak activites of Dermacentor ond Haemaphysalis spp. Under continental climate in Hungary. Vet. Parasitol. 163, 366-369. http://dx.doi.org/10.1016/j.vetpar.2009.03.048 PMid:19410373

21. Janković, M. (1973). Biljni svet prirodnih ekosistema SR Srbije. SANU, referati naučnog skupa »Čovek i životna sredina«, Beograd. PMCid:PMC1423154

22. Janković, M., Pantić, N., Mišić, V., Diklić, N., Gajić,M.(1984).VegetacijaSRSrbije.SANU,Beograd. PMCid:PMC1009372

23. Jongejan, F., Uilenberg, G. (2004). The global importance of ticks. Parasitol. 129, Suppl. S3-14.

24. Kapustin, F.U. (1955). Atlas parazitov krovi životnih i klešćei iksodid. Gasudarstvenoe izdetejlstvo seljskohazjajstvenoi literaturi. Moskva PMid:13313366

25. Kolonin, G.V. (2009). Fauna of ixodid ticks of the world (Acari:Ixodidae), Moscow. http://www.kolonin.org/3.html.

26. L'Hostis, M., Dumon, H., Dorchies, B., Biosdron, F., Gorenflot, A. (1995). Seasonal incidence and ecology of the ticks Ixodes ricinus (Acari: Ixodidae) on grazing pastures in Western France. Exp. Appl. Acarol. 19, 211-220. http://dx.doi.org/10.1007/BF00130824 PMid:7641568

27. Maroli, M., Khouzy, C., Frusteri, L., Manila, G. (1996). Distribution of dogs ticks (Rhipicephalus sanguineus Latreille, 1806) in Italy: a public health problem. Ann. Inst. Super. Sanita. 23, 387-397.

28. Mihalca, A.D., Dumitrache, M.O., Magdaş, C., Gherman, C.M., Domşa, C., Mircean, V., Ghiral. V., Pocora, V., Ionescu, D.T., Sikó Barabási, S., Cozma, V., Sándor, A.D. (2012). Synopsis of the hard ticks (Acari: Ixodidae) of Romania with update on host associations and geographical distribution. Exp. Appl. Acarol. 58, 183-206. http://dx.doi.org/10.1007/s10493-012-9566-5 PMid:22544174

29. Milutinović, M. (1992). Ekološka istraživanja krpelja (Acarina,Ixodidea,Ixodia) Srbije, PhD disertation, Biology faculty University in Belgrade, Serbia

30. Milutinović, M., Petrović, Z., Bobić, B., Pavlović. I. (1996). Ecological notes on ticks colected in West Serbia Yugoslavia. Parasitol.Hung 29/30: 67-74.

31. Milutinović, M., Aleksić-Bakrač, N., Pavlović, I. (1997). Ticks (Acari: Ixodidae, Argasidae) in the Belgrade area. Acta. Entom. Serb. 2, 77-85.

32. Milutinović, M., Aleksić-Bakrač, N., Pavlović, I. (1998). Faunistic and ecological notes on ticks (Acari: Ixodidae,Argasidae) in the extended area of Belgrade. Mag. Allator. Lapja 120, 434-436.

33. Milutinović, M., Aleksić-Bakrač, N., Pavlović, I. (1998). Reserch of tick population (Acari: Ixodidae) in Eastern part of Serbia. Ars Vet. 14, 227-234.

34. Milutinović, M., Petrović, Z., Miščević, Z. (1987). Fauna i ekologija krpelja (Acarina, Ixodoidea, Ixodidae) severoistočnog dela SR Srbije. Zbornik V jugoslovenski konkres infektologov, (pp.140-145), Ljubljana, Yugoslavia.

35. Miščević, Z., Milutinović, M., Biševac, Lj. (1990). Tick fauna (Acarina, Ixodidea, Ixodidae) of northeast Serbia with special emphasis on the species Ixodes ricinus. Acta Vet. 40, 143-150.

36. Nieder, M., Bojkovski, J., Pavlović, I., Savić, B., Elezović, M., Silaghi, C. (2013). Studies on the occurence of granulocytic anaplasmosis in cattle and on biodiversity of vectors (ixodid ticks) in Serbia. Zbornik kratkih sadržaja 18.godišnjeg savetovanja doktora veterinarske medicine Republike Srpske sa međunarodnim učešćem, pp. 25, Teslić, Republika Srpska, BiH

37. Papazahariadou, M.G., Saridomichelakis. M.N., Koutinas, A.F., Papadopoulos. E.G., Leontides, L. (2003). Tick infestation of dogs in Thessaloniki, northern Greece. Med. Vet. Entomol. 17, 110-113. http://dx.doi.org/10.1046/j.1365-2915.2003.00404.x PMid:12680933

38. Pavlović, I., Kulišić. Z., Nešić, D., Romanić, S. (1995). Ectoparasites of sheep and goats in Prizren district. Proceeding of 3rd Internat Conference Sheep and Goat Production, (pp.101-105), Ohrid, Macedonia

39. Pavlović, I., Milutinović, M., Kulišić, Z., Dimitrić. A., Pavlović, V. (1999). Prisustvo artropoda od biomedicinskog značaja na zelenim površinama grada Beograda. Zbornik radova II Gradske konferencije o suzbijanju štetnih artropoda i glodara sa međunarodnim značajem, (pp. 81-87), Belgrade, SRYugoslavia

40. Pavlović, I., Milutinović, M, Petković, D., Terzin, V., Terzin, D. (2002). Epizootiological research of canine babesiosis in the Belgrade district. J. Protozool. Res. 12 (1-2): 10-15.

41. Pavlović, I., Savić, B., Ivetić, V., Radanović, O., Žutić, M, Jakić-Dimić, D., Bojkovski, J. (2009). The effect of parasitic infections to production results of sheep. IV Balkan Conf Animal Sci BALNIMALCON 2009, Proceeding of Challanges of the Balkan Animal industry and the Role of science and Cooperation, (pp. 389-391), Stara Zagora, Bulgaria

42. Pavlović, I., Petković, D., Kukovska, V., Stamenković. V., Jovčevski, S., Pavlović, M., Jovčevski, St., Elezović, M. (2012). Most important food-borne disease of dogs caused by ticks and its control. Proceeding of 3rd International Scientific Meeting Days of Veterinary Medicine, (pp. 34-37), Ohrid, Macedonia

43. Pavlovic, I., Ivanovic, S., Zujovic, M. (2013). Tick fauna of goat and sheep in Belgrade area. Sci Works Series C Vet Med LIX (1), 51-53.

44. Pavlović, I., Jovčevski, S., Jovčevski, St., Kukovska, V., Dimitrić, A. (2014). Tick fauna of sheep and cattle at Kumanovo arae (Macedonia). Lucr.Ştii. Med.Vet. XLVII (3), 88-95.

45. Petrović, Z., Milutinović, M., Pavlović, I. (1996). Istraživanja krpelja (Acari: Ixodidae, Argasidae) u Jugoslaviji. In. Z.Petrović (Ed.) Akademik Čedomir P. Simić, Naučni skup posvećen 100-godišnjici rođenja (pp. 96-101). Beograd: SANU Odeljenje mecidinskih nauka i Jugoslovensko društvo parazitologa

46. Pomerancev, B.L. (1950). Fauna SSSR. Paukoobraznie. Iksodidovie kleščei (Ixodidae). Akadema Nauk SSSR, Moskva-Leningrad

47. Rivosecchi, L., Khoury, C., Lezzerini, C., Dell Uomo, G. (1980). Osservazioni su Rhipicephalus sanguineus (Ixodidae) nella periferia di Roma. Riv. Parasitol. 41, 273-276.

48. Tovornik, D. (1976). Seasonal and diurnal periodicity of the tick Ixodes ricinus L. in the Pannonian tick-borne encephalitis focus (Stara Ves). JAZU, Razred za medicinske znanosti 99-103.

49. Zahler, M., Gothe, R. (1995). Effect of temperature and humidity on egg hatch, moulting and longevity of larvae and nymphs of Dermacentor reticulatus (Ixodidae). Appl. Parasitol. 36, 53 -65. PMid:7780450

21

FIRST RESULTS FROM INSEMINATION WITH SEX-SORTED SEMEN IN DAIRY HEIFERS IN MACEDONIA

Ljupche Kochoski[1], Zoran Filipov[2], Ilcho Joshevski[2], Stevche Ilievski[2], Filip Davkov[2]

[1]*Faculty of Biotechnical Sciences Bitola, University "St. Kliment Ohridski" – Bitola, Partizanska bb, 7000 Bitola, Macedonia*
[2]*ZK Pelagonija Bitola, Boris Kidrik 3, 7000 Bitola, Macedonia*

ABSTRACT

Science has been searching for a long time for a reliable method for controlling the sex of mammalian offspring. Recently, the application of specific modern cellular methodologies has led to the development of a flow cytometric system capable of differentiating and separating living X- and Y-chromosome-bearing sperm cells in amounts suitable for AI and therefore, commercialization of this sexing technology. The aim of this work was to present the first results of heifers that introduce bovine AI with sex sorted semen, for the first time in Macedonia. Insemination with sex sorted cryopreserved semen (2×10^6 spermatozoa per dose) imported from the USA was done at two dairy farms in ZK Pelagonija. In total, 74 heifers (Holstein Friesian) were inseminated. Inseminations were carried out in a timely manner following a modified OvSynch protocol. During the insemination, the sperm was deposited into the uterine horn ipsi lateral to the ovary where a follicle larger than 1.6 cm was detected by means of transrectal ultrasound examination. Pregnancy was checked by ultrasound on day 30 after the insemination. Overall, the average pregnancy rate in both farms was 43,24% (40,54% and 45,95%, for farm 1 and farm 2, respectively). All pregnant heifers delivered their calves following a normal gestation length (274,3 days in average) and of the 32 born calves, 30 (93,75%) were female. In conclusion, since the first results from inseminations with sex-sorted semen in dairy heifers in Macedonia are very promising, the introduction of this technique may bring much benefit to the local dairy sector. Average pregnancy rate seems similar with results obtained following 'regular' inseminations, notwithstanding the relatively low number of spermatozoa per insemination dose. Due to the latter, we however recommend inseminations only to be carried out by experienced technicians followinga TAI protocol and ultrasound examinations of the ovaries prior to insemination.

Key words: sperm sexing, heifer, ultrasound, artificial insemination

INTRODUCTION

For a long time, people were searching for a methodology that would be able to predetermine the sex of the offspring (13,15,16). For dairy cattle, this means production of female calves. Until recently, it was not possible to do that with a high accuracy.

In 1989, a major breakthrough in sperm sexing was reported. The USDA Beltsville Research Center group reported production of live offspring

Corresponding author: Prof. Ljupche Kochoski, PhD
E-mail address: ljupce.kocoski@uklo.edu.mk
Present address: Faculty of Biotechnical Sciences, Bitola
University "St. Kliment Ohridski" – Bitola
Partizanska bb, 7000 Bitola Macedonia

from sex-sorted, rabbit sperm (1). This was the first report of the birth of offspring of which the gender had been predetermined at conception by the use of living sperm sorted into the respective X- and Y-chromosome-bearing sperm cells. Sperm cells were stained with Hoechst 33342, sorted according to their DNA content, and subsequently deposited into the oviducts of rabbits (1). Insemination with sex-sorted Y-chromosome-bearing sperm resulted in 81% males (17/21), whereas insemination with X-chromosome-bearing sperm resulted in 94% females (15/16).

It is now possible to predetermine the sex of the offspring before fertilization in a number of species. The reported accuracy regarding the birth of offspring of the predetermined sex varies from 85 to 95% (2, 3, 4, 5).

Mature male gametes are small, haploid cells that can be accurately analyzed for DNA content because they are stable in healthy sperm. High resolution measurement of the DNA content of sperm was first achieved by flow cytometric analysis of demembranated spermatids or sperm nuclei (6, 7). The precision of this DNA measurement is such that the difference in DNA content between mammalian X- and Y-chromosome bearing sperm is detectable in a variety of species (7, 8). The initially used preparation process, however, severely damaged the sperm cells due to the aggressive removal of the tail and the membranes surrounding the nuclei prior to the staining with the membrane impermeable dye, 40-6-diamidino-2-phenylindole (DAPI) (7). It was only when the membrane permeable bisbenzimidazole DNA-binding dye, Hoechst 33342, was employed that accurate measurement of the DNA content was successfully achieved in living sperm (9). Precise measurement of the difference in DNA content between X- and Y-chromosome-bearing sperm of mammals has provided an effective means of separating viable gametes carrying either the X- or Y-chromosome with an accuracy of 85–95%. Flow cytometric sex-sorting of sperm according to their DNA content is patented (10) and has been sub-licensed for non-human mammals to XY Inc., through Colorado State University.

In domestic cattle, the chromatin of each somatic cell contains 60 chromosomes. Male gametes contain half that number because the haploid X-chromosome-bearing sperm that produces females carry 29 autosomes plus the X-chromosome. The haploid Y-chromosome-bearing sperm have the same 29 autosomes plus the male determining Y-chromosome. According to Moruzzi (11), the difference in total length of the bovine chromosomes than those from bulls and cows is approximately 4.2%.

Commercialization of sexed semen in the United States started in 2003 with a license granted to Sexing Technologies (ST). In February 2003, the first ST sexing laboratory started operations in Navasota, Texas.

Since Macedonia is still a country largely dependent on the import of female replacements for the further expansion of the dairy industry, our aim is to introduce bovine AI using sex sorted semen, in order to increase the number of internally raised heifers. The specific aim of the present paper was to report the results of the first inseminations using sex sorted semen in dairy heifers in Macedonia.

MATERIAL AND METHODS

Inseminations were performed on two dairy farms in ZK Pelagonija, using sex-sorted semen imported from the USA. As claimed by the company, each dose of sex-sorted semen contained 2.0×10^6 frozen spermatozoa. For that purpose, a total of 107 Holstein Friesian heifers were initially selected. Farms were large scale, with 500 cows each, and average milk production of 6200 liters per year. Cows and heifers in both farms are managed by routine husbandry procedures. The heifers included in the insemination schedule with sex-sorted semen were 15 months of age with at least 380 kg weight. Before the start of the estrus synchronization, all heifers were evaluated for their body development according to their age, and for ovarian functionality. Only 87 of the initially selected heifers were submitted to an OvSynch protocol before insemination with sex-sorted semen. Shortly, the protocol consisted of a basic GnRH treatment, followed by ultrasound examination (12) and PGF treatment (the latter only for heifers in which a functional CL – a CL with a diameter > 25 mm - could ultrasonographically be detected) and adding a second GnRH injection 60 hours after the PGF injection. This second GnRH injection induces ovulation of the dominant follicle recruited after PG-induced luteolysis. Before the second GnRH injection, another ultrasound examination was performed, and animals with follicles ≥ 16 mm were inseminated immediately, while the rest of them were checked again with ultrasound and inseminated at 12 hours after the second GnRH injection. Inseminations on both farms were carried out by the same experienced inseminator.

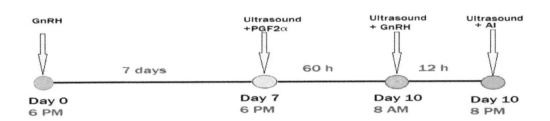

Figure 1. Modified OvSynch protocol for TAI of the heifers intended to be inseminated with sex-sorted semen

Out of 87 synchronized heifers, a total of 74 were inseminated. Heifers bearing small follicles <5 mm (n=13) on day 10 of the protocol, were considered as non-reactive to the treatment and were not inseminated. Insemination was done into the uterine horn ipsilateral to the ovary where a follicle larger than 16mm was ultrasonographically detected. Pregnancy was checked by ultrasound on day 30 after the insemination.

RESULTS

Data showing pregnancy rates for the heifers at both farms are presented in Table 1.

Reasonable pregnancy rates have been achieved with low-dose sex-sorted, cryopreserved sperm. The results varied between 25,00% to 71,43%, with individual variations within the farms from 0,00% to 71,43%. The only group with no pregnancy was on farm 1 during the winter season. We have to underline that within that group half of the prepared heifers were not inseminated due to problems with their condition or based on an unsatisfactory response to the treatment. The average conception rate for all groups was 43,24%, which is lower than the conception rate following insemination with conventional semen containing 20×10^6 spermatozoa. At the same farms, heifers inseminated with conventional semen achieved an average pregnancy rate of 63,33%.

Table 1. Total results from insemination of heifers with sex sorted semen at 2 farms in Macedonia during the period of June 2012 – March 2013

Month	Total prepared heifers	Total treated heifers	Total inseminated heifers	Total pregnant heifers	% pregnant from inseminated
June	10	10	7	5	71,43 %
October	7	7	7	3	42,85%
November	14	9	8	2	25,00%
December	12	12	12	5	41,66 %,
January	10	6	6	3	50,00%
February	31	20	15	3	42,86%
March	23	23	19	11	50,00%
Total	107	87	74	32	43,24%

Table 2. Percentage of the female calves from the calved heifers inseminated with sex-sorted semen during June 2012 – March 2013

Month	Total inseminated heifers	Total pregnant heifers	% pregnant from inseminated	Born female calves	% females
June	7	5	71,43 %	5	100%
October	7	3	42,85%	3	100%
November	8	2	25,00%	2	100%
December	12	5	41,66 %,	5	100%
January	6	3	50,00%	3	100%
February	15	3	42,86%	2	66,66%
March	19	11	50,00%	10	90,90%
Total	74	32	43,24%	30	93,75%

All the pregnant heifers delivered their calves following a normal gestation length and 30 of the 32 (93,75%) born calves were female (Table 2).

From a total of 32 pregnant heifers inseminated with sex-sorted semen, 30 gave birth to a female calf, while only 2 of the calves were males. The latter implies an accuracy of the gender prediction of 93,75% (ranged from 66,66 to 100,00%).

DISCUSSION

The results mentioned in the present report, are as predicted by the semen company (pregnancy rate >40% and >90% female calves), and are similar with results mentioned by other authors (13, 14, 17).

Seidel and Garner (13) reported on their large scale experiment (371 heifers were inseminated during 3 days) an average pregnancy rate of 53%, using two different doses of sexed spermatozoa ($1,5 \times 10^6$ and $4,5 \times 10^6$ frozen spermatozoa per insemination dose), with no significant difference.

Results from several trials conducted by XY, Inc. in Colorado (2) show that pregnancy rates with unsexed control semen were 74% at pregnancy examinations carried out at 30 to 33 d after insemination and 69% at reexaminations at 64 to 67 d after insemination. Pregnancy rates with sexed semen at 30 to 33 d after insemination ranged from 48 to 55%, but the effects of sperm concentration (1.5 vs. 3 million per straw) and semen placement (uterine horn vs. uterine body) were minimal. Pregnancy loss between 30 and 33 d and 64 and 67 d after insemination with sexed semen, ranged from 2 to 7%, and was similar to the rate observed using conventional semen. These results are similar with our results although we observed a variation in final pregnancy rates from 25,00% to 71,43 %. This rather big variation could mainly be attributed to problems with one group of the heifers. In that particular group, 18,75% of the originally selected animals were excluded even before the implementation of the OvSynch protocol, while a further 31,25% were not inseminated due to poor development of the follicles. When this group should be excluded, the pregnancy rate was on a satisfactory level. The same conclusion was obtained from Garner and Seidel (14). In their review on the history of the commercialization of sexed semen for use in cattle, they pointed out that among 25 herds, where more than 100 doses of sexed semen were used (608 - 122 inseminations/herd), conception rates averaged 48.2% and ranged from 33 to 72%. They argued that these rather large variations in results between different herds indicate that differences in management level at the herd are of decisive importance in realizing satisfactory results.

CONCLUSION

In the present paper we report the first results obtained from inseminations with sex-sorted semen in dairy heifers in Macedonia.These results are very promising and will have much benefit to the further development of the local dairy sector.

Average pregnancy rate was as could be expected taking into acountthe relatively low number of spermatozoa per insemination dose.

Due to this fact, we recommend inseminations only to be carried out by experienced technicians applying the TAI protocol and under strict ultrasound control of the ovaries prior to insemination.

REFERENCES

1. Johnson, LA., Flook, JP., Hawk, HW. (1989). Sex preselection in rabbits: live births from X and Y sperm separated by DNA and cell sorting. Biol Reprod., 41, 199–203.
http://dx.doi.org/10.1095/biolreprod41.2.199
PMid:2804212

2. Seidel, Jr GE., Schenk, JL., Herickhoff, LA., Doyle, SP., Brink, Z., Green, R.D., Cran, D.G. (1999). Insemination of heifers with sexed sperm. Theriogenology 52, 1407–1420.
http://dx.doi.org/10.1016/S0093-691X(99)00226-5

3. Welch, GR., Johnson, LA. (1999). Sex preselection: laboratory validation of the sperm sex ratio of flow-sorted X- and Y-sperm by sort reanalysis for DNA. Theriogenology 52, 1343–1352.
http://dx.doi.org/10.1016/S0093-691X(99)00221-6

4. Johnson, LA. (2000). Sexing mammalian sperm for production of offspring: the state-of-the-art. Anim. Reprod. Sci., 60–61, 93–107.
http://dx.doi.org/10.1016/S0378-4320(00)00088-9

5. Kočoski Lj., Kitanvoski D., Najdovski Z. (2011) Application of sex-sorted semen in bovine reproduction. Mac. Vet. Rev., Vol 34, No. 2, 59 - 98.

6. Otto, FJ., Hacker, U., Zante, J., Schumann, J., Göhde, W., Meistrich, ML. (1979). Flow cytometry of human sperm. Histochemistry 62, 249–254.
http://dx.doi.org/10.1007/BF00508445

7. Pinkel, D., Lake, S., Gledhill, BL., Van Dilla, MA., Stephenson, D., Watchmaker, G. (1982). High resolution DNA content measurements of mammalian sperm. Cytometry 3, 1–9.
http://dx.doi.org/10.1002/cyto.990030103
PMid:6180870

8. Garner, DL., Gledhill, BL., Pinkel, D., Lake, S., Stephenson, D., Van Dilla, MA., Johnson, LA. (1983). Quantification of the X- and Y-chromosome-bearing spermatozoa of domestic animals by flow cytometry. Biol Reprod, 28, 312–321.
http://dx.doi.org/10.1095/biolreprod28.2.312
PMid:6682341

9. Johnson, LA., Flook, JP., Look, MV. (1987). Flow cytometry of X- and Y-chromosome-bearing sperm for DNA using an improved preparation method and staining with Hoechst 33342. Gamete Res, 17, 203–212.
http://dx.doi.org/10.1002/mrd.1120170303
PMid:3507347

10. Johnson, LA. (1991). Method to preselect the sex of offspring. United States Patent #5 135, 759.

11. Moruzzi, JF. (1979). Selecting a mammalian species for the determination of X- and Y-chromosome-bearing sperm. J Reprod Fertil, 57, 319–323.
http://dx.doi.org/10.1530/jrf.0.0570319
PMid:513021

12. Atanasov, B., Mickov, Lj., Esmerov, I., Ilievska, K., Nikolovski, M., Dovenski, T. (2014). Two possibile hormonal treatment methods for inducing follicular growth in dairy cows with inactive - static ovaries. Mac Vet Rev., 37 (2): 171-177.
http://dx.doi.org/10.14432/j.macvetrev.2014.09.023

13. Seidel, Jr GE., Garner, DL. (2002). Current status of sexing mammalian spermatozoa. Reproduction 124, 733–743.
http://dx.doi.org/10.1530/rep.0.124073
PMid:12537000

14. Garner, D.L., Seidel, G.E. Jr. (2008). History of commercializing sexed semen for cattle. Theriogenology 69, 886–895.
http://dx.doi.org/10.1016/j.theriogenology.2008.01.006
PMid:18343491

15. Macedo, G. G., de Sá Filho, M. F., Sala, R. V., Mendanha, M.F., de Campos Filho, E.P., Baruselli, P.S. (2013). The use of sex-sorted sperm for reproductive programs in cattle. In Alemayehu Lemma (Ed.), Success in artificial insemination - quality of semen and diagnostics employed (pp. 39-61). Intech Open Access.
PMid:23380037

16. Klinc, P., Rath, D. (2006). Application of flow cytometrically sexed spermatozoa in different farm animal species: a review. Arch. Tierz., Dummerstorf 49(1): 41-54.

17. Otava, G. (2010). Comparative study of conception rate on heifers artificially inseminated with sexed and conventional semen. Lucrari Stiinlifice Medicina Veterinara Vol. XLIII (2), Timisoara 46-51.

22

FREE-ROAMING DOGS CONTROL ACTIVITIES IN ONE ITALIAN PROVINCE (2000-2013): IS THE IMPLEMENTED APPROACH EFFECTIVE?

Shanis Barnard[1], Matteo Chincarini[1], Lucio Di Tommaso[2],
Fabrizio Di Giulio[2], Stefano Messori[1], Nicola Ferri[1]

[1]Istituto Zooprofilattico Sperimentale dell'Abruzzo e del Molise 'G. Caporale',
Campo Boario, 64100 Teramo, Italy
[2]Servizio Sanità Animale Dipartimento di Prevenzione della ASL di Pescara,
Via Paolini 47 65100 Pescara, Italy

ABSTRACT

In Italy, standards for the management of free-roaming dogs (FRDs) are defined by regional norms, generating a high variability of approaches around the country. Despite efforts carried out by the competent authorities, FRDs are still a reality impacting upon animal health and welfare and public costs. A similar scenario can be found in many other Mediterranean and Balkan counties. Here we present 14 years of data (2000–2013) retrieved from the admission dog registry of a public shelter (PS) responsible for the collection of stray dogs from one Italian province. The aim of this retrospective study was to describe the local FRD population, identifying its source and to evaluate the effectiveness of the actions implemented by the local authorities. In the investigated period, 7,475 dogs were admitted to the PS. Despite the intense sterilisation plan (mean 381.7 sterilisations per year), the overall number of dogs entering PS did not decrease consistently across the years. Results highlighted a lack of responsibility of owners by failing to sterilise and identify their dogs and allowing intact animals to roam free, therefore producing uncontrolled and unwanted litters. The current dog population management strategy, based on both sheltering and capture-neuter-release programmes, is insufficient to tackle the straying phenomenon. Educational and sterilisation programmes should be an integral part of a successfully implemented FRD control plan. Our results provide further insight on free-roaming dog population dynamics and control systems, and may have important implications for many other local contexts across Europe trying to overcome the straying phenomenon.

Key words: dog, free-roaming, prevention, public health, shelter, welfare

INTRODUCTION

Free roaming dogs (FRDs) can represent an ecological, medical and social hazard in several ways to property, wildlife and farm animals (1). They can be reservoir of diseases transmissible to humans (zoonosis), attack people and other animals, cause accidents and can be responsible for nuisances and fouling (2, 3). Targeted actions addressing the issue are implemented by intergovernmental organisations (e.g. OIE, FAO), as well as by the European Commission and the national competent authorities (4). Despite these efforts, FRDs still raise many animal welfare and public health issues and have an impact on public costs in many countries, especially in the Mediterranean and Balkan areas (5-7). At the first OIE regional Seminar on stray dog population management for the Balkan countries for example, 60% of the represented countries reported experiencing increasing trends in national stray dog populations in the past three years and all but two reported rabies in wildlife and domestic animals (8). The OIE offers detailed and complete guidelines on how to control stray dog populations (9). However, in most countries the legislation regulating dog population management and surveillance is promulgated at national or even local level, offering a scattered and un-harmonised framework. Although the drivers are very similar, authorities provide different implementation strategies. These are established on the basis of socio-economic,

Corresponding author: Dr. Shanis Barnard, PhD
E-mail address: shanis.barnard@gmail.com
Present address: Istituto Zooprofilattico Sperimentale
dell'Abruzzo e del Molise 'G. Caporale',
Campo Boario, 64100 Teramo, Italy

cultural and political components, but an effective and univocal formula for eradicating the problem has not been found (4-6).

The Italian national framework law 281/1991 on companion animals and stray dog prevention promotes dog identification and registration, birth control actions and protects stray and abandoned animals. This law forbids the euthanasia of stray animals unless they are seriously ill, incurable or proven dangerous (10). However, this national framework law does not provide standards for the managing and keeping of stray dogs, which are defined by the Regions. This has generated a high variability of approaches around the country, as can be also found in other European countries (6). The Abruzzi Region in central Italy for example, allows trap-neuter-release (TNR) programmes on the territory, whereas other Regions do not. At the municipality level, the Local Veterinary Health Unit (LVHU) is responsible for the capture and management of FRDs. All captured animals must be hosted in the local public shelter (PS) for health screening. Facilities such as PS can function as epidemiological observatories, systematically collecting valuable information on the structure, size and characteristics of the local FRD population.

Data gathered over a period of 14 years (2000 – 2013) from the admission registry of dogs at the PS of Pescara was retrieved. Pescara province (over 300 thousand inhabitants) is located in Central Italy in the Abruzzi Region, and was used as case study to understand local dog population dynamics and to investigate if it was possible, through a retrospective analysis, to identify causes and risk factors associated with the FRDs phenomenon and to identify ameliorative solutions. Although the eradication of the straying phenomenon might be an ambitious objective, a deeper insight into the population dynamics and the identification of gaps in the actions in place can help similar local contexts to implement more targeted and effective actions, thus improving overall public health and animal welfare.

MATERIAL AND METHODS

Background information

The LVHU managing the PS included in this study is responsible for the control and management of FRDs covering 46 municipalities of the Pescara province (including Pescara municipality). According to the Italian National Institute of Statistics (ISTAT www.istat.it, 2011), the territory of action of this LVHU (1,224 km²) is divided in three areas: coastal/inland plain, hills and mountains.

The PS provides temporary housing for animals while they are checked and treated, if necessary, before deciding their destination. Dogs are caught from the streets after reports from police officers, animals' rights associations or citizens. According to the National Law 281/1991 (10), dogs in Italy have to be identified and registered. Owned dogs found roaming without a microchip are identified (with a transponder) by the shelter veterinarians before returning them, and a fine is applied to the owner following law prescriptions. Stray and abandoned animals are identified and registered, neutered and usually entrusted to rescue shelters for adoption. The regional law of Abruzzi also allows TNR programmes. Dogs under this programme are identified and registered as "community dogs" and are under the responsibility of the mayor of the municipality where the dog is released. These dogs are reintroduced to the territory under specific conditions i.e. the dog is sterilised, harmless and accepted by the community. Biting dogs which are reported for aggression, are kept under clinical (for rabies control) and behavioural observation for 10 days. They are kept either at the owner's house or if the dog is unknown, at the PS. If the dog is diagnosed as being dangerous, it has to be kept in the shelter or euthanized according to the national framework recommendations, otherwise it can be adopted or returned to its territory.

Data collection

All dogs entering the PS are registered in an electronic database, compiled by the two public veterinarians managing the facility. For this study, we retrieved the data recorded from January 2000 to December 2013. For each dog, information about sex, size, breed, age (estimate), place of capture, electronic identification, neutering/spaying status, general health status, stay time (days) and destination, were logged in. Since the shelter policy slightly changed during the investigated period, some data were not recorded across all years. When this was the case, missing data have been pointed out in the results section.

Statistical analysis

A descriptive screening of the data was carried out to investigate the variation in the variables across time or between groups of dogs entering the PS. Associations between variables were evaluated by applying the Chi-squared test and variations in time were analysed using linear regression models. Spearman correlation test was used to compare the number of caught dogs per municipality and the human population. Kruskal-Wallis test was applied to compare the dog/inhabitant ration in the different type of territory (plain, mountain, and hill). Wilcoxon test was used to compare the age of sterilised versus non-sterilised animals entering the PS. Alpha value was set for = 0.05. All analyses were carried out using R® version 2.15.3 software package for Windows 7.

RESULTS

Sex, size and breed

The total number of dogs included in the study was 7,475 and on average, the number of dogs

The dog population was represented by large (15% > 26 kg), medium (46% 16-25 kg) and small (39% <15 kg) (11) size dogs (total n=7,423).

Stay time in PS was on average 11 days (median=9 days) with the minimum being 1 day and the maximum being 195 days. After the first clinical check, dogs were either returned to their owner or sent to an adoption centre. Long stays were associated with dogs that needed surgery or special care due to severe injuries or sickness.

The majority (77%) of captured dogs were mongrels (i.e. not ascribable to any breed, n=5,643). On average 403±68.3sd (median=413.5) mongrels

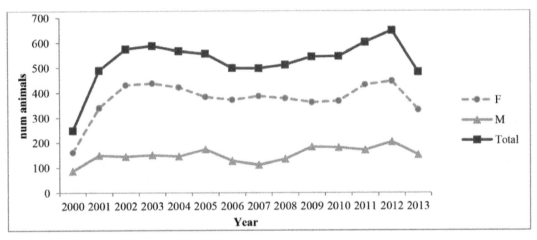

Figure 1. Number of shelter entries - Males (M), females (F) and total number of dogs entering the PS yearly between 2000 and 2013

entering the shelter annually was 530.1. In 54 cases, sex was not reported in the PS registry. Of the remaining 7,421 dogs, a higher proportion of female dogs (71%) entered the PS compared to male dogs (29%) (Fig. 1).

entered each year in similar proportion. A further 12% (n=883) were cross-breeds with a morphology clearly associated to a breed (mean±sd=62.1±30.1, median=61.5). Finally, 12% (n=865) were pure breed dogs (mean±sd=61.4±13.5, median=61.5) (see Table 1 for breeds details).

Table 1. Six most represented pure breeds and cross breeds in the sample entering the PS (proportions are calculated within each category)

Pure breed (n=883)	n	% +	Cross-breed (n=865)	n	%
German Shepherd	209	24.5%	Abruzzi Sheepdog cross	245	27.9%
Abruzzi Sheepdog	162	18.9%	German Shepherd cross	186	21.2%
Hound	83	9.7%	Hound cross	70	8.0%
Pit Bull	82	9.6%	Siberian Husky cross	44	5.0%
Rottweiler	75	8.8%	Setter cross	42	4.8%
Setter	66	7.7%	Spitz cross	30	3.4%

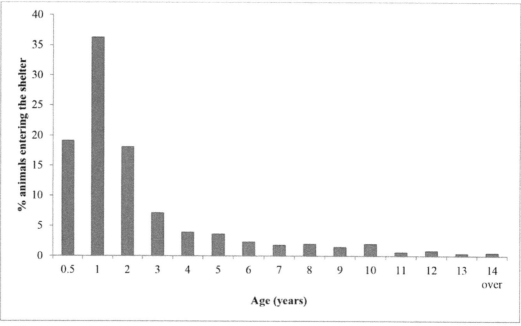

Figure 2. Age of animals entering the PS - Percentage of animals per age, entering the public shelter during the study period (2002-2013)

Age

Age was estimated by the veterinarians on the basis of the animals' dentition and general status (e.g. reproductive status) (12). The age range of the dogs entering the PS was variable, including puppies of few days old to dogs over 18 years old (mean 2.3; median 1.04; Q_1=0.7; Q_3=2.6 years-old). It was not possible to retrieve the data about the age of the dogs in the years 2000-2001, so age data refer to the period 2002-2013. As showed in Fig. 2, the age distribution is skewed to the left, with a peak at around one year-old (38% of total animals entering the shelter).

The linear regression analysis highlighted a significant decrease in the average age of the dogs entering the shelter across the years (b= -0.11, p>0.0001; Fig. 3).

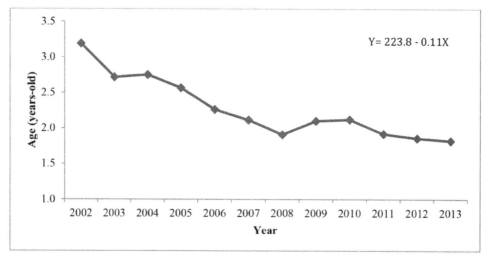

Figure 3. Average age of dogs entering the PS - Average age of dogs entering the public shelter each year, during the period of study (2002-2013)

Type of dogs entering the shelter and geographical origin

During the study period, 879 puppies (12.8% of the total population), usually arriving in litters, entered the PS. However, most of the dogs captured from the territory were healthy adult FRDs (67.3%;

disease (e.g. gastro-enteric or respiratory disorders, mange, alopecia); and 1% (n=63) included abused animals, or dogs reported to predate livestock or other small animals. The majority of FRDs entering the PS were stray-unowned dogs (91%), the remaining 9% (n=667) were owned dogs that

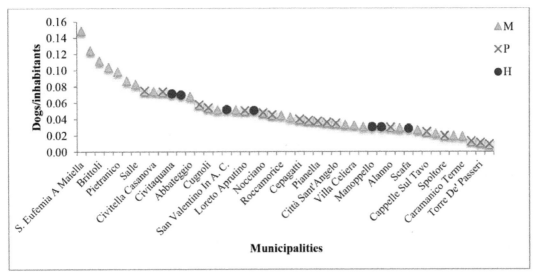

Figure 4. Geographical distribution of FRDs FRDs/inhabitant ratio per municipality associated to the type of territory (M=mountain; P= plain/costal; H= hill), municipalities are ordered according to the FRDs/inhabitant ratio

average year entrance=359.3, median=347.5 dogs). The remaining fifth of the population was represented by 6.7% (n=463) of dangerous dogs, that either showed aggressive behaviours or had attacked people; 7.1% (n=487) of injured animals (e.g. car accident); 5.2% (n=356) were found with a

escaped or that were left free to roam unsupervised on the territory.

A significant positive correlation emerged between the number of captured dogs in each municipality and the human population (R=0.87, p<0.0001). The 10 municipalities where most of

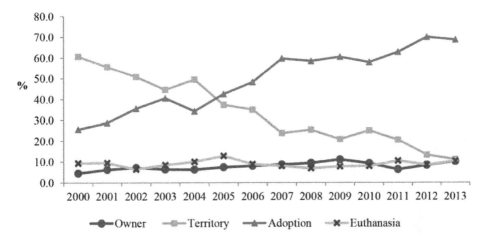

Figure 5. Destination of dogs after sheltering – Destination of dogs per year (i.e. return to the owner, return to the territory under TNR program, admission to an adoption program and euthanasia)

the dogs were collected (64% of all dogs) were the 10 municipalities with more inhabitants, also these were predominantly plain or coastal areas. When looking at the FRDs/inhabitants ratio instead, the 10 municipalities with the highest ratio were in the mountains (Fig. 4) although no significant difference emerged comparing the different types of territories among them (H= 2.9, p =0.23).

Destination of dogs after sheltering

After veterinary check-up, dogs could have different destinies. In the current study, 7.9% owned dogs returned to their owners, 50.8% unowned dogs were adopted or housed in rescue shelter for adoption, 32.3% were released on the territory as 'community dogs', and 8.9% of the total either died or were euthanized for reasons in compliance with the national law. The remaining 9 dogs (0.1%) escaped from the PS. While a low percentage of dogs were returned to owners or euthanized, with rather constant numbers across the years, a clear increase in the number of animals destined for adoption can be seen with an opposite reduction in the number of dogs released on the territory (Fig. 5). Comparing these two groups (adoptions and territory) using a chi-square test revealed that before 2006 the number of animals destined for adoption was significantly below that expected by chance, while after 2006, it was significantly higher than would be expected by chance (χ^2=762.9; p<0.0001).

Bite/attack events

A total of 463 dogs entered the PS of Pescara due to being involved in aggressive attacks or bite events. Of these, 65 (14%) were owned dogs, whilst the remaining 398 were strays. The association between aggressive events and ownership was found to be significant (χ^2=15.3; p<0.0001). In particular, the observed frequencies of aggressive owned dogs were significantly higher than the expected frequencies for this group.

Looking at breed types, 59.8% were mongrels (not ascribed to any specific breed) 7.6% were *Abruzzi sheepdog* cross-breeds, 5.2% were *Abruzzi sheepdog* (pure breed), 5.2% *German shepherd dog* cross breed, 5% Pit Bull type, 3.9 and 3.7% were *German shepherd dog* and *Rottweiler* respectively. Other breeds were represented by around 1% or below. After an accurate anamnesis and behavioural consultations most dogs were reintroduced on the territory, given up for adoption or returned to their owner (n=350). The remaining dogs (21%) were declared dangerous and euthanized in accordance with law prescriptions.

Sterilisation

Sterilisation events were not reported in the record forms of the PS before 2002. During the remaining years, Pescara PS veterinarians performed 4,580 sterilisations, 85.6% on females. Among dogs entering in the PS, 289 were already neutered and among these, only 28 were owned out of a total of 667 (4.2%) owned dogs. The average number of sterilisations per year between 2002 and 2013 was 381.7 (median 382; Q_1=360.3; Q_3=407.5).

Looking only at owned dogs, a highly significant association emerged between sex and neutering status (χ^2= 21.7; p<0.0001). A significantly higher proportion of neutered female (85.7%), compared to neutered male dogs (14.3%), entered the shelter. On average, 350 ±29.4 (mean±SD) entire stray females and 17±7.1 (mean±SD) entire owned females dogs entered the PS each year. A significant difference also emerged when comparing the age of sterilised animals entering the PS, these being older than non-sterilised dogs (sterilised: mean= 5.9 y.o.; non-sterilised: mean= 2.0; p<0.0001)

Identification

A total of 515 FRDs captured from the territory were "community dogs" (under the TNR programme), therefore had an identification code (i.e. microchip). No free-roaming dog that had already been identified entered the PS in 2000 and only two did so in 2001. Between 2002 and 2013 a mean of 42.8±8.3SD already identified dogs per year entered the PS (8.9% of the average yearly entrance rate of unowned FRD entering the shelter), of which 42.5% were injured, ill or involved in attacks or bite events. According to their status, 28.3% dogs were returned to their territory, 19.2% died or were euthanized and 52.6% were adopted or committed to a rescue shelter for adoption. Among owned dogs (n=667), 61.8% had a transponder. The remaining 38.2 % of owned dogs, which did not have a transponder, were not in compliance with the law. A chi-square test highlighted a significant association between the types of FRD (owned or stray) with the presence/absence of an identification code (χ^2=1605.8; p<0.0001). In particular, it emerged that observed frequencies of identified owned dogs were significantly higher than expected frequencies. PS veterinarians inoculated 5904 transponders to FRDs during 14 years.

DISCUSSION

Demographic data

Estimating the FRD population size and understanding its source is recognised to be the first step needed to gain a picture of the baseline situation to plan targeted and effective actions, and to understand the amount of resources required to tackle this problem (8, 9, 13).

It is reported that a 70% sterilisation rate is necessary to block dog population growth (14). Unfortunately, no reliable estimates of the FRD population in the province of Pescara is available at the moment, but since all dogs reported to the LVHU are captured and sterilised, it can be supposed that almost all FRD on the streets are eventually caught. TNR programmes in place for many years, as in this case study, should lead to a reduction of the reproduction rate and consequently to a progressive aging of the stray population. The present results highlight a high entrance rate of sub-adult animals (around 1 y.o., Fig. 2) and a rejuvenation of the population across the years (Fig. 3). Thus, the FRDs captured on the territory are new dogs, either born in the street or derived from abandoned and unwanted litters. This, together with the constantly high entrance rates at the PS (Fig. 1) are important symptoms of a failure in the dog population management system, which appears not to be targeting the source of new FRDs. It is important to consider the costs that a high capture and sterilisation activity entails for LVHU: sterilisation 70€/dog plus capture, medical and maintenance costs (around 200€/dog).

Although the more densely populated areas were those were the higher number of dogs were caught, on average a higher FRD-to-inhabitants ratio was found in mountain areas, being mostly rural or semi-rural (Fig. 4). The distribution of FRDs in the different geographical areas (plain, hill and mountain), however, did not differ statistically. As it also emerged in other dog surveys (15), in rural areas owners leave the dog free to roam, probably due to the higher tolerance by the community. In Abruzzi mountain areas pastoralism is common; farm stockperson often leave their dogs, mainly not sterilised, free to roam. Moreover, herders may abandon herding dogs that are not good for working thus contributing to the free roaming population of shepherd breed dogs (16). This behaviour could explain the higher prevalence of German Shepherds and Abruzzi Sheepdogs, both pure breed and their crosses, entering the PS (Table 1). Awareness and free microchipping campaigns targeting citizens may not reach farmers that rarely walk their working dogs to town. Targeted actions, such as door-to-door campaigns in rural areas and incentivising the sterilisation of non-working animals, would help in enforcing the law on identification and registration. This strategy, applied to the present and similar scenarios, could substantially reduce one of the sources of FRDs.

A certain ecological niche attracts animals according to the resource availability. Each niche has a carrying capacity therefore limiting the entrance of new individuals when resources are already taken. Reintroducing neutered dogs on the territory contributes to filling certain niches and is therefore one of the strategies applied to control FRD populations. The LVHU strategy has changed over the years, decreasing the number of dogs released on the territory as community dogs and increasing the number of animals destined for adoption (either direct or through rescue shelters; Fig. 5). Nevertheless, whichever was the primary DPM (dog population management) strategy used (i.e. TNR or sheltering), the average number of dogs entering the PS did not vary accordingly, suggesting once more that targeting only the 'symptom' of a problem and not the source has no effect in reducing the population size.

Public health and animal welfare

Dog bites to people are a serious issue for public safety, involving a high number of citizens every year in many countries all over the world, including Europe (17, 18). A total of 463 dogs entered the PS of Pescara because of involvement in aggressive attacks or bite events during the 14 years analysed here. Although observed frequencies of aggression events by owned dogs were higher than expected by chance alone, unowned animals represented the higher proportion of aggressive dogs entering the shelter. This result is in line with previous work carried out in Belgrade by Vučinić et al. (19) which also found that stray dogs caused a significantly higher number of bites to humans than owned dogs, although another study carried out in Italy show the opposite trend (20). Nevertheless, cases of attacks from dogs whose owner is unknown are known to be over-reported as compared to attack events from owned dogs. This may be due to people being more concerned about strays as carriers of diseases or conversely, because only serious bites are likely to be reported by victims of a family dog (17, 21). Also, previous works have highlighted how the reduction of the number of domestic animals roaming in the community could considerably help in preventing most bite injuries (19, 22).

Over one third of the population entering PS included injured, sick or abused animals, abandoned litters or biting animals. This data confirms that free roaming conditions in urban environments entail a range of risks to the dogs, potentially compromising their health and welfare, as well as being a potential threat for public safety as has also been reported elsewhere (3). A rather constant percentage of the caught animals were 'community dogs' (i.e. strays with an identification code), being recaptured every year. The re-catching of these animals implies costs as well, and this should be considered when deciding whether to implement TNR as a dog population management action.

Responsible ownership

Dog overpopulation can be a consequence of human behaviours, identified as deficiencies in pet maintenance and pet sterilisation (23, 24). Responsible ownership is a key factor in the control of FRD populations. In our study, 667 owned dogs were collected while roaming in the streets without supervision. This demonstrates irresponsible behaviour by dog owners in the province of Pescara. It was reported that dogs kept outside the house are less likely to be neutered, therefore increasing the probability of producing unwanted litters (24, 25).

Results from the PS show that a very low percentage of owned dogs caught from the street were sterilised (4.2%), especially male dogs. Slater et al. (26) found similar results in Teramo, another province of the Abruzzi region, implying that cultural norms may underlie this phenomenon, as it has also been referred to in other papers (27, 28). In addition to owned dogs, just fewer than 400 entire female stray dogs were captured every year. These numbers are alarming when taking into account the number of litters and pups per litter that they could potentially generate if not neutered in time, thus the increase could be exponential. In accordance with other authors, we agree that methods to reduce the number of dogs that require rescue care should include increasing peoples' awareness of responsible ownership and also the provision of educational activities in schools. A significantly higher number of entire fertile animals were young dogs (i.e. around 2 y.o.), compared to sterilised dogs entering the shelter that were older animals. An increase in neutering rates, preferably at early stages of the dogs' life, may be necessary to reduce the risk of unwanted litters (29-31). This is also in line with OIE recommendations to promote responsible dog ownership, as it can significantly reduce the number of stray dogs. Also, due to dog ecology being linked to human activity effective control of dog populations has to be accompanied by changes in human behaviour (8). Høgåsen et al. (7) demonstrated through a deterministic model that the nuisance and costs associated with FRD population management can be effectively reduced by acting on dog ownership, decreasing the proportion of free roaming owned dogs and of abandonments, rather than by increasing kennel capacity. This model would allow significant savings, including reducing neutering costs at PS.

Since 2003, the Italian national law requires compulsory electronic dog identification and registration in the Regional Canine Registry (RCR) (32). An efficient traceability system plays a key role in dog population size and composition estimation. It also provides a tool to evaluate and monitor animal health, helping in disease outbreak management and surveillance (including zoonosis), vaccination programmes and welfare monitoring (33). However, the accuracy of the RCR also relies on the owners' diligence in registering and removing dogs after death, which has often proven to be lacking (34). For example, in a town of the Abruzzi region (Teramo), Slater and colleagues (26) found that 72% of the owners were aware about the RDR, but only half of them correctly registered their dogs. Voslárová and Passantino (6) highlighted that the province of Pescara was one of the most successful areas concerning dog identification compared to other Italian provinces. Despite this, in the present study, one third of caught owned dogs were not identified. Although a general yearly increase in the overall proportion of identified owned dogs could be discerned, there is still a good margin for improvement. A recent telephone interview study on dog ownership in the Pescara province confirms this data: 25.4% of owners did not identify their pet dog, although of these, only 3% admitted to being aware of the existence of the RDR (35). This data stresses once more the lack of awareness of the importance of an efficient traceability system for pet animals, and the need to increase citizens' knowledge on this topic.

CONCLUSION

Stray dog overpopulation is a serious public concern in several countries and difficulties in coping with FRDs are often consequences of limited eco-epidemiological data, poor planning, weak multidisciplinary and inter-sectorial collaboration and also a lack of resources (6). The condition of straying itself also entails risks for both dog health and welfare. Hence, actions targeted at preventing the causes that lead to the animals abandonment, such as overpopulation and behavioural problems, should be implemented (36). There is a need to find solutions that are economically sustainable, whilst bearing in mind the severe restriction in state-funding available regarding FRDs. The data presented in this paper adds to our understanding of dog population trends in the Pescara area. This may provide a basis for making policy decisions about effective methods to control overpopulation. The implemented neutering plan alone, targeting

FRDs, appears to be insufficient in controlling the local dog population. Veterinary services involved in DPM should consider these aspects of their local contexts when setting strategies to control FRD populations in their country.

ACKNOWLEDGMENTS

A special thanks to Dr. Fabrizio De Massis for his precious suggestions that helped improving this work and to Dr. Mary Friel for language revision.

REFERENCES

1. Slater, M. R. (2001). The role of veterinary epidemiology in the study of free-roaming dogs and cats. Preventive veterinary medicine 48(4): 273-286 http://dx.doi.org/10.1016/S0167-5877(00)00201-4

2. Kato, M., Yamamoto, H., Inukai, Y., Kira, S. (2003). Survey of the stray dog population and the health education program on the prevention of dog bites and dog-acquired infections: A comparative study in Nepal and Okayama prefecture, Japan. Acta Medica Okayama 57(5): 261-266. PMid:14679405

3. Vučinić, M., Đorđević, V., Radisavljević, K., Atanasijević, N., Nedeljković-Trailović, J. (2011). Feeding behavior of stray dogs in a municipal shelter. Acta veterinaria 61(1): 99-105. http://dx.doi.org/10.2298/AVB1101099V

4. Dalla Villa, P., Matthews, L. B., Alessandrini, B., Messori, S., Migliorati, G. (2014). Drivers for animal welfare policies in Europe. Revue Scientifique Et Technique-Office International Des Epizooties 33(1):,39-46.

5. Dalla Villa, P., Kahn, S., Stuardo, L., Iannetti, L., Di Nardo, A., Serpell, J. A. (2010). Free-roaming dog control among OIE-member countries. Preventive veterinary medicine 97(1): 58-63 http://dx.doi.org/10.1016/j.prevetmed.2010.07.001 PMid:20709415

6. Voslářvá, E., Passantino, A. (2012). Stray dog and cat laws and enforcement in Czech Republic and in Italy. Annali dell'Istituto superiore di sanita 48(1): 97-104.

7. Hogasen, H. R., Er, C., Di Nardo, A., Dalla Villa, P. (2013). Free-roaming dog populations: a cost-benefit model for different management options, applied to Abruzzo, Italy. Preventive veterinary medicine 112(3-4): 401-413. http://dx.doi.org/10.1016/j.prevetmed.2013.07.010 PMid:23973012

8. OIE (2014). 1st OIE regional workshop on stray dog population management for Balkan countries. Bucharest, RO, 17-19 June

9. OIE (2014). Terrestrial Animal Health Code. 23rd ed. Paris

10. Italian law (1991). Legge n.281 of 4 Agosto 1991. In materia di animali d'affezione e prevenzione al randagismo. Gazzetta Ufficiale, n. 203, 30 agosto 1991

11. Diesel, G., Pfeiffer, D. U., Brodbelt, D. (2008). Factors affecting the success of rehoming dogs in the UK during 2005. Preventive Veterinary Medicine 84(3): 228-241 http://dx.doi.org/10.1016/j.prevetmed.2007.12.004 PMid:18243374

12. Fraser, Clarence M. (1986). The Merck veterinary manual. No. Ed. 6. Merck & Co.

13. FAO (2014). Dog population management. Report of the FAO/WSPA/IZSAM expert meeting - Banna, Italy - 14-19 March 2011. Animal Production and Health Report. No. 6. Rome, Italy

14. Jackman, J., Rowan, A. N. (2007). Free-roaming dogs in developing countries: The benefits of capture, neuter, and return programs. Animal studies repository. In D.J. Salem & A.N. Rowan (Eds.), The state of the animals 2007 (pp. 55-78). Washington, DC: Humane Society Press

15. Brickner, I. (2002). The impact of domestic dogs (Canis familiaris) on wildlife welfare and conservation: a literature review

16. Namgail, T., Fox, J. L., Bhatnagar, Y. V. (2007). Carnivore-caused livestock mortality in Trans-Himalaya. Environmental Management 39(4): 490-496. http://dx.doi.org/10.1007/s00267-005-0178-2 PMid:17318699

17. Butcher, R. L., De Keuster, T. (2013). Dog-associated problems affecting public health and community well-being. Dogs, Zoonoses and Public Health, 2nd Ed., 24-42. http://dx.doi.org/10.1079/9781845938352.0024

18. Santoro, V., Smaldone, G., Lozito, P., Smaldone, M., Introna, F. (2011). A forensic approach to fatal dog attacks. A case study and review of the literature. Forensic Science International 206(1-3): E37-E42. http://dx.doi.org/10.1016/j.forsciint.2010.07.026 PMid:20719439

19. Vučinić, M., Dordevic, M., Brana, R.-D., Ljiljana, J., Mirilovic M. (2008). Bites to humans caused by stray and owned dogs in Belgrade. Acta Veterinaria-Beograd 58(5-6): 563-571. http://dx.doi.org/10.2298/AVB0806563V

20. Fedele, V., Gnaccarini, M., Laurenti, P., Marino, M., Meia, B. (2008). Monitoraggio delle morsicature nel pinerolese negli anni 1998 - 2008. Argomenti 4, 53-59.

21. Overall, K. L., Love, M. (2001). Dog bites to humans - demography, epidemiology, injury, and risk. Journal of the American Veterinary Medical Association 218(12): 1923-1934
http://dx.doi.org/10.2460/javma.2001.218.1923
PMid:11417736

22. Sinclair, C. L., Zhou, C. (1995). Descriptive epidemiology of animal bites in Indiana, 1990-92 a rationale for intervention. Public Health Reports 110(1): 64-67.
PMid:7838946 PMCid:PMC1382076

23. Fournier A. K., Geller E. S. (2005). Behavior analysis of companion-animal overpopulation: A conceptualization of the problem and suggestions for intervention. Behav. Soc. 13, 51-68.
http://dx.doi.org/10.5210/bsi.v13i1.35

24. Fielding, W. J. (2010). Dog breeding in New Providence, The Bahamas, and its potential impact on the roaming dog population I: planned and accidental. Journal of applied animal welfare science: JAAWS. 13(3): 250-260.

25. Slater, M. R., Di Nardo, A., Pediconi, O., Dalla Villa, P., Candeloro, L., Alessandrini, B., Del Papa, S. (2008). Free-roaming dogs and cats in central Italy: Public perceptions of the problem. Preventive veterinary medicine 84(1): 27-47
http://dx.doi.org/10.1016/j.prevetmed.2007.10.002
PMid:18055046

26. Slater, M. R., Di Nardo, A., Pediconi, O., Villa, P. D., Candeloro, L., Alessandrini, B., Del Papa, S. (2008). Cat and dog ownership and management patterns in central Italy. Preventive veterinary medicine 85(3-4): 267-294.
http://dx.doi.org/10.1016/j.prevetmed.2008.02.001
PMid:18374434

27. Levy, J. K., Crawford, C., Appel, L. D., Clifford, E. L. (2008). Comparison of intratesticular injection of zinc gluconate versus surgical castration to sterilize male dogs. American journal of veterinary research 69(1): 140-143.
http://dx.doi.org/10.2460/ajvr.69.1.140
PMid:18167099

28. McKenzie, B. (2010). Evaluating the benefits and risks of neutering dogs and cats. CAB Reviews: Perspectives in agriculture, veterinary science, nutrition and natural resources 5(045).
http://dx.doi.org/10.1079/PAVSNNR20105045

29. Clark, C. C. A., Gruffydd-Jones, T., Murray, J. K. (2012). Number of cats and dogs in UK welfare organisations. Veterinary Record 170(19): 493.
http://dx.doi.org/10.1136/vr.100524
PMid:22589036

30. Di Nardo, A., Candeloro, L., Budke, C. M., Slater, M. R. (2007). Modeling the effect of sterilization rate on owned dog population size in central Italy. Preventive veterinary medicine 82(3-4): 308-313.
http://dx.doi.org/10.1016/j.prevetmed.2007.06.007
PMid:17692414

31. Voith, V. L. (2009). The impact of companion animal problems on society and the role of veterinarians. Vet Clin N Am-Small., 39(2): 327.

32. Italian law (2003). Accordo del 6 Febbraio 2003 tra il Ministro della salute, le regioni e le province autonome di Trento e di Bolzano in materia di benessere degli animali da compagnia e pet-therapy. Gazzetta Ufficiale, n. 51, 03/03/2003

33. Dalla Villa, P., Messori, S., Possenti, L., Barnard, S., Cianella, M., Di Francesco, C. (2013). Pet population management and public health: a web service based tool for the improvement of dog traceability. Preventive veterinary medicine 109(3-4): 349-353
http://dx.doi.org/10.1016/j.prevetmed.2012.10.016
PMid:23182028

34. Caminiti, A., Sala, M., Panetta, V., Battisti, S., Meoli, R., Rombola, P., Spallucci, V., Eleni, C., Scaramozzino, P. (2014). Completeness of the dog registry and estimation of the dog population size in a densely populated area of Rome. Preventive veterinary medicine 113(1): 146-151.
http://dx.doi.org/10.1016/j.prevetmed.2013.10.003
PMid:24188820

35. Magnani, D., Barnard, S., Messori, S., Di Bonaventura, I., Giovannini, A., Dalla Villa, P., Ferri, N. (2015). Investigation on responsible ownership in two different urban context. Proceedings 2nd International conference on dog population management; Istanbul, Turkey, 3-5 March (p.63)

36. Verga, M., Michelazzi, M. (2009). Companion animal welfare and possible implications on the human-pet relationship. Ital J Anim Sci., 8(1s): 231-240.
http://dx.doi.org/10.4081/ijas.2009.s1.231

23

CLINICAL TESTING OF COMBINED VACCINE AGAINST ENZOOTIC PNEUMONIA IN INDUSTRIAL PIG FARMING IN BULGARIA

Roman Pepovich[1], Branimir Nikolov[2], Ivo Sirakov[4], Krasimira Genova[3], Kalin Hristov[2], Elena Nikolova[4], Radka Hajiolova[5], Boika Beltova[5]

[1]Department of Infectious Pathology & Hygiene, Technology and Control of Food of Animal Origin, Faculty of Veterinary Medicine, University of Forestry, Sofia, Bulgaria
[2]Department of Obstetrics, Gynecology, Biotechnology of Reproduction & Pathological Anatomy and Biochemistry, Faculty of Veterinary Medicine, University of Forestry, Sofia, Bulgaria
[3]Department of Animal Breeding Science, Faculty of Veterinary Medicine, University of Forestry, Sofia, Bulgaria
[4]Department of Virology and Viral Diseases, National Diagnostic and Research Veterinary Institute, Sofia, Bulgaria
[5]Department of Pathophysiology, Faculty of Medicine, Medical University, Sofia, Bulgaria

ABSTRACT

In the pig farm with signs of a respiratory disease complex and laboratory confirmed enzootic pneumonia, the prophylactic efficacy of the combination vaccine (*M. hyo+PCV2*), a single injection administered intramuscularly 21 days after birth, at a dose of 2 ml was tested. The clinical condition, pathological changes in the lungs and some epidemiological and economic results were reported. It was found that vaccinated pigs are in a better clinical condition in comparison with the control group. Morbidity in the rearing period was reduced from 16.3% in the control group to 6.0% in vaccinated pigs, and in the fattening period, respectively, from 30.6% in the control group to 10.0% in the vaccinated group. Pathological features in the lung characteristic for the enzootic pneumonia in the vaccinated pigs were reduced from 25.5%±7.24 to 4.0%±2.44, and PCVI - from 13.0%±4.66 to 0%. Vaccination of pigs has been received and a higher average daily gain in groups for rearing (0.624 kg) and for fattening (0.723 kg) was recorded.

Key words: Enzootic pneumonia, *Mycoplasma hyopneumoniae*, pigs, vaccination

INTRODUCTION

Porcine enzootic pneumonia (EP) is a chronic respiratory disease caused by *Mycoplasma hyopneumoniae* (*M. hyopneumoniae, M. hyo*) (13). This is one of the most common respiratory diseases in swine and causes considerable economic losses worldwide as a result of poor feed efficiency, growth retardation, higher morbidity and mortality, emergency slaughter and prophylaxis and treatment costs (2, 5, 11).

Immunoprophylaxis is a key tool in the overall infection control program. Although the existing vaccines do not prevent lung colonization by *M. hyo*, what they do provide is partial protection against pathological changes in organs (9). Vaccination has a marked positive effect: improvement of clinical signs, reduced severity of pathological lesions in the lungs, improvement in mean daily gain, shorter fattening period, and last but not least, lower mortality (3, 10, 12, 14, 15).

Eggen et al. (4) studied the effect of different combinations of *M. hyo* and porcine circovirus type 2 (*PCV2*) vaccines in swine and reported that

Corresponding author: Dr. Roman Pepovich, PhD.
E-mail address: rpepovich@abv.bg
Present address: Department of Infectious Pathology & Hygiene, Technology and Control of Food of Animal Origin, Faculty of Veterinary Medicine, University of Forestry, Sofia, Bulgaria

following single-dose vaccination, the lung lesions decreased with 53% to 61% and the antibody titer against *PCV2* continued to increase up to 10 weeks of age. The authors suggest that there is no immunological interference between *M. hyo* and *PCV2* in the tested combinations and that there is little difference in the antibody titer against *PCV2* between the groups given a single combined vaccine and those given the two vaccines separately.

The aim of the present study was to assess and analyze the prophylactic effect of a combined vaccine against enzootic pneumonia in industrial pig farming in Bulgaria.

MATERIAL AND METHODS

Animals

The study was carried out on a pig-breeding and fattening farm where manifestations of porcine respiratory disease complex (PRDC) – with enzootic pneumonia as the main etiological agent–had been noted. The study included 100 animals at the same age and live weight. They were equally divided into two groups:

Group 1: Pigs (n=50) were given a single dose of the combined inactivated vaccine (*M. hyo+PCV2*) on day 21 after birth. The vaccine was administered intramuscularly (IM) at a 2 ml dose, according to the manufacturer's instructions.

Group 2: Pigs (n=50) were not vaccinated and served as a control group.

The animals from the two groups were reared under the same conditions.

Clinical examinations

All animals were subjected to clinical examinations during the experimental period. The examinations included overall condition (febrility, conjunctivitis, appetite, discomfort, nutritional status) and clinical signs characteristic of porcine respiratory infections (respiratory distress, cough, discharge from nostrils). The clinical condition of the animals was evaluated on the basis of a four-point scale: very good (++++); good (+++); satisfactory (++) and poor (+).

Pathological lesions

Autopsy was performed on animals that died during the experiment. At the end of the fattening period the lungs of all animals were examined and the size, type and severity of the lung lesions were scored. The severity of macroscopic changes in lung-specific enzootic pneumonia was determined by quantification of the damage described by Kristensen et al. (8). Individual lobes represent

a percentage of the total area of the lungs: right apical lobe (10%); right cardiac lobe (10%); right diaphragmatic lobe (35%); right accessory lobe (5%); left apical lobe (5%); left cardiac lobe (5%); left diaphragmatic lobe (30%).

Serological analyses

Before vaccination, a total of 16 blood samples were taken (8 samples per group) and were analyzed by blocking ELISA (Oxoid) for the presence of antibodies against *M. hyopneumoniae* glycoprotein 74 KDa. Two negative and two positive controls were included, according to the manufacturer's instructions. Optical density (OD) was measured monochromatically at 450 nm.

DNA extraction and Polymerase Chain Reaction (PCR)

DNA was extracted from 20–50 mg lung tissue samples. The samples were incubated with 20 μL of proteinase K (10 mg/mL) and 400 μL of reagent B (10 m MTris, 1 mM EDTA and 0.1 M NaCl) at 50° C for at least 3 h or overnight. Following centrifugation for 3 min at 3000 rpm, 400 μL of the supernatant were mixed with 400 μL of reagent C (Tris-saturated phenol and chlorophorm : isoamyl alcohol (24:1) in a 1:1 ratio), vortexed and centrifuged at 13 000 rpm for 5 min. The supernatant was pipetted into another microtube and an equivalent amount of chlorophorm/isoamyl alcohol (at a 24:1 ratio) was added. After vortexing and centrifugation for 5 min at 13 000 rpm, the supernatant was again pipetted into a new microtube and mixed with 100% ethanol (Merck, Germany) in a 1:2 ratio; and 5 μL of 7 M ammonium citrate (Sigma, USA) were added. The samples were then left to precipitate for 30 min at -20° C, and were centrifuged at 13 000 rpm for 15 min. The resulting supernatant was discarded and the pellet was washed with cold 70% ethanol and centrifuged at 13 000 rpm for 2 min. The resulting pellet was dried for 7 min and dissolved in 20–50 mL distilled water.

PCR reactions were performed with the primers and protocol described by Villarreal et al. (15) with modifications (annealing at 53.5°C for 40s). The reaction mixtures contained: 3.0 μL of DNA, 10 pmol of each primer, 12.5 μL of 2x PCR Master Mix (Geneshun Biotech co. ltd, China) and distilled water to a volume of 25 μL.

The quantity and quality of the extracted DNA and the PCR products were analyzed by 2% agarose gel electrophoresis (Geneshun Biotech co. ltd, China), with 10 mg/mL ethidium bromide (Sigma, USA) staining and a 100 bp DNA Ladder (Geneshun Biotech Co. ltd, China), at 120 V for 40 min.

Statistical analysis

All results were processed statistically by the use of computer software StatMost (StatMost 3.6, Dataxiom Software, 2003). The results are presented as mean with standard error (*mean±SE*), after application of the one-way ANOVA statistic. Statistically significant differences were accepted at *p<0.05.*

RESULTS

During the suckling period –from birth to weaning– no clinically infected pigs were observed. One pig from the control group died and the pathoanatomical examination showed lesions typical for EP and *Actinobacillus pleuropneumoniae* (APP). In the group of animals which were administered the combined vaccine (*M. hyo+PCV2*), there was a 0.538 kg (p<0.01) higher weight gain (Table 1).

All the animals from group 1 (n = 50) as well as 49 animals from group 2 continued into the growing period (Table 2), which continued for 73 days. During the growing period, there were no deaths, but the morbidity of the control group increased sharply to reach 16.3% in comparison to 6% in the group of the vaccinated animals. In this period, the vaccinated animals showed higher mean daily gain (up to 0.624 kg) than the non-vaccinated ones (0.512 kg).

Table 1. Business and economic outcomes in experimental piglets vaccinated with combination vaccine (*M. hyo+PCV2*) and unvaccinated

Parameters	Units	I group (M. hyo+PCV2)	II group (Control)
1. Pigs in the group	number	50	50
2. Average live weight at birth	кg	1. 200±2.23*	1. 200±1.89
3. Stay in group "piglets"	days	35	35
4. Diseased	number	0	0
	%	0	0
5. Died from PRDC	number	0	1
	%	0	2
6. Average live weight at the end of the period	кg	9.090±2.58**	8.552±3.02
	%	106.3	100
7. Derived growth period	кg	7.890	7.352
	%	107.3	100
8. Average daily gain	кg	0. 225	0. 210
	%	107.2	100

 * $p < 0.05$ ** $p < 0.01$ *** $p < 0.001$

Table 2. Business and economic outcomes in the experimental weaners pigs vaccinated with combination vaccine (*M. hyo+PCV2*) and unvaccinated

Parameters	Units	I group (M. hyo+PCV2)	II group (Control)
1. Pigs in the group	number	50	49
2. Average live weight at beginning of period	кg	9.090±2.58*	8.552±3.02
3. Stay in weaners	days	73	73
4. Average live weight at the end of the period	кg	54. 634±3.07*	45. 905±3.64
	%	119	100
5. Diseased	number	3	8
	%	6	16.3
6. Died from PRDC	number	0	0
	%	0	0
7. Derived growth period	кg	45.544	37.353
	%	121.9	100
8. Average daily gain	кg	0. 624	0. 512
	%	121.9	100

 * $p < 0.05$ ** $p < 0.01$ *** $p < 0.001$

During the fattening period (94 days), the mean live weight was 8.729 kg higher in the group of vaccinated pigs than in the control (non-vaccinated) group. There were also no deaths. However, clinical signs of a respiratory infection were evident in 10% of the vaccinated pigs and in 30.6% of the control ones. The live weight measured at regular slaughter of animals from both groups was shown to be 19.6 kg ($p<0.05$) higher in the vaccinated animals as compared to the non-vaccinated ones (Table 3).

Details about the overall and the clinical condition of the pigs during the growing and the fattening period are given in Table 4 and Table 5.

Table 6 presents the results from the pathoanatomical examinations and the observed lesions in the vaccinated and non-vaccinated pigs. The pathoanatomical findings in the lungs of both groups of animals were similar: for EP, APP and PCVI. In the vaccinated animals, the number of lesions characteristic of EP was reduced from 25.5 %±7.24 ($p<0.01$) to 4%±2.44 ($p<0.01$), and of PCVI, from 13 %±4.66 ($p<0.05$) in the control group to 0% ($p<0.05$) in the vaccinated group. The lesions typical for APP amounted to 11.5%±7.67 in the control group, but were reduced to 2.0%±1.10 owing to the vaccination.

Table 3. Business and economic outcomes in the experimental fattening pigs vaccinated with combination vaccine (*M. hyo+PCV2*) and unvaccinated

Parameters	Units	I group (M. hyo+PCV2)	II group (Control)
1. Pigs in the group	number	50	49
2. Average live weight at beginning of period	кg	54.634±3.07*	45.905±3.64
3. Stay in group fattening	days	94	94
4. Average live weight at the end of the period	кg	122.6±2.06*	103.0±1.98
	%	119	100
5. Derived growth period	кg	68.0	57.0
	%	119.3	100
6. Average daily gain	кg	0.723	0.607
	%	119.1	100
7. Diseased	number	5	15
	%	10	30.6
8. Died from PRDC	number	0	0
	%	0	0
9. Slaughtered «economic foreshore»	number	1	4
	%	2	8

* $p < 0.05$ ** $p < 0.01$ *** $p < 0.001$

Table 4. Total and clinical state of the experimental pigs in the two groups during the period of «rearing» vaccinated with combination vaccine (*M. hyo+PCV2*) and unvaccinated

Clinical condition of the experimental pigs	Rearing - first period (8 – 12 кg)				Rearing - second period (12 – 40 кg)			
	I group (M. hyo+PCV2) n=50		II group (Control) n=49		I group (M. hyo+PCV2) n=50		II group (Control) n=49	
	number	%	number	%	number	%	number	%
Very good (++++)	28	56	11	22.4	22	44	8	16.3
Good (+++)	17	34	21	42.9	23	46	22	44.9
Satisfactory (++)	3	6	12	24.5	4	8	16	32.7
Poor (+)	2	4	5	10.2	1	2	3	6.1
Mean ±SE	12.5 ±6.19	25.0*** ±12.39	12.3 ±3.30	25.0*** ±6.74	12.5 ±5.80	25.0 ±11.61	12.3 ±4.21	25.0 ±8.60

* $p < 0.05$ ** $p < 0.01$ *** $p < 0.001$

Table 5. Total and clinical state of the experimental pigs in the two groups during the period of "fattening" vaccinated with combination vaccine (*M. hyo+PCV2*) and unvaccinated

Clinical condition of the experimental pigs	Fattening - first period (40 – 70 кг)				Fattening - second period (70 – 105 кг)			
	I group (M. hyo+PCV2) n=50		II group (Control) n=49		I group (M. hyo+PCV2) n=50		II group (Control) n=49	
	number	%	number	%	number	%	number	%
Very good (++++)	20	40	6	12.2	26	52	5	10.2
Good (+++)	23	46	19	38.8	22	44	15	30.6
Satisfactory (++)	2	4	9	18.4	1	2	25	51
Poor (+)	5	10	15	30.6	1	2	4	8.2
Mean ±SE	12.5 ±5.26	25.0 ±10.53	12.3 ±2.92	25.0 ±5.98	12.5 ±6.68	25.0 ±13.37	12.3 ±4.92	25.0 ±10.03

*$p < 0.05$ **$p < 0.01$ ***$p < 0.001$

Table 6. Results of pathology examinations at regular slaughter of pigs in experimental groups

№ of pigs	I group vaccinated with "M. hyo+PCV2"			II group unvaccinated "Control"		
	% of changes in the lungs			% of changes in the lungs		
	EP	APP	PCVI	EP	APP	PCVI
1	0	0	0	50	0	0
2	0	0	0	75	30	0
3	25	0	0	30	0	0
4	5	0	0	30	0	20
5	5	0	0	20	10	25
6	5	0	0	0	0	0
7	0	5	0	0	0	40
8	0	0	0	20	75	0
9	0	5	0	10	0	25
10	0	10	0	20	0	20
Mean ±SE	4.0 %** ±2.44	2.0 % ±1.10	0 %* ±0	25.5 %** ±7.24	11.5 % ±7.67	13.0 %* ±4.66

*$p < 0.05$ **$p < 0.01$ ***$p < 0.001$

DISCUSSION

The efficacy of a single dose of the combined inactivated vaccine (*M. hyo+PCV2*) on day 21 after birth of the pigs was demonstrated by the date of the vaccination in a farm, where manifestations of PRDC with enzootic pneumonia as the main etiological agent had been noted.

The results related to the overall and the clinical condition of the pigs during the growing and the fattening period indicate that, as a whole, the vaccinated pigs were in a better condition and with better health than those in the control group. The vaccination led to a reduction in the percentage of animals with signs associated with poor clinical outcomes.

The results of the serological tests before vaccination show that the studied serum 16 (8 sera from both groups) in pigs in the experimental group did not show specific antibodies against *M. hyopneumoniae*, and in the control group 6 samples reacted positive (75%). When examining the antibody titers against *M. hyopneumoniae*, three weeks after application of the combined vaccine it was found that of the test samples 17 - 13 (76.5%) reacted positive. These animals had an intense and protective immune response. In the sera of 3 pigs (17.6%) vaccine antibodies were not detected, in a pig from group 1 (5.9%) the results are questionable. In the control group of 17 analyzed samples, 16 samples (94.1%) had negative titers and in 1 sample (5.9%) they were dubious. Analysis of the results of serological tests on samples obtained at the end of the fattening period, shows that in pigs vaccinated with a combination vaccine, out of 6 samples in 2 (33.3%) there were antibodies against *M. hyo*. In the control group the results are similar. In conclusion, we can say that high titers of maternal antibodies induced by infection or vaccination, have had a negative effect on vaccination of pigs, which is confirmation of the data exported from Jayappa et al. (7) and Hodgins et al. (6).

Since established pathomorphological changes are characteristic and typical for enzootic pneumonia, but not specific, then contact differentiating them from changes caused by other participants in the PRDC, especially swine influenza (SI) was established through conducting a molecular biological research. Of the 14 examined lungs with lesions typical of EP by a conventional PCR, the DNA of *M. hyopneumoniae* was detected in 5 samples (35.7%). 4 samples (28.6%) are suspicious and 5 samples (35.7%) were negative.

Aiguo et al., (1) demonstrated the improvement of productivity in a Chinese farm with a continuous production system by implementing combination vaccine (*M. hyo+PCV2*). The vaccines are mixed before using and thus they save labor and reduce stress for the piglets. Similar to our results, they established that total mortality and the culling rate during the nursery and fattening period was reduced (5.26% in the vaccinated group), as well as the clinical signs.

Our results demonstrate that the combined vaccine against *M. hyo* and *PCV2* has good prophylactic efficacy not only in terms of reduction of clinical signs and good overall condition of the animals, but in higher mean daily gain in the growing (0.624 kg) and the fattening period (0.723 kg). The vaccination also contributed to the decrease in the degree and severity of the pathoanatomical lesions characteristic of EP and PCVI in the lungs of slaughtered pigs. These results are in agreement with other investigations (3, 10, 12, 14) who report a good prophylactic effect of vaccination, despite the fact that it does not render pigs completely immune against *M. hyo* infection.

ACKNOWLEDGMENTS

This research work was carried out with the support of University of Forestry and the project BG051PO001-3.3.06-0056 "Support for the development of young people in the University of Forestry", Operational Programme "Human Resources Development" financed by the European Social Fund of the European Union.

REFERENCES

1. Aiguo, W., Yanlong Li, Longquan Yao, Liande Zhu, Tan Tao. (2013). Efficacy of Ingelvac Mycoflex®.

2. In a chinese farm. The 6th Asian Pig Veterinary Society Congress Ho Chi Minh City, Vietnam, September 23-25, 2013. PO35.

3. Dawson, A., Harvey, R.E., Thevasagayam, S.J., Sherington, J. (2002). Studies of the field efficacy and safety of a single-dose Mycoplasma hyopneumoniae vaccine for pigs. Vet. Rec., 151, 535-538. http://dx.doi.org/10.1136/vr.151.18.535 PMid:12448490

4. Eggen, A., Schmidt, U., Raes, M., Witvliet, M. (2010). One-dose vaccination against M. hyo and PCV2. Pig Progress, 23.

5. Georgakis, A.D., Bourtzi-Hatzopoulou, E., Kritas, S.K., Balkamos, G.C., Kyriakis, S.C. (2002). A study on the Porcine Respiratory Disease Syndrome (PRDC): Update review and proposed measures for its control. J Hellenic Vet Med Society 53, 265-271.

6. Hodgins, D., Shewen, P., Dewey, C. (2004). Influence of age and maternal antibodies on antibody responses of neonatal piglets vaccinated against Mycoplasma hyopneumoniae. J. Swine Hlth. Prod. 12, 10-16.

7. Jayappa, H., Davis, B., Rapp-Gabrielson, V., Wasmoen, T., Thacker, E. (2001). Evaluation of the efficacy of Mycoplasma hyopneumoniae bacterin following immunization of young pigs in the presence of varying levels of maternal antibodies. In: Proc. 32nd Annual Meeting Am. Assoc. Swine Vet., Nashville, Tennessee, 237-241.

8. Kristensen, Ch., Vinther, J., Svensmark, B., Baekbo, P. (2014). A field evaluation of two vaccines against Mycoplasma hyopneumoniae infection in pigs. Acta Veterinaria Scandinavica, 56, 24, 1-7. http://dx.doi.org/10.1186/1751-0147-56-24

9. Maes, D., Deluyker, H., Verdonck, M., Castryck, F., Miry, C., Vrijens, B., Verbeke, W., Viaene, J., De Kruif, A. (1999). Effect of vaccination against Mycoplasma hyopneumoniae in pig herds with an all-in/all-out production system. Vaccine. 17, 1024-1034. http://dx.doi.org/10.1016/S0264-410X(98)00254-0

10. Maes, D., Verbeke, W., Vicca, J., Verdonck, M., De Kruif, A. (2003). Benefit to cost of vaccination against Mycoplasma hyopneumoniae in pig herds under Belgian market conditions from 1996 to 2000. Livestock Production Science. 83, 85-93.
http://dx.doi.org/10.1016/S0301-6226(03)00039-3

11. Maes, D., Segales, J., Meyns, T., Sibila, M., Pieters, M., Haesebrouck, F. (2008). Control of Mycoplasma hyopneumoniae infections in pigs. Vet. Microbiol. 126, 297-309.
http://dx.doi.org/10.1016/j.vetmic.2007.09.008
PMid:17964089

12. Pallares, F.J., Gomez, S., Munoz, A. (2001). Evaluation of zootechnical parameters of vaccinating against swine enzootic pneumonia under ield conditions. Vet. Rec. 148, 104-107.
http://dx.doi.org/10.1136/vr.148.4.104
PMid:11232924

13. Thacker, E. L (2006). Mycoplasmal diseases. In: Leman, A.D., Straw, B.E., D'Allaire, S., Mengeling, W.L., and Taylor, D.J., (Ed.), Diseases of Swine, 9th ed. The Iowa State University Press, Ames, IA, [701-717.

14. Wallgren, P., Vallgarda, J., Lindberg, M., Eliason-Selling, L. (2000). The efficacy of different vaccination strategies against Mycoplasma hyopneumoniae. In Proc. of the 16-th IPVS Congress, Melbourne, Australia, 461.

15. Villarreal, I., Vranckx, K., Duchateau, L., Pasmans, F., Haesebrouck, F., Jensen, J., Nanjiani, L., Maes, D. (2010). Early Mycoplasma hyopneumoniae infections in European suckling pigs in herds with respiratory problems: detection rate and risk factors. Veterinarni Medicina. 55, 7, 318–324.

24

JOINT DISEASES IN ANIMAL PALEOPATHOLOGY: VETERINARY APPROACH

Oliver Stevanović[1], Maciej Janeczek[2], Aleksander Chrószcz[2], Nemanja Marković[3]

[1]PI Veterinary Institute of Republic Srpska „Dr. Vaso Butozan" Branka Radičevića 18, 78000 Banja Luka, Bosnia and Herzegovina
[2]Department of Biostructure and Animal Physiology, Department of Veterinary Medicine Wroclaw University of Environmental and Life Sciences, Kożuchowska 1/3 51-531, Poland
[3]Institute of Archaeology, Kneza Mihaila 35/IV, 11000, Belgrade, Serbia

ABSTRACT

Animal paleopathology is not a very well known scientific discipline within veterinary science, but it has great importance for historical and archaeological investigations. In this paper, authors attention is focused on the description of one of the most common findings on the skeletal remains of animals - osteoarthropathies. This review particularly emphasizes the description and classification of the most common pathological changes in synovial joints. The authors have provided their observations on the importance of joint diseases in paleopathology and veterinary medicine. Analysis of individual processes in the joints of the animals from the past may help in the understanding of diseases in modern veterinary medicine. Differential diagnosis was made a point of emphasis and discussion, so that this work could have practical significance for paleopathology and veterinary medicine.

Key words: joint diseases, paleopathology, veterinary medicine, archaeozoology

INTRODUCTION

Animal bones are common archaeological finds and it is well-recognised that their detailed study provides important information about past human activities (7, 8, 9).The major part of faunal assemblages are domestic animals skeletal remains (27). The identification and correct description of pathological changes plays significant role in understanding of the human-animal interactions in daily life in the past (15). Usually, osteological changes observed in the past within animal bones are the result of human activity and the character of animal utilization. The interpretation should be related with socio-cultural aspects (18, 20, 21). For example, the characteristic changes in the distal parts of the limbs in cattle coming from the territory of the Roman Republic and Empire are in close relationship with the Roman economy, dietary tradition and animal utilization (1, 4, 11, 26). In this context, the possible interpretations should follow this direction. Some skeletal pathologies typical for the animals from the past are not observed nowdays, because of wide technological, social and other factors strongly influencing the animal herding and utilization methods.

The first pathological changes in joints in domestic animals were detected in Roman-British dog remains (13). Following these widely reported cases, many surveys since have been demonstrating the high prevalence of arthropathies in archaeozoological material (2, 32, 33). According to these first systematic studies in animal paleopathology, it was concluded, that arthropathies was a commonly observed condition in the working animals, such as draught cattle and horses. This phenomenon was explained by mechanical stress

Corresponding author: Oliver Stevanović, MSC, DVM
E-mail address: oliver.stevanovic@virsvb.com
Present address: PI Veterinary Institute of Republic Srpska
„Dr Vaso Butozan" Branka Radičevića 18,
78000 Banja Luka, Bosnia and Herzegovina

(common in working animals), as a one of the most important predisposing factor that can lead to osteoarhropathies. This was probably the crucial point in joint anomalies interpretation in animal paleopathology.

The development of new diagnostic methods and procedures in modern veterinary medicine allows for the possibility of numerous etiopathogenic factors analysis, which are responsible for many disorders of the skeletal system of animals. In fundamental pathology, "new" joint diseases descriptions can be found, thus forming a separate clinical entity in veterinary medicine. Literature data from animal paleopathology is mainly focused on interpretation and recording methodologies of osteoarthropathies (10, 15).

In respect to similar investigations, the aim of this paper is to describe joint diseases recorded in paleopathology, using the classification and nomenclature methods of fundamental veterinary pathology (12, 31).

CLASSIFICATION OF OSTEOARHROPATHIES IN ANIMAL PALEOPATHOLOGY

There is no complete classification of anomalies in veterinary pathology. The same conclusion can be made for joint diseases, but in the case of paleopathology, there are several other complicating factors. Diagnostic methods in paleopathology are often limited to gross examination (paleoradiological and histopathological investiagations were described in some surveys) of animal bone materials revealed during archaeological explorations. In most cases, analysis is performed on fragmented skeletal components, because whole and complete animal skeletons are a rarity (15, 26, 27). Moreover, many paleopathogists are not professional veterinarians or veterinary pathologists, which significantly limit their ability for correct identification, description, diagnosis and interpretation of the observed pathological changes. The most important factor is the many differences and inconsequences in the nomenclature of pathological conditions that can be found in the veterinary pathology textbooks. Namely, these textbooks are the source material for paleopathological diagnosis. Finally, the last factor is the lack of abnormalities classification in paleopathology. All these factors can lead to misdiagnosis and wrong interpretation of pathomorphological lesions in osteological animal remains.

The best way to recognize the significance and nature of the disease process is to apply a systematic approach to the pathological conditions. It is necessary to localize and describe pathological changes and develop a list of etiological factors (cause-result relation) and differential diagnosis. This reduces the possibility of mistakes in diagnosis, but it is essential to have correct classification with systematization of nomenclature in paleopathology. Some attempts for professional description and typisation of animal paleopathologies can be indicated in the available literature (2, 3, 4, 16).

Osteoarthropathies are one of the most commonly studied aspects of animal paleopathology (14, 15, 24, 32). It was stated that joint diseases are the most prevalent pathological changes in cattle remains (14, 32). Nevertheless, changes in the joints are also described in the skeletal remains of dogs (32), sheep/goat (2,3), pigs and some birds (3).

On the basis of anatomical localization, pathological processes can affect joints of the axial and appendicular skeleton, but depending on the type of joint some changes can be localized in various parts of the joints (12, 31). In this review we present a classification of joint diseases according to general veterinary pathology:
1. Developmental diseases of joints
2. Degenerative diseases of joints
3. Inflamatory diseases of joints
4. Traumatic diseases of joints
5. Tumors and tumor-like lesions of joints

1. Developmental diseases of joints
Developmental abnormalities of joints and bones are less frequently detected in bone animal remains than in other acquired pathological changes. Regardless, in order to facilitate the better understanding of the complexity in arthropathology, we shall show here only those anomalies that can be detected in archaeofauna. Etiology is the same as for the development of diseases in other organs, namely: unknown, multifactorial, monogenic, chromosomal and teratogenic. A great number of developing joint diseases are known in pathology: osteochondrosis (eg. hip dysplasia), developmental dislocations/subluxations, arthrogryposis, congenital torticollis, etc. (12, 31).

The best example of developmental abnormalities of the joints is canine hip dysplasia, also diagnosed in horses and cattle. The disease has polygenetic and multifactorial etiology with influence of the environmental factors. Clinical symptoms usually affect older dogs of large dog breeds. The changes start with synovitis and erosions on the articular cartilage. The femur head loses the round contour, creating severe degeneration of the articular surfaces with periarticular exostoses. The acetabulum is shallow and fills new osseous mass. The neck of the femur is wider than usual due to the new-created osteophytes. In palaeopathology, data on hip dysplasia is scarce, but this condition is expected to be found in the bones of dogs (23).

Another example of developmental anomalies of the joints is osteochondrosis. It is a frequent osteoarthropathy of pigs, horses and large dog's breeds. Cattle and sheep are rarely affected. Young and fast growing animals are predisposed to it. It occurs due to the disorders of endochondral ossification. Synonyms for this disorder are *osteochondritis dissecans* and *osteochondrosis dissecans*. The primary lesion occurs in the articular surface and is characterized by aseptic degradation of the articular cartilage and subchondral bone. Macromorphological diagnosis of osteochondrosis is difficult, because it needs well-preserved osteological material. Taphonomical changes and osteoarthritis can hinder the diagnosis of this pathology (24). The insertions in the articular surface can be found due to defragmentation of the subchondral bone. Osteochondrosis is common in palaeopathology, but it is often the cause of degenerative osteoartropathies which have much more pronounced changes. However, Sapir-Hen et al. (28) claim to have diagnosed osteochondrosis in talus of cattle from the archaeological site of Tel Megadim, Israel. Y. Telldahl (30) reports, that the articular depressions may be a sign of osteochondrosis or *osteochondritis dissecans*. However, articular depresions have often been seen in animal bone remains. According to Baker and Brothwell (2), articular depresions occurs in 7-13% of cases of all pathological changes. Earlier, it was believed, that the articular depressions are not pathological changes. It is easy to diagnose these changes. Noticeably, there are different types of incissions on articular facets and it is obvious, that the changes are identical to those in osteochondrosis of the joints.

2. Degenerative diseases of joints

Osteoarthrosis (degenerative osteoarthritis, degenerative joint disease, degenerative osteoarthropathy) is an abnormal condition of the joints, which is paleopathologicaly characterized by: grooving on the articular surface, eburnation, extension of the articular surface and peripheral exostoses (Fig. 1) (2).

These are the accepted criteria for diagnosis of osteoarthrosis in paleopathology. As previously mentioned, the great number of findings indicates this disease of the joints. The pathological image

of lesions in the joint depends on the period of process development. Based on the etiological and pathological aspects of this joint pathology, there is a primary and secondary osteoarthrosis. Primary osteoarthrosis can develop in cases when there are no external predisposing factors that can lead to disease. Aging is the only predisposing factor that leads to primary osteoarthrosis in animals, thus it is possible to question this kind of change when we observe archaeozoological material. Reduced blood flow in the joints of the animals leads to ischemic necrosis of the cartilage, which is the initial factor for further degenerative change (31).

Secondary osteoarthrosis is the consequence of a developmental disease of the joints (osteochondrosis) or, more frequently, some exogenous predisposing factors (trauma, physical burdening), which directly influence the formation of lesions within the articular cartilage. Traumatic changes, eg. impact in the joint region, can lead to instability, which causes degenerative lesions in cartilage. Necrosis, fractures, metabolic diseases of the joints, septic arthritis are changes which can cause secondary degenerative joint diseases (31).

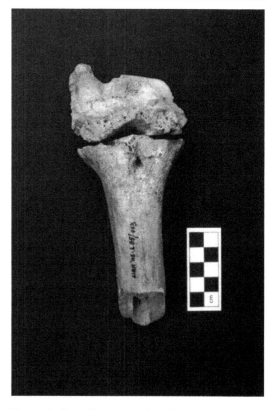

Figure 1. Ostearthrosis (spavin) of the tarso-metatarsal joint in cattle from Sirmium (Late Antiquity), Serbia (22)

Morphological changes in the joints are identical, regardless the primary or secondary osteoarthrosis. The primary changes are the erosion of the cartilage in those parts of the articular surface where the highest load bearing occurs. Articular cartilage is ulcerative, rough and macroscopically there is visible fibrillation. Linear-grooves on the articular surface, as a result of fibrillation, are seen most commonly in horses. The pathological process is extending to the subchondral bone that suffers sclerosing changes causing eburnation. In some rarer cases (due to eburnation) subchondral formation of cysts can be formed (24). Finally, after 7 days in the margin of articular surface exostoses can be seen (12, 31). Marginal osteophytes or exostoses are of different size, depending on the period of the occurrence of the process. Sclerosis of the subchondral bone may be the initial lesion in degenerative joint disease. However, the whole process is ending with extension of the articular surface. All described changes can be found on the skeletal remains of animals and almost always point to osteoarthrosis.

Osteorthrosis in paleopathology is common, especially in cattle and horses, which was concluded on the basis of the observations of many authors (4, 10, 11). This is a pathology of "working" animals. According to Baker and Brothwell (2), the first archaeozoological reports from the nineteenth and twentieth centuries have pointed to the high prevalence of osteoarthrosis in horses and cattle. Constant exploitation is the main explanation in archaeozoology used for this interpretation (2, 3, 14, 26). Bartosiewicz et al. (4) stated that joint pathology in cattle is the best "indicator" of exploitation on the basis of the similarities between the pathomorphological changes observed in cattle skeletal remains and modern Romanian draught oxen abnormalities.

Also, Bartosiewicz et al. (3, 4) had provided a comparative analysis of the osteological material, especially on metapodial bones and phalanges, in cattle from the Roman period and the Middle Ages with the same bone remains of prehistoric cattle. Lesions of the bones and joints in metapodials and phalanxes ocuured more often in cattle from the Roman period and the Middle Ages. This can be explained by the increased use of the animal species by man in the later period, as it was during the development of agriculture in ancient World civilizations (Roman Empire) and later, in medieval times. The systematic conducted survey of distal skeletal elements of bovine limbs remains from Eketorp (Sweden) has shown that there are no major changes in the prevalence of pathological lesions between animals of the Iron Age and the Middle Ages (30). However, the most prevalent degenerative joint diseases that can be found in archaeozoological material are bone spavin and ring bone (Fig. 2) in horses and cattle. The etiology of the bone spavin and ring bone is similar to ostearthrosis generally. Rather, there is almost no paleopathological survey in which this joint abnormalities are not described. What is interesting is the fact that bone spavin and ring bone even today have a high clinical importance in veterinary orthopedy of sport horses.

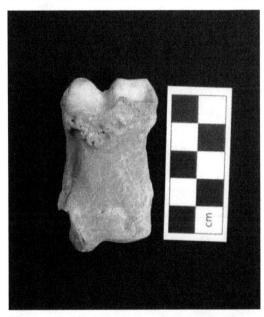

Figure 2. Proximal exostoses and lipping observed on phalanx prima from Sirmium - ringbone (Late Antiquity), Serbia (22)

Spondylosis chronica deformans is a degenerative disease of joints characterized by a fusion of the vertebrae (Fig. 3). Modern veterinary medicine knows many degenerative diseases of the spine (disc protrusion, fibrocartilage embolism), which can not be diagnosed in the dry bones form archaeological sites. Spondylosis is given special attention in paleopathology. This disease occurs in all domestic animals, but higher prevalence of occurrence of the disease was observed in older dogs (31). The exact cause of the disease is unknown, but traumatic lesions of *nucleus pulposus* have a crucial importance for the etiopathogenesis of spondylosis (12, 31). It is interesting that the skeletal remains of spondylitis or spondylosis, in the form of osteophyte formation, are usually diagnosed in horse remains. A wide range of "back problems" is observed in horse's remains, too. Paleopathology has reveald that spondylosis in horses occurs most likely due to over-riding or when using an improper saddle (5, 17, 19). The "kissing spine syndrome" as a fusion of 17 vertebrae in the spinal remains in the so-called "shaman" horse was described by Bökönyi (6). Bartosiewicz and Bartosiewicz (5) reported a severe form of spondylosis in the spine of the Migration period horse from the necropoly located in Hungary. This was a very severe case, maybe a terminal stage of spondylotic process, which authors compared with Bechterev´s diseases in humans. According to that, the frequent reports of vertebral fusion in animal paleopathology in the majority of the cases could be interpreted as a result of spine overloading and improper utilization of young animals (17, 29).

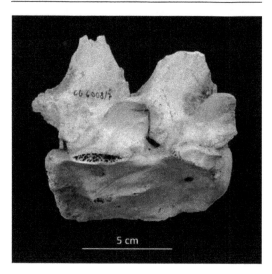

Figure 3. Vertebral column pathologies of horse – fussion of T18 – L1 verterbrae. Unpublished material from Caričin Grad (*Justiniana Prima*), early Byzantine period, Serbia

3. Inflamatory diseases in joints

Inflammatory diseases or inflammations of the joints in the literature cited below are synonims for arthritis and synovitis (12, 31). It should be stated that the inflammatory process is not the same as the infectious process - in this case arthritis. Secondary inflammation is a common alteration in degenerative joint diseases - osteoarthrosis, which in many cases can make a diagnosis difficult. Following this fact, inflammatory diseases of joints can be divided into: infective - with the presence of infectious microorganisms, and non - infective with the absence of microorganisms.

Many biological agents, including bacteria, viruses and fungi can be the cause of infectious arthritis of domestic animals. Septic arthritis caused

by bacteria is common (in contrast to viruses or fungi) in large and slaughter animals as a sequel of septicemia. Therefore many bacterial species can become a cause of arthritis. Probably the most important are pyogenic bacterias such as: *Arcanobacter pyogenes, Staphylococcus aureus, Streptococcus spp., Actinobacillus spp.* etc. *Salmonella spp. Escherichia coli, Mycoplasma spp., Brucella spp., Erysopelotrix rhusiopathie, Klebsiella spp.* can cause a joint infection in domestic animals (31), but species determination of bacteria in bone lesions from animal remains was not reported.

Animal skeletal remains of disarticulated joints had shown the sign of infection (2, 3, 24). According to the literature, in one study, 30% of the phalanges originating from cattle (Viking Age) showed destruction of the articular surface, which may be the result of infection (24). Baker and Brothwell (2) report a number of cases of joints infection (axial and appendicular skeleton) in all domestic animals, mostly among the remains from the British sites. Osteolytic changes in the form of cavitation and sinuses are a sign of supurative processes (abscesses) within bone tissues. Degradation of the articular surface with the periosteal reaction and the formation of marginal osteophytes are also present in articular infection. Articular extension and eburnation are rare findings in cases of joint infection. Irregular bone proliferation can lead to complete joint ankylosis. Such terminal pathological changes detected in tibia, talus, calcaneus, tarsal and metatarsal bones horse from Nitra – Chrenova site (Slovakia) (Fig. 4) are one of the most advanced joint and bone infections documented recently in animal paleopathology (15). The osteolytic changes were diagnosed in the distal phalanx of sheep and cattle, which are characteristic for footrot (2).

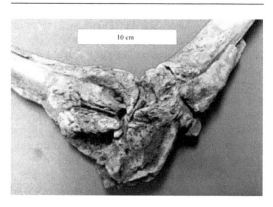

Figure 4. Infection of horse tarsal joint from Roman period, Nitra-Chrenova site, Slovakia (15)

Aseptic arthritis occurs without the involvement of microorganisms. A typical example is the rheumatoid arthritis in dogs and cats. Unfortunately, the accessible literature lacks any reports on animal bone assemblage from archaeological sites, because of the macroscopic differential diagnosis difficulties.

4. Traumatic diseases of joints

The most important traumatic injuries of the joints are *distorsio, luxatio* and *subluxatio*. According to the clinical status, they are divided into acute and chronic traumatic osteoarthropathy. The causes and archaeological significance of traumatic joints injuries of the joints are identical to those of bone trauma (2, 3). Traumatic joints injuries in paleopathological surveys have been observed (2). Some changes, dislocations/subluxations are difficult to distinguish from degenerative osteoarthritis or from some stages of degenerative joint disease (24). Spectacular post-traumatic changes are observed in sites dating from the Roman Republic and the Roman Empire. It is clear, that traumas of the skeletal system were caused by human intentional activities, Roman sports like chariots racing (22, 26).

5. Tumors and tumor-like lesions of joints

Neoplasms or tumors of joints are rare in archaeozoological findings. As with other bone tumors, macroscopic diagnosis and differential diagnosis of certain joint tumours types is almost impossible on the basis of unearthed animal bones. Paleopathological reports on these joint changes in animals are scarce, but some neoplastic alterations were found in dog skeletal remains. Onar et al. (25) described tumor in dog's humerus coming from Urartian fortress Van Yoncatepe. The tumor was described in the pelvis of the sacriefed monkey from Tuna El-Gebel (Egypt) by Angela von den Driesch et al. (33). The latter work formed a source of many arthropaties proofs, which were interpreted as results of traumas, hypovitaminosis (vitamine D metabolism disorder because of lack of sunlight) and technopaties (33).

CONCLUSION

Osteoarthropathies belong to the most frequent pathological conditions, which can be detected on animal skeletal remains. The most common joint defects are degenerative changes, which may be a sign of the intense use of animals by human populations in the past. According to the available literature (2, 3) and the authors' experiences in this field, it can be concluded that the ethiopathogenic factors that lead to osteoarthropathies are complex and multifactorial. In cases of palepathological surveys, it is preferred that joint malformations undergo paleoradiological and histological analysis. These techniques can confirm macroscopic diagnosis, which is in some cases subjective. This paper applied the classification and systematization of fundamental pathology of joint disease. These methods of classification can in certain circumstances be applied in animal paleopathology.

REFERENCES

1. Albarella, U., Johnstone, C., Vickers, K. (2008). The development of animal husbandry from the Late Iron Age to the end of the Roman period: a case study from South-East Britain. J. Archaeol. Sci. 35, 1828-1848 http://dx.doi.org/10.1016/j.jas.2007.11.016

2. Baker, J., Brothwell, D. (1980). Animal diseases in archaeology. Academic Press, London

3. Bartosiewicz, L . (2013). Shuffling nags, lame ducks: The archaeology of animal disease. Oxbow Books, Oxford

4. Bartosiewicz, L., Van Neer, W., Lentacker, A. (1997). Draught cattle: their osteological identification and history. Annales du Musée Royal de l'Afrique Centrale, Sciences Zoologiques, Tervuren, 281, 9-121.

5. Bartosiewicz, L, Bartosiewicz, G (2002). "Bamboo spine" in a migration period horse from Hungary. J Archaeol Sci. 29, 819-30. http://dx.doi.org/10.1006/jasc.2001.0715

6. Bokonyi, S. (1974). History of domestic mamals in Central and Eastern Europe, Akademiai Kiado. Budapest

7. Chrószcz, A., Krupska, A., Janeczek, M., Pospieszny, N., Jaworski, K., Pankiewicz, A. (2010). Animal remains from the archaeological excavation at Gromnik Hill (Rummelsberg) in Poland. Acta Scien. Pol. 9, 19-32.

8. Chrószcz, A., Janeczek, M., Miklikova, Z. (2010). Animal remains from Liptovská Mara, Northern Slovakia: A preliminary report. In: J. Beljak, G. Březinová, V. Varsik (Eds.), Archeólogia Barbarov 2009, (pp. 225 - 237). Achaeologica Slovaca Monographiae

9. Chrószcz, A., Janeczek, M. (2012). Wstępna ocena szczątków kostnych zwierząt ze stanowiska archeologicznego przy ul. Katedralnej 4 na Ostrowie Tumskim. In: A. Pankiewicz (Ed.), Wratislavia Antiqua 17, Nowożytny cmentarz przy kościele św. Piotra i Pawła na Ostrowie Tumskim we Wrocławiu (1621-1670), (pp. 205- 222). Instytut Archeologii UWr

10. Chrószcz, A., Janeczek, M., Pasicka, E., Bielichova, Z., Zawada, Z., Klećkowska-Nawrot, J., Szarek, A. (2014). Paleopathology of brown bear (Ursus arctos, L. 1758) from Liptovská Mara, Northern Slovakia. Res. Opin. Anim. Vet. Sci. 4, 35-39.

11. De Cupere, B., de Lentacker, A., van Neer, W., Waelkens, M., Verslype, L. (2000). Osteological evidence for the draught exploitation of cattle: First application of a new methodology. Int. J. Osteoarchaeol. 10, 254-267.
http://dx.doi.org/10.1002/1099-1212(200007/08)10:4<254::AID-OA528>3.0.CO;2-#

12. Dzietz, O., Huskamp, B. (2008). Parktyka kliniczna: Konie. Galaktyka, Łódź

13. Harcourt, R.A. (1967). Osteoarthritis in a Romano-British dog. J Small Anim Pract. 8, 521-522.
http://dx.doi.org/10.1111/j.1748-5827.1967.tb06774.x

14. Harcourt, R. A. (1971). The palaeopathology of animal skeletal remains. Vet. Rec. 89, 267-272.
http://dx.doi.org/10.1136/vr.89.10.267
PMid:5106361

15. Janeczek, M., Chrószcz, A., Miklikova, Z., Fabis, M. (2010). The pathological changes in the hind limb of a horse from the Roman Period. Vet. Med. Czech. 55, 331-335.

16. Janeczek, M., Chrószcz, A. (2011). The occipital area in medieval dogs and the role of occipital dysplasia in dog breeding. Turk. J. Vet. Anim. Sci. 35, 453-458.

17. Janeczek, M., Chrószcz, A., Onar, V., Henklewski, R., Piekalski, J., Duma, P., Czerski, A., Całkosiński, I. (2014). Anatomical and biomechanical aspects of the horse spine: the interpretation of vertebral fusion in a medieval horse from Wroclaw (Poland). Int. J. Osteoarchaeol. 24, 623–633.
http://dx.doi.org/10.1002/oa.2248

18. Köpke, N., Baten, J. (2008). Agricultural specialization and height in ancient and medieval Europe. Explorations in economic history. 45, 127-146.
http://dx.doi.org/10.1016/j.eeh.2007.09.003

19. Levine, AM., Whitwell, EK., Jeffcott, B.L. (2005). Abnormal thoracic vertebrae and the evolution of horse husbandry. Archaeofauna 14, 93-103.

20. Makowiecki, D. (2003). The usefulness of archaeozoological research in studies on the 'reconstruction' of the natural environment. Archaeozoologia 21, 121-134.

21. Marciniak, A. (2003). What is 'natural' in the archaeozoological animal bone assemblage? Taphonomic and statistical arguments. Archaeozoologia 21, 103-120.

22. Marković, N., Stevanović, O., Nešić, V., Marinković, D., Krstić, N., Nedeljković, D., Radmanović, D., Janeczek, M. (2014). Palaeopathological study of cattle and horse bone remains of the Ancient Roman city of Sirmium (Pannonia / Serbia). Rev Med Vet. 175, 77-88.

23. Murphy, EM. (2005). Animal palaeopathology in prehistoricand historic Ireland: a review of the evidence. In: Davies J, Fabis M, Mainland I, Richards M, Thomas R. (Eds.), Diet and health in past animal populations: current research and future directions. (pp. 8-23). Oxbow, Oxford
PMid:16045800 ; PMCid:PMC1215510

24. O'Connor, T. (2008). On the differential diagnosis of arthropathy in bovids. In: G. Grupe, G. McGlynn, J. Peters (Eds.), Limping together through the ages: joint afflictions and bone infections. Documenta Archaeobiologiae 6. (pp. 165 - 186). Verlag Marie Leidorf GmbH, Rahden/Westf.

25. Onar, V., Armutak, A., Belli, O., Konyar, B. (2002). Skeletal remains of dogs unearthed from the Van-Yoncatepe necropolises. Int. J. Osteoarchaeol. 12, 317-334.
http://dx.doi.org/10.1002/oa.627

26. Onar, V., Alpak, H., Pazvant, G., Armutak, A., Chrószcz, A. (2012). Byzantine horse skeletons of Theodosius harbour: 1. Paleopathology. Rev Med. Vet. 163, 139-146.

27. Reitz, E. J., Wing, E. S. (2001). Zooarchaeology. University Press Cambridge

28. Sapir – Hen, L., Bar – Oz, G., Hershkovitz, I., Raban-Gerstel, N., Marom, N., Dayan, T. (2008). Paleopathology survey of ancient mammal bones in Israel. Vet Med Zoot, 42, 62 – 70.

29. Stevanović, O., Marković, N. (2013). Traces of pathological changes on horses bones in past: paleopathological study. 4. Proceedings of the International fair and horse breeding – Horseville, pp. 132 - 138. Novi Sad (Serbia).

30. Telldahl, Y. (2002). Can paleopathology be used as evidence fo draught animals? In: Davies, J., Fabis, M., Mainland, I., Richards, M., Thomas, R. (Eds.), Diet and health in past animal populations. Current research and future directions (pp. 63-67). Proceedings of the 9th ICAZ Conference, Durham.

31. Thompson, K. (2007). Bones and joints. In: Grant, Jubb, Kennedy & Palmer's M (Eds.), Pathology of domestic animals. 5th ed. (pp. 2-180). Elsevier.

32. Von den Driesch, A. (1975). Die Bewertung pathologisch-anatomischer Veränderungen an vor- und frühgeschichtlichen Tierknochen. In: A. T. Clason (Ed.), Archaeozoological Studies. (pp. 413-425). North-Holland/American Elsevier, Amsterdam

33. Von den Driesch, A., Kessler, D., Peters, J. (2004). Mummified baboons and other primates from the Saitic-Ptolemaic animal necropolis of Tuna El-Gebel, Middle Egypt. Doc. Archaeobiol. 2, 231-278.

25

EFFECTS OF EXPERIMENTAL *TRYPANOSOMA CONGOLENSE* INFECTION ON SPERM MORPHOLOGY IN YANKASA RAMS

Oluyinka O. Okubanjo[1], Victor O. Sekoni[2], Ologunja J. Ajanusi[1], Adewale A. Adeyeye[3]

[1]Department of Veterinary Parasitology and Entomology, Faculty of Veterinary Medicine, Ahmadu Bello University, Zaria-Nigeria
[2]Department of Veterinary Public Health and Reproduction, College of Veterinary Medicine, Federal University of Agriculture, Abeokuta-Nigeria
[3]Department of Theriogenology and Animal Production, Faculty of Veterinary Medicine, Usmanu Danfodiyo University, Sokoto-Nigeria

ABSTRACT

The objective of the study was to determine the effect of *T. congolense* on the sperm morphology of Yankasa rams (YKR). Nine YKR aged 24-30 months-old were assigned into two groups of 6 infected and 3 uninfected control and were monitored for 7 weeks. The infected group of YKR was each inoculated with 1×10^6 *T. congolense* through the jugular vein, while the control group remained uninfected. The entire infected group developed trypanosomosis post infection (pi) characterized by sperm morphological abnormalities in the semen. There were significant (P<0.001) increases in the mean percentage of acrosomal, head, middle piece and tail abnormalities. Proximal and distal droplets as well detached heads were also significantly (P<0.001) increased post infection (pi). Acrosomal abnormalities, distal droplet and tail abnormalities increased from week 1 pi till the end of the study, while head abnormalities and detached heads increased from week 2 pi. Middle piece abnormalities and proximal droplets increased from week 3 and 4 pi till the end of the study respectively. The high incidence of morphological defects caused by *T. congolense* is capable of causing infertility from the first week pi thereby making the rams unfit for breeding at the end of the study.

Key words: infertility, sperm abnormalities, spermatogenesis, *Trypanosoma congolense*, Yankasa rams

INTRODUCTION

Sheep is a major source of animal protein in Nigeria (21), playing an important role in the livelihood of most Nigerians (26). Their distribution is majorly affected by socio-economic and environmental factors, such as availability of feeds, animal traction, marketing systems, cultural preferences and disease (8), which is a major constraint to livestock production in Nigeria (15).

Corresponding author: Dr. Adewale A. Adeyeye, DVM
E-mail address: adewale.adeyeye@udusok.edu.ng
Present address: Department of Theriogenology and Animal Production, Faculty of Veterinary Medicine, Usmanu Danfodiyo University, Sokoto-Nigeria

Trypanosomosis is an economic and zoonotic disease caused by protozoa of the genus *Trypanosoma* (20). It affects the cardiovascular, nervous, respiratory, digestive and reproductive systems of the body (12).

In the male reproductive tract, pathological disorders attributed to trypanosomosis include testicular degeneration, scrotal inflammation, penile protrusion, prepucial inflammation, testicular odema, epididymitis and abnormal spermatogenesis (1, 33, 34, 35). In the female, there is abortion, irregular oestrus cycle, cystic degeneration of the ovary, follicular cyst, flaccidity of the uterine horn, decreased conception rate, low birth-weights and neonatal death (10, 13, 16, 28). In addition, pregnant animals infected by trypanosomes may die before or after parturition (4, 6).

Trypanosoma congolense has a wide host range (11, 19). It is transmitted biologically (17) although mechanical (12) as well as congenital transmissions (14) have been reported. Infection of males with

T. congolense causes severe testicular degeneration, penile protrusion, haemorrhage, prepucial inflammation, decreased testosterone levels, increased cortisol concentration, depressed pituitary and adrenocortical functions in sheep, cattle and pig (18, 31, 35). Although Adeyemo et al. (3) studied the pathogenesis of *T. congolense* and *T. brucei* infections on West African Dwarf ram, while Sekoni (33) the effect of *T. vivax* on sperm morphology in Yankasa rams, there is no study on the effect of *T. congolense* on reproduction in Yankasa rams to the best of our knowledge. Aspects of the study involving genital lesions, reaction time, and semen characteristics have been described elsewhere (23, 24). This paper therefore reports on the effect of *T. congolense* on the incidence of sperm morphology of Yankasa rams.

MATERIAL AND METHODS

The study was carried out at the experimental animal house, Faculty of Veterinary Medicine, Ahmadu Bello University Zaria, Nigeria. Nine mature healthy Yankasa rams from an initial flock of sixteen rams purchased from local markets around the study facility were used. Their age was 24 – 30 months old and they were fed on legume hay (*harawa*), ground nut, maize offal, concentrate (100gm/head/day) multi-mineral nutrient block and fresh pasture. Water was also provided *ad libitum* throughout the experiment. The animals were acclimatized for 4 months in fly and tick proof pens. *Trypanosoma congolense* used for this study was obtained from the Nigerian Institute for Trypanosomiasis Research (NITR) Vom, Nigeria. This trypanosome was initially isolated from cattle but inoculated into mice and maintained by continuous passage until use. The study was approved by the ethical board of the Faculty of Veterinary Medicine, Ahmadu Bello University, Zaria and adequate measures were taken to minimize pain or discomfort.

The rams were divided into 2 groups of six infected and three uninfected control. They infected group of six (6) animals were inoculated with 1 x 10^6 *Trypanosoma congolense* through the jugular vein. All the rams were closely monitored for clinical signs suggestive of trypanosomosis. Semen was collected weekly from each ram, for seven weeks using electro-ejaculator and evaluated according to the methods of Chemineau and Cagnie (9). Sperm morphological abnormalities were estimated by dilution of semen sample with buffered formal saline and by staining with eosin-nigrosin stain then counting at least 500 sperms per slide as described by Sekoni et al. (29). Data obtained were analyzed using unpaired student *t*-test on SAS computer package. Values of P<0.001 were considered statistically significant.

RESULTS

The parasites were detected in the infected Yankasa rams within 7-11 days post infection (pi). There was a steady increase in mean acrosomal abnormalities of the infected Yankasa rams from 0.43 % to between 1.66 % and 12.25 % pi. These values were significantly increased (P<0.001) from week 1 pi compared to the control group, that ranged from 0.33 % - 1.25 % pi (Fig. 1).

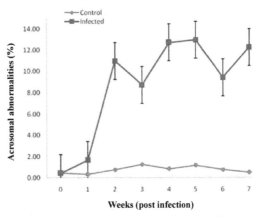

Figure 1. Mean percentage acrosomal abnormalities of Yankasa rams experimentally infected with *T. congolense*

The mean head abnormalities rose from 0.04 % pre-infection to a pi value of 0.88 % - 9.55 % for the infected group, which were significantly (P<0.001) increased compared to the control group (0.67 % - 1.00 %) from week 2 pi (Fig. 2).

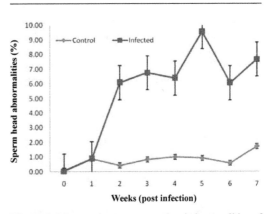

Figure 2. Mean percentage sperm head abnormalities of Yankasa rams experimentally infected with *T. congolense*

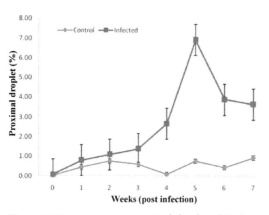

Figure 3. Mean percentage proximal droplet of Yankasa rams experimentally infected with *T. congolense*

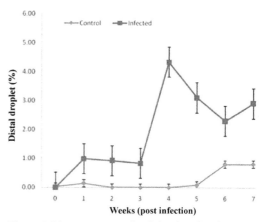

Figure 4. Mean percentage distal droplet of Yankasa rams experimentally infected with *T. congolense*

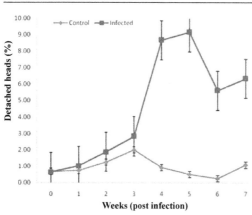

Figure 5. Mean percentage detached heads of Yankasa rams experimentally infected with *T. congolense*

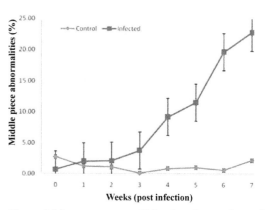

Figure 6. Mean percentage middle piece abnormalities of Yankasa rams experimentally infected with *T. congolense*

The mean proximal droplet values of infected Yankasa rams (0.33 % - 6.15 %) were significantly increased (P<0.001) compared to the control (0.08 % - 0.92 %) from week 4 pi till the end of the study (Fig. 3). There was also significant increase (P<0.001) in the mean distal droplet of the infected group (0.83 % - 4.33 %) compared to the control group (0.00 % - 0.42 %) from week 1 pi till the end of the study (Fig. 4). The mean percentage of detached sperm heads of control and infected rams is presented in Figure 5. There was a significant (P<0.001) increase in the mean detached heads of the infected rams (1.02 % - 9.15 %) compared to the control (0.25 % - 2.00 %) from week 2 pi till the end of the study. The middle piece abnormalities of the infected rams (1.98 % - 22.79 %) were significantly (P<0.05) increased compared to rams in the control group (0.08 % - 3.63 %), from week 3 pi till the end of the study (Fig. 6).

Tail abnormalities also significantly (P<0.05) increased, but from week 1 pi till the end of the study in the infected rams (13. 99 % - 44.75 %) compared

to rams in the control group (6.72 % - 16.72 %) (Fig. 7). Sperm tail abnormalities were more prominent in infected rams than abnormalities associated with the sperm head.

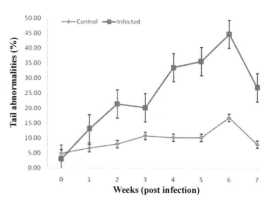

Figure 7. Mean percentage tail abnormalities of Yankasa rams experimentally infected with *T. congolense*

DISCUSSION

The infection of Yankasa rams with *T. congolense* showed some clinical signs (fluctuating, pyrexia, ruffled hair coat, dullness, weight loss and pallor of the mucous membrane) that have been published in our previous investigations (24).

In this study we demonstrated the adverse effect of *T. congolense* infection on the sperm morphology of Yankasa rams. The morphological abnormalities seen were acrosome abnormalities, sperm head abnormalities, proximal droplet, distal droplet, middle piece abnormalities, detached head and tail abnormalities. Sperm morphology is one of the factors determining semen quality besides sperm motility and concentration (27). The occurrence of sperm morphological abnormalities in the semen of animals is associated with infertility and sterility (30). From the first week of infection, substantial acrosomal, tail and distal droplets defects were observed. This was capable of compromising acrosomal reaction and sperm motility and by extension the fertility of infected animals. Other morphological abnormalities were seen in the second (sperm head and detached head abnormalities); third (middle piece) and fourth (proximal droplet) weeks post infection. However, signs of infertility in the infected rams would have been evident as early as the first week and will continue to increase till the end of the study. This progressive increase in abnormalities for the 7 weeks study period, which is also the duration for a spermatogenic cycle in rams, suggest that *T. congolense* infection in Yankasa rams may not just affect the spermatogenesis in the testicles alone, but also the maturation process at the tail of the epididymis. This is supported by the lesions observed in the epididymis and the testis in our earlier study (23). The sperm morphological abnormalities seen in this study are also similar to those reported by Sekoni (33) in *T. vivax* infected Yankasa rams where abnormalities were seen from the second week post infection. However, in this study, abnormalities were seen from the first week post infection. The variation in trypanosome specie maybe responsible for this, since its infectivity and pathogenesis depends on the specie and strain of the trypanosome (22). This may suggest that *T. congolense* in more virulent than *T. vivax* in Yankasa rams. Previous studies in bulls have also supported this fact (32, 34). Osaer et al. (25) observed minor morphological abnormalities following infection of Djallonke rams with *T. congolense*. They also observed return of sperm morphology to their pre-infection state as the infection progressed in this breed of sheep. This is contrary to the report in this study, which may have been influenced by

breed difference. The Djallonke sheep is a West Africa Dwarf sheep found in Gambia and are generally known to be trypanotolerant surviving in tsetse infested areas (7). In contrast, the Yankasa breed used in this study are highly susceptible to trypanosomosis (2, 5, 33).

CONCLUSION

The *T. congolense* used in this study is pathogenic to Yankasa rams with substantial percentage of sperm morphological abnormalities. The outcome of this on Yankasa rams in field situation may increase the incidence of infertility which is detrimental to sheep production.

REFERENCES

1. Adamu, S.; Fatihu, M. Y., Useh, N. M., Mamman, M., Sekoni, V. O., Esievo, K. A. N. (2007). Sequential testicular and epididymal damage in Zebu bulls experimentally infected with *Trypanosoma vivax*. Veterinary Parasitology, 143(1): 29-34. http://dx.doi.org/10.1016/j.vetpar.2006.07.022 PMid:16935425

2. Adenowo, T. K, Njoku, C. O., Oyedipe, E. O., Sannusi, A. (2004). Experimental trypanosomiasis in Yankasa ewes: the body weight response. African Journal of Medicine and Medical Sciences, 33(4): 323-326. PMid:15977439

3. Adeyemo, O.; Oyejide, A., Agbedana, O. (1990). Plasma testosterone in *Trypanosoma congolense* and *Trypanosoma brucei* infected West African dwarf rams. Animal Reproduction Science, 22, 21-26. http://dx.doi.org/10.1016/0378-4320(90)90034-D

4. Anene, B. M., Omamegbe, J. O. (1984). Abortion associated with *Trypanosoma brucei* infection in an Alsatian bitch: A case report. Tropical Veterinarian, 2, 211-213.

5. Audu, P. A., Esievo, K. A. N., Mohammed, G., Ajanusi, O. J. (1999). Studies on infectivity and pathogenicity of an isolate of *Trypanosoma evansi* in Yankasa sheep. Veterinary Parasitology, 86, 185-190. http://dx.doi.org/10.1016/S0304-4017(99)00141-7

6. Bawa, E. K., Sekoni. V. O., Olorunju. S. A. S., Uza, D. V., Ogwu, D., Oyedipe, E. O. (2005). Comparative clinical observations on *Trypanosoma vivax* infected pregnant Yankasa and West African Dwarf ewes. Journal of Animal and Veterinary Advances, 4 (7): 630-636.

7. Bengaly Z., Clausen, P. H., Boly, H., Kanwe, A., Duvallet G. (1993). Comparison of experimental trypanosomiasis in various breeds of small ruminants in Burkina Faso. Revue d'Elevage et de Medcine Veterinaire des Pays Tropicaux, 46(4): 563-570. PMid:7915427

8. Blench, R. M. (1999). Traditional livestock breeds: geographical distribution and dynamics in relation to the ecology of West Africa. Retrieved November, 28, 2010 from http://www.odi.org.uk/resources/download/2041.pdf.

9. Chemineau, P., Cagnie, Y. (1991). Training manual on artificial insemination in sheep and goats. FAO Animal Production and Health Paper: 83.

10. Dalal, S. M., Amer, H. A., Rwaida, M. R. (2008). Pathological and some biochemical studies on pregnant ewes experimentally infected with *Trypanosoma evansi*. Egyptian Journal Comparative Pathology and Clinical Pathology, 21, 372- 400.

11. Desquesnes, M. (2004). Livestock Trypanosomoses and their Vectors in Latin America (English translation). Published by World Organization for Animal Health (OIE). PP. 8-19.

12. Desquesnes, M., Dia, M. L. (2003). Mechanical transmission of *Trypanosoma congolense* in cattle by the African tabanid Atylotus agrestis. Experimental Parasitology, 105: 226–231. http://dx.doi.org/10.1016/j.exppara.2003.12.014 PMid:14990316

13. Faye, D., Sulon, J., Kane, Y., Beckers, J. F., Leak, S., Kaboret, Y., Sousa, N. M., Losson, B., Geerts, S. (2004). Effects of an experimental *Trypanosoma congolense* infection on the reproductive performance of West African Dwarf goats. Theriogenology, 62: 1438-1451. http://dx.doi.org/10.1016/j.theriogenology.2004.02.007 PMid:15451252

14. Griffin, L. (1983). Congenital transmission of *Trypanosoma congolense* in mice. Journal of Comparative Pathology, 93(3): 489-492. http://dx.doi.org/10.1016/0021-9975(83)90036-1

15. Lamorde, A. G. (1996). The role of veterinarians in a developing economy. Nigerian Veterinary Journal (Special Edition), 1(1): 106-111.

16. Leigh, O. O., Fayemi, O. E. (2013). The effect of experimental *Trypanosoma brucei* infection on hormonal changes during the oestrous cycle, pregnancy and pregnancy outcome in West Africa Dwarf does. Wayamba Journal of Animal Science, ID 1365263763.

17. Mbaya, A. W., Kumshe, H., Nwosu, C. O. (2012). The mechanisms of anaemia in trypanosomosis: A Review. In: Anemia, (D. Silverberg editor.). Published by InTech. pp. 276. http://dx.doi.org/10.5772/29530

18. Mutayoba, B. M., Eckersall, P. D., Seely, C., Gray, C. E., Cestnik, V., Jeffcoate, I. A., Holmes, P. H. (1995). Effects of *Trypanosoma congolense* on pituitary and adrenocortical function in sheep: responses to exogenous corticotrophin-releasing hormone. Research in Veterinary Science, 58, 180-185. http://dx.doi.org/10.1016/0034-5288(95)90074-8

19. Office of the International Epizootic (OIE) (2009). Trypanosomosis (Tsetse-transmitted). Retrieved from www.oie.int/fileadmin/...in.../TRYPANO_TSETSE_FINAL.pdf.

20. Office of the International Epizootic (OIE) (2013). *Trypanosomosis - tsetse* transmitted. In: OIE Terrestrial Manual. pp. 1-11.

21. Opasina B.A., David-West K.B. (1987). Position paper on sheep and goat production in Nigeria. In: Proceedings of an FAO seminar on Sheep and goat meat production in the humid tropics of West Africa held in Yamoussoukro, Côte d'Ivoire. PMid:3424454

22. Ogunsanmi, A. O., Akpavie, S. O., Anosa, V. O. (1994). Haematology changes in ewes experimentally infected with *Trypanosoma brucei*. Revue d"Elevage et de medicine Veterinaire des pays Tropicaux, 47(1): 53-57.

23. Okubanjo, O. O.; Sekoni, V. O.; Ajanusi, O. J., Nok, A. J., Adeyeye, A. A. (2014). Testicular and epididymal pathology in Yankasa rams experimentally infected with *Trypanosoma congolense*. Asian Pacific Journal of Tropical Disease, 4(3): 185-189. http://dx.doi.org/10.1016/S2222-1808(14)60502-8

24. Okubanjo, O. O., Sekoni, V. O., Ajanusi, O. J., Adeyeye, A. A. (2014). Semen characteristics and reaction time of yankasa rams experimentally infected with *Trypanosoma congolense*. Global Veterinaria, 13 (3): 297-301.

25. Osaer S., Goossens, B., Sauveroche, B., Dempfle, L. (1997). Evaluation of the semen quality and reproductive performance of trypanotolerant Djallonké rams following an artificial infection with *Trypanosoma congolense*. Small Ruminant Research, 24(3): 213–222. http://dx.doi.org/10.1016/S0921-4488(96)00944-3

26. Otchere E. O. (1986). Small ruminant production in tropical Africa. In: Proceedings an FAO expert consultation held in Sofia, Bulgaria, 8–12 July 1985. Paper 58.

27. Podstawski Z., Kosiniak-Kamysz K., Bittmar A. (2007). Relationship between some enzymes activity, sperm morphology and stallion semen quality. Zootehnie şi Biotehnologii, 40(1): 152-156.

28. Rodrigues, C. M. F., Olinda, R. G., Silvaa, T. M. F., Valea, R. G., Da Silvaa, A. E., Limaa, G. L., Garciab, H. A., Teixeirab, M. M. G., Batista, J. S. (2013). Follicular degeneration in the ovaries of goats experimentally infected with *Trypanosoma vivax* from the Brazilian semi-arid region. Veterinary Parasitology, 191, 146–153. http://dx.doi.org/10.1016/j.vetpar.2012.08.001 PMid:22921989

29. Sekoni, V. O.; Gustafsson, B. K., Mather, E. C. (1981). Influence of wet fixation staining techniques and storage time on bull sperm morphology. Nordisk Veterinaer Medicin, 33, 161-166.
PMid:6172775

30. Sekoni, V. O., Gustafsson, B. K. (1987). Seasonal variations in the incidence of sperm morphological abnormalities in dairy bulls regularly used for artificial insemination. British Veterinary Journal, 43, 312-317.
http://dx.doi.org/10.1016/0007-1935(87)90064-9

31. Sekoni, V. O.; Njoku, C. O.; Kumi-Diaka, J., Saror, D. I . (1990a). Pathological changes in male genitalia of cattle infected with *Trypanosoma vivax* and *Trypanosoma congolense*. British Veterinary Journal, 146, 175-180.
http://dx.doi.org/10.1016/0007-1935(90)90011-Q

32. Sekoni V. O., Saror D. I., Njoku C. O., Kumi-Diaka J. (1990b). Elevation of morphological abnormalities of spermatozoa in the semen of Zebu bulls consequent to *Trypanosoma vivax* and *Trypanosoma congolense* infections. Theriogenology, 33(4): 925-936.
http://dx.doi.org/10.1016/0093-691X(90)90827-G

33. Sekoni V. O. (1993). Elevated sperm morphological abnormalities of Yankasa rams consequent to *Trypanosoma vivax* infection. Animal Reproduction Sciences, 31(3-4): 243–248.
http://dx.doi.org/10.1016/0378-4320(93)90009-G

34. Sekoni, V. O., Rekwot, P. I., Bawa, E. K. (2004). Effects of *Trypanosoma vivax* and *Trypanosoma congolense* infections on the reaction time and semen characteristics of Zebu (Bunaji) x Friesian crossbred bulls. Theriogenology, 61, 55-62.
http://dx.doi.org/10.1016/S0093-691X(03)00183-3

35. Victor I.; Sackey A. K. B., Natala A. J. (2012). Penile protrusion with hemorrhages and prepucial inflammation in pigs experimentally infected with *Trypanosoma congolense*. Journal of Animal Production Advances, 2(6): 297-302.

26

OBSERVATION OF PHYSIOLOGICAL CHANGES AFTER DETOMIDINE ADMINISTRATION IN PATERI GOAT

Ahmed Tunio[1], Shamasuddin Bughio[1], Jam Kashif Sahito[1],
Muhammad Ghiasuddin Shah[1], Mahdi Ebrahimi[2], Shazia Parveen Tunio[3]

[1]*Faculty of Animal Husbandry and Veterinary Sciences,
Sindh Agriculture University, Tandojam 70060, Pakistan*
[2]*Faculty of Veterinary Medicine, Universiti Putra Malaysia*
[3]*Social Science Research Institute, Tandojam, Pakistan*

ABSTRACT

The objective of this study was to determine the physiological effects of detomidine on Pateri goats. A total of six female Pateri goats were randomly treated with three different dose rates of Detomidine at 40 µg, 50 µg and 60 µg/kg body weights. The effects of Detomidine on respiratory and heart rate, rectal temperature and serum glucose level were investigated. Following detomidine intravenous administration in goats, it produced dose dependent effect on physiological parameters. Respiratory and heart rate decreased after intravenous administration in all goats. The heart rate decreased at 5 min with all dose rates and returned to the base line at 60 min. This change in heart rate was dose dependent and there was no significant (P>0.05) change observed with 40 µg and 50 µg/kg of Detomidine. However, there was significant difference (P<0.05) at 75 min between the 40 µg and 60 µg/kg of Detomidine in all goats. However, significant (P<0.01) increase in serum glucose level occurred with all dose rates at 30 min compared with control groups. It is concluded that Detomidine has produced no adverse effect on physiological parameters.

Key words: Pateri goat, detomidine, respiratory rate, heart rate, glucose

INTRODUCTION

Goats undergo many surgical procedures, such as hernia, dystocia and traumatic injuries. Presently, Detomidine is used to provide good sedation and analgesia in horses (1, 2) at a dose rate of 10-20 µg/kg in horses (3). It is a highly potent drug, used for sedation in all animals, but has significant effect on physiological parameters. Results of several studies on the use of Detomidine have shown some impact on physiological parameters, with detomidine decreasing the heart rate, respiratory rate and then vital parameters returning to normal level slowly (4).

Corresponding author: Prof. Ahmed Tunio, PhD
E-mail address: ahmedtuniodvm2009@gmail.com
Present address: Faculty of Animal Husbandry and
Veterinary Sciences, Sindh Agriculture University
Tandojam, 70060, Pakistan

Meanwhile, Detomidine with 40 µg/kg decreases the respiratory rate, heart rate and rectal temperature, when used in sheep and goats respectively (5, 6). Beside this it increases the serum glucose level in goats (7, 8). Generally, goats kept for milk purpose on which various surgical procedures are performed and they need safe pre-anesthetics (9). Sedative and analgesics are used on goats for minor surgery, in order for animals to get relief from pain. Our practice suggests that application of Detomidine is a good choice for minor operations in goats. To our knowledge, there are limited reports available concerning the assessment of the physiological effects of Detomidine in goats. The purpose of this study was to assess whether Detomidine can be used in goats and have limited effects on physiological parameters. The hypothesis was that goats receiving Detomidine may have minimal effects on their physiological parameters in the case of minor and major clinical surgical procedures. The physiological effects of Detomidine are investigated to learn about the side effects and for future application.

MATERIAL AND METHODS

This study was carried out in the Department of Surgery and Obstetrics, Faculty of Animal Husbandry and Veterinary Sciences, Sindh Agriculture University Tandojam. Six healthy Pateri female goats, aged between 6 to 8 months with body weight of 23.03±3.50 kg (mean ± SE) were used. All animals were purchased from the local market for this experiment. Goats received routine physical examination and they were found to be bright, alert and responsive during the study time. All animals were fed bursem grass and provided fresh water *ad libitum*. They were ear tagged from 1 to 6 for identification and were adapted for two weeks. The goats were randomly treated with three different dose rates of Detomidine (Dermosidan, 10mg/ml, Farmos Group ltd, Turku, Finland) as 40µg/kg, 50µg/kg and 60µg/kg body weights. Each goat received three dose rates with 10 days interval between each treatment. After weighing the goats, hairs around left and right jugular vein sites were clipped using automatic hair clipper and prepared aseptically. The left jugular vein was used for intravenous administration of the drug using an 1 ml disposable syringe. The right jugular vein was used for blood sample collection using a 3 ml disposable syringe, transferred into plain tube and labeled as a control (before treatment) and treatment sample at intervals after drug administration. Physiological parameters were recorded before and after treatment, i.e., respiratory rate (RR) breaths/min were examined by counting thoracic movement in one minute, heart rate (HR) beats/min was taken from the left side of the thorax using a stethoscope and taken from all animals five minutes before the experiment as a control and then at 5, 15, 30, 45, 60, 75, 90, 105 and 120 min. after treatment in all goats. The rectal temperature ^0C (RT) was obtained from each animal at five minutes before and then every 15 min. up to 120 min. post Detomidine administration using a clinical thermometer. For determination of the glucose level, venous blood samples 3 ml were collected each time from the jugular vein as a control and then at 30, 90 and 1440 min. after the administration of Detomidine. The blood samples were centrifuged at 4000 revolutions/min for 15 minutes and then the serum glucose was determined using a reflotron glucose test strip (Boehringer Mnnheim, Germany) on Reflotron Plus blood chemistry machine (Boehringer Mannheim Diagnostics, Germany).

Statistical analysis

The results obtained were analyzed using one way analysis of variance (ANOVA) with Tukey-Kramer multiple comparison test. All statistical tests were conducted at 95% confidence level.

RESULTS

Respiratory rate (RR)

The mean control values of respiratory rate (RR) breathe/min with three treatments were 18.66±0.98, 19.33±1.11 and 18.66±0.98 in all goats respectively (Table 1). The Control values were not significantly different, respectively. RR decreased significantly at 30, 15 and 5 minutes after administration of 40µg/kg, 50µg/kg and 60µg/kg of Detomidine, respectively in all goats. The maximum decrease in RR occurred at 30 min. in all dose rates. Then RR slowly returned to the base line by 60 min., 90 min. and 105 min. after treatment of 40µg/kg, 50µg/kg and 60µg/kg of Detomidine respectively, in all goats (Table 1).

Table 1. Mean (±SE) respiratory rate with various dose rates of Detomidine in goats

Time (minutes)	Detomidine dose rates		
	40µg/kg	50µg/kg	60µg/kg
0	18.66±0.98	19.33±1.11	18.66±0.98
5	16.83±1.01	15.66±0.95	13.33±0.98**
15	14.83±0.65	14.66±0.95*	12.00±0.51**
30	13.00±0.51**	12.00±0.51**	11.33±0.42**
45	13.50±0.50**	13.66±0.80**	11.66±0.61**
60	14.83±0.40	14.00±0.73**	12.00±0.73**
75	15.50±0.50	14.66±0.66*	12.66±0.71**
90	17.00±0.44	15.00±0.85	14.16±0.90*
105	18.00±1.03	18.00±0.89	15.33±1.08
120	18.66±0.98	19.00±1.00	18.66±0.98

* =Significant difference at (P<0.05) between the values and corresponding control
** = Significant difference at (P<0.01) between the values and corresponding control

Table 2. Mean (±SE) heart rate with various dose rates of Detomidine in goats

Time (minutes)	Detomidine dose rates		
	40µg/kg	50µg/kg	60µg/kg
0	76.33±1.58	81.66±2.10	76.16±2.59
5	50.16±4.24[aa]	48.33±2.10[aa]	47.33±1.60[aa]
15	51.33±3.16[aa]	50.83±2.34[aa]	47.33±1.14[aa]
30	54.66±2.44[aa]	53.33±3.49[aa]	43.50±0.88[aa]
45	57.33±2.40[aa]	56.16±3.16[aa]	47.50±1.02[aa]
60	62.50±3.33[aa,bb]	58.50±3.32[aa]	49.50±1.08[aa,bb]
75	66.66±2.95[bb]	64.00±3.81[aa,c]	51.50±1.08[aa,bb,c]
90	69.00±3.64[bb]	68.66±3.56[a,cc]	57.16±1.01[aa,bb,cc]
105	74.00±2.42[b]	71.66±3.40	62.50±1.25[aa,b]
120	76.33±1.58	78.33±2.27	76.16±1.60

a   = Significant difference at (P<0.05) between the values and corresponding control
aa   = Significant difference at (P<0.01) between the values and corresponding control
b   = Significant difference at (P<0.05) between the values of 40µg/kg and 60µg/kg at corresponding time
bb   = Significant difference at (P<0.01) between the values of 40µg/kg and 60µg/kg at corresponding time
c   = Significant difference at (P<0.05) between the values of 50µg/kg and 60µg/kgat corresponding time
cc   = Significant difference at (P<0.01) between the values of 50µg/kg and 60µg/kg at corresponding time

Heart rate (HR)

The mean control values of heart rate (HR) beats/min in goats were 76.33±1.58, 81.66±2.10 and 76.16±2.59 per min. respectively. Table 2 shows that mean control values were not different significantly from each other. However, PR decreased at 5 min. with all doses and returned to base line at 60 min., 90 min. and 105 min. after 40µg/kg, 50µg/kg and 60µg/kg administration of Detomidine respectively. Detomidine showed that there was no significant difference in the PR rate in goats after all the treatment, but   significant difference (*P*<0.01) was observed from 60 to 90 min. and at 105 min. a significant difference (P<0.05) was observed between 40µg/kg and 60µg/kg of Detomidine respectively.

Rectal temperature (°C)

Mean control values of rectal temperature (RT) were 39.26±0.01°C, 39.31±0.1°C, 39.30±0.0°C in all goats respectively (Table 3). There were no significant difference observed between 40µg/kg, 50µg/kg and 60µg/kg of Detomidine in all goats respectively.

Serum glucose level

There was no significant difference in corresponding control values between all groups. However, there was significant difference (P<0.05) in the serum glucose level after Detomidine administration because this increase of glucose was dose dependent. Maximum increase in the serum glucose happened at 30 minutes when using all

Table 3. Mean (±SE) rectal temperature (°C) in goats after Detomidine administration at difference dose rates

Time (minutes)	Detomidine dose rates		
	40µg/kg	50µg/kg	60µg/kg
0	39.26±0.01	39.31±0.1	39.30±0.0
15	39.10±0.1	39.05±0.1	38.96±0.1
30	38.90±0.1	38.80±0.1	38.58±0.2
45	38.85±0.1	38.48±0.3	38.26±0.2
60	38.91±0.1	38.30±0.3	37.98±0.19
75	38.85±0.2	38.18±0.3	37.98±0.19
90	38.85±0.2	38.26±0.2	38.16±0.31
105	38.85±0.2	38.65±0.3	38.20±0.3
120	39.01±0.1	39.15±0.1	39.13±0.14

Table 4. Mean (±SE) glucose level after administration of Detomidine in goats

Time (minutes)	Detomidine dose rates		
	40µg/kg	50µg/kg	60µg/kg
0	66.91±2.32	64.80±2.39	64.01±2.70
30	125.67±3.75 [aa, dd]	139.33±4.39 [dd]	154.83±4.56 [aa, dd]
90	83.56±3.01[b, d, ññ]	101.52±2.49 [b, ññ, dd]	127.17±5.80 [dd, dd, mm]
1440	65.50±2.23	63.96±2.69	62.13±2.42

aa = Significant difference at (P<0.01) between the values of 40µg/kg and 60µg/kg at corresponding time
b =Significant difference at (P<0.05) between the values of 40µg/kg and 50µg/kg at corresponding time
d = Significant difference at (P<0.05) corresponding control
dd = Significant difference at (P<0.01) corresponding control
mm = Significant difference at (P<0.01) between the values of 40µg/kg and 60µg/kg at corresponding time
ññ = Significant difference at (P<0.01) between the values of 50µg/kg and 60µg/kg at corresponding

three doses and then the serum glucose level started to return gradually from 90 minutes up-to 24 hours. The mean values for the serum glucose level were significantly decreased at 30 minutes (P<0.05) with 40µg/kg as compared to values with 50µg/kg of Detomidine (Table 4). Similarly mean values were significantly lower at 30 minutes (P<0.01) and 90 minutes with 40µg/kg as compared to values with 50µg/kg of Detomidine. Similarly mean values were significantly lower at 30 min. (P<0.01) and 90 min. with 40µg/kg as compared to corresponding values with 60µg/kg of Detomidine. Mean values were significantly lower at 90 min. (P<0.01) with 50µg/kg as compared to corresponding values with 60µg/kg of Detomidine.

DISCUSSION

Data on the physiological effects of detomidine in goat is limited. The respiratory rate (RR) decreased significantly in all goats in this study, which is similar to the findings observed in goats (6), in horses (4, 10, 11) and in calves (12). However, on the other hand in sheep it was observed that Detomidine had accelerated the respiratory rate in the first 15 min. with Detomidine (5, 7). The heart rate decreased after Detomidine administration of 40µg/kg, 50µg/kg and 60µg/kg in all goats. Similarly, decrease in the heart rate has been reported in horses (4, 10, 13) as well in sheep's (5) and in buffalo's (14). While rectal temperature in this study slightly decreased after administration of Detomidine, this decrease was not significant compared to the control values. Previous study by Singh et al. (6) reported that in goats rectal temperature decreased with 40µg/kg of Detomidine. In other animals Detomidine also had an effect on body temperature, with decreases in calves (12) and in sheep's (7).

In this study increase in serum glucose occurred in all goats and this increase of the serum glucose is also in agreement with results published by Ambrósio, A. M. et al. (15), where serum glucose increased because Detomidine has an anti-insulin effect and stimulates the alpha-2 receptors in pancreas resulting in increased blood glucose level. This effect on the blood glucose was due to Detomidine in this study. Similarly it was reported that glucose increased in sheep with Detomidine at 30µg/kg, 60µg/kg and 90µg/kg dose rates (7). Increase in the serum glucose level was also reported by other recherches in goats (6, 8).

CONCLUSION

The study revealed that Detomidine has no adverse effects on physiological parameters. In addition, the effects on physiological parameters remained dose dependent, proving Detomidine is useful for goats. Further physiological study is needed to confirm these findings.

REFERENCES

1. Grimsrud, K. N., Mama, K. R., Thomasy, S. M., Stanley S. D. (2009). Pharmacokinetics of detomidine and its metabolites following intravenous and intramuscular administration in horses. Equine Vet J. 41 (4): 361-365.
http://dx.doi.org/10.2746/042516409X370900
PMid:19562897

2. Mama, K. R., Grimsrud, K., Snell, T., Stanley, S. (2009). Plasma concentrations, behavioural and physiological effects following intravenous and intramuscular detomidine in horses. Equine Vet J. 41 (8): 772-777.

3. Hall, L.W., Clarke, K.W. (1991). Veterinary anesthesia. 9th ed, Bailler Tindall. 191-193.
PMid:1889172

4. Jochle, W. (1990). Dose selection for Detomidine as a sedative and analgesic in horses with colic from controlled and open clinical studies. J. Equine. Vet. Scs. 10 (1): 6-11.
http://dx.doi.org/10.1016/S0737-0806(06)80075-4

5. Komar, E. (1989). Detomidine as a sedative in sheep. Folia Veterinaria 33, 9-17.

6. Singh, A. P., Peshin, P. K., Singh, J., Sharifi, D., Patil, D. B. (1990). Evaluation of detomidine as a sedative in goats. Acta Veterinaria Hungarica 39 (3-4): 109-114.

7. Singh, J., Singh, A. P., Peshin, P. K., Sharifi, D., Patil, D. B. (1994). Evaluation of Detomidine as a sedative in sheep. Indian J Ani Sci. 63 (3): 237-238.

8. Dilip, K.D., Sharma, A. K., Gupta O. P. (1997). Studies on hematological and biochemical changes induced during alpha adrenoreceptor against sedation in goats. Indian Vet.J. 74 (6): 496-498.

9. Zeedan, K. I., El-Malky, O. M., El-Ella, A. A. (2014). Nutritional, physiological and microbiological studies on using biogen-zinc on productive and reproductive performance of ruminants. 2-productive performance, digestion and some blood components of Damascus goats. Egyptian J Sheep and Goat Sci. 9 (3): 49-66.

10. Aguiar, A. J., Hussni, C. A., Luna, S. P., Castro, G. B., Massone, F., Alves, A. L. (1993). Propofol compared with propofol V guaiphenesin after detornidine premedication for equine surgery. Vet Anaes Analg. 20 (1): 26-28.
http://dx.doi.org/10.1111/j.1467-2995.1993.tb00105.x

11. Skarda, R. T., Muir, W. W. (1996). Comparison of antinociceptive, cardiovascular, and respiratory effects, head ptosis, and position of pelvic limbs in mares after caudal epidural administration of xylazine and detomidine hydrochloride solution. American J Vet Res. 57 (9): 1338-1345.
PMid:8874730

12. Garcia, O.H., Errecalde, C., Prieto, G. (1991). Clinical evaluation of intravenous detomidine hydrochloride in calves. Veterinary argent. 8 (74): 248-251.

13. Short, C.E. (1992). The response to the use of Detomidine (Domosedan) in the horse. Wiener-Tieraztliche-Monatsschrift 79 (1): 2-12.

14. Silva, D.D.N., Dangolla, A., Silva, L.N.A. (1991). Preliminary studies on sedative analgesic effects of Detomidine (dermosidan) in buffalo calves. Srilanka Vet. J. 38, 26.

15. Ambrósio, A. M., Casaes, A. G., Ida, K. K., Souto, M. T., Silva, L. da. Furtado, P. V., Fantoni, D.T. (2012). Diferenças no aumento da glicemia entre equinos recebendoxilazina e detomidina para procedimento sclínico scirúrgicos e não-cirúrgicos. Braz J Vet Res Ani Sci. 49 (6): 493-499.
http://dx.doi.org/10.11606/issn.1678-4456.v49i6p493-499

27

ASSESSMENT OF REAGENT EFFECTIVENESS AND PRESERVATION METHODS FOR EQUINE FAECAL SAMPLES

Eva Vavrouchova, Stepan Bodecek, Olga Dobesova

University of Veterinary and Pharmaceutical Sciences,
Faculty of Veterinary Medicine, Equine Clinic, Brno, Czech Republic

ABSTRACT

The aim of our study was to identify the most suitable flotation solution and effective preservation method for the examination of equine faeces samples using the FLOTAC technique. Samples from naturally infected horses were transported to the laboratory and analysed accordingly. The sample from each horse was homogenized and divided into four parts: one was frozen, another two were preserved in different reagents such as sodium acetate-acetic-acid–formalin(SAF) or 5% formalin. The last part was examined as a fresh sample in three different flotation solutions (Sheather's solution, sodium chloride and sodium nitrate solution, all with a specific gravity 1.200). The preserved samples were examined in the period from 14 to 21days after collection. According to our results, the sucrose solution was the most suitable flotation solution for fresh samples (small strongyle egg per gram was 706 compared to 360 in sodium chlorid and 507 in sodium nitrate) and the sodium nitrate solution was the most efficient for the preserved samples (egg per gram was 382 compared to 295 in salt solution and 305 in sucrose solution). Freezing appears to be the most effective method of sample preservation, resulting in minimal damage to fragile strongyle eggs and therefore it is the most simple and effective preservation method for the examination of large numbers of faecal samples without the necessity of examining them all within 48 hours of collection. Deep freezing as a preservation method for equine faeces samples has not, according to our knowledge, been yet published.

Key words: horse, flotation solution, small strongyles, freezing, formalin

INTRODUCTION

The FLOTAC technique was developed as a new multivalent copromicroscopic technique for veterinarians and was then adapted for human parasitology (1). The apparatus, three FLOTAC techniques and types of reagents are described in detail elsewhere (2). The FLOTAC technique allows quantification of eggs and larvae of nematodes, trematodes and cysts or oocysts of intestinal protozoa in as little as 1 gram of faeces.

Many papers have compared the FLOTAC technique with the standard Kato-Katz (3-5)

Corresponding author: Dr. Štěpán Bodeček, PhD
E-mail address: bodeceks@vfu.cz
Present address: Equine Clinic, Faculty of Veterinary Medicine University of Veterinary and Pharmaceutical Sciences Brno Palackého 1/3, 612 42 Brno, Czech Republic

and the ether concentration method used in human parasitology. The FLOTAC technique has superior diagnostic sensitivity when compared to multiple Kato-Katz thick smears and to the ether concentration method (2, 6), especially for samples with a lower EPG (eggs per gram) content.

FLOTAC techniques have also been successfully used for the diagnosis of *Aelurostrongylus abstrusus* larvae in cats (7), *Crenosoma vulpis* (8), *Ancylostoma caninum* (9), *Angiostrongylus vasorum* (10) in canine faecal samples and *Dicrocoelium dendriticum* (11) in sheep, as well as produced promising results for the diagnosis of pinworm in rabbits (12) and whipworm infection in simians (13).

Many factors may influence the performance of FLOTAC such as parasitic elements, flotation solutions and different methods of faecal preservation. Several preservation methods including freezing, 10% and 5% formalin, modified PVA (polyvinylchloride alcohol) and special commercial reagents such as SAF (sodium acetate-acetic acid formalin), Ecofix, Parasafe, Proto-fix, STF (streck tissue fixative) are used in parasitology

(14). The majority of published articles describe preservation with formalin or SAF rather than freezing which can damage fragile eggs.

Experience has shown that the use of fresh faeces produces the most accurate results, but FLOTAC techniques can be performed on faeces stored for 1-3 days at 4°C and on preserved faecal samples stored in 5 or 10% formalin or SAF for several weeks or months (1). Five percent formalin produced more accurate results than other faecal preservatives (1). Sheather's solution, saturated sodium chloride, sodium nitrate (NaNO₃) and Rinaldi's solution (sucrose and potassium iodomercurate) were recommended in Cringoli's article for the assessment of common intestinal parasites in horses.

MATERIAL AND METHODS

Based on our previous screening of several farms in South Moravia, the selection of a proper breeding farm for this study was made according to the number of horses available, good cooperation with owners, more than 200 egg per gram (EPG) count for strongyles by McMaster and the anticipated occurrence of *Parascaris equorum* in young horses. Twenty naturally infected horses were included in the study. The young horses were pastured together, whereas the adults were stabled in individual boxes and weanlings were group housed.

Twenty fresh samples were collected in January 2012 (17 samples from adults and three from weanlings born the previous spring). Each sample was individually packed and numbered. Samples were immediately transported to the laboratory where they were homogenized using a manual mixing from a larger faecal sample, weighed and either prepared for immediate use, or preserved by freezing or placed in an appropriate reagent. For preservation by freezing, 10 g were removed and placed in plastic tubes in a deep freezer (-80°C). Samples which were intended for preservation in different reagents (SAF or 5% formalin), one gram was removed and added to 10 ml of the preservative solution. Tubes with samples preserved in reagent were stored in a fridge (4°C) for period 14 to 21 days before examination.

The three flotation solutions (Sheather's solution, sodium chloride and sodium nitrate, all with specific gravity 1.200) selected for use in our study were the most efficient according to a previous study of strongyle, *Parascaris equorum* and *Anoplocehpala perfoliata* egg detection in horses. They were prepared using the standard methods (1). Sodium chloride solution was identified as the least

suitable for the fresh samples as it gave the lowest EPG count and therefore was eliminated from further processing. The remaining two flotation solutions (Sheather's and sodium nitrate) were used for examination of preserved samples.

Fresh, defrosted (in laboratory temperature 20 °C) and reagent preserved samples were placed in the FLOTAC® which permits a maximum magnification of 400. The FLOTAC double technique which is based on simultaneous examination of two different faecal samples from two different hosts using a single FLOTAC apparatus was used (1).

Statistical analysis

A linear regression model was selected to assess any relationship within the data due to the low number of samples and character of the data. Initially a suitable method had to be chosen to modify the data prior to the use of the linear regression model. This was carried out in accordance with the principle "round-robin" and by obtaining comparative data. This method was based on descriptive statistics and correlation coefficients. Subsequently, metric values were used to compare the different flotac media and to indentify the most suitable.

The input data consisted of twenty independent samples in four separate files (a separate file for fresh samples, frozen samples and samples preserved in 5% formalin or SAF). Each of these files contained a triplet of independent measurements for every sample which differed only in the reagent used. Files for 5% formalin and SAF preservation contained only data recorded using the sodium nitrate or Sheather's flotation solutions.

RESULTS

Examination of fresh samples

All the faeces samples were positive for strongyle eggs and three samples (13, 14, 15) were positive for *Parascaris equorum* eggs. The most efficient flotation reagent for detection of strongyle eggs and *Parascaris equorum* in fresh samples was Sheather's solution (s. g. 1.200). In comparison with sodium chloride (s. g. 1.200) and sodium nitrate (s.g. 1.200), the EPG values in the Sheather's solution were higher in 17 cases (85%, the exceptions being samples No. 1, 2 and 12).

Frozen samples

A different situation was found in the defrosted samples. Half of the samples (10; 50%) had the highest strongyle EPG values when floated in a sodium nitrate solution, whilst eight samples (40%) had the highest EPG values in Sheather's solution and two samples (10%) in a salt solution. The salt solution was shown to be the least suitable and was thus eliminated from the next procedure.

Preserved samples

A higher strongyle EPG value was found in samples preserved in 5% formalin and floated in a sodium nitrate solution (15 cases, 75%) than in Sheather's solution (only five cases, 25%). From the samples which had been preserved in a SAF reagent, 7 (37%) had a higher EPG in a sodium nitrate solution. In ten samples (50%), the results from both solutions (sodium nitrate and Sheather's) were comparable.

from -80°C and in each of the different flotation solutions showed a higher faecal egg count when compared with those from the two preservation reagents. In seven cases (35 %) the values of EPG were higher than from fresh samples in sodium nitrate solution and in three cases (15%) higher than those in fresh samples floated in Sheather's solution.

Eggs of *Parascaris equorum* were least visible after preservation in SAF, while after freezing and preservation in 5% formalin, the number of eggs had decreased to approximately one third of that in the fresh samples floated in Sheather's solution. When samples were floated in sodium nitrate solution, the

Table 1. Value of roundworms egg per gram in three positives samples

Sample	NaCl		NaNO$_3$			Sheather's			
	fresh	fresh	frozen	formalin	SAF	fresh	frozen	formalin	SAF
13	54	40	66	28	44	90	30	26	24
14	30	34	24	14	0	30	10	8	0
15	14	2	2	4	2	10	0	4	0

NaCl – sodium chloride, SAF - sodium acetate-acetic acid formalin, NaNO$_3$ - sodium nitrate solution

Flotation reagent

Sodium nitrate was shown to be the most suitable flotation reagent for preserved samples. Values of small strongyle EPG were higher than in the Sheather's solution for all methods of preservation, not only with respect to the average and median values, but also for the maximum and minimum values.

Comparison

The most suitable preservation method in our study appeared to be freezing. Samples defrosted

EPG value for *Parascaris equorum* eggs showed no correlation with fresh, frozen or samples preserved in 5% formalin (Table 1).

Summary

Descriptive statistic analysis of this data, i.e. average, variance, median, minimum and maximum values are contained in Table 2 for each flotation solution and for each preservation method.

The average value of recorded eggs in the file for fresh samples could be considered as the natural base for distinguishing the capability of flotation

Table 2. Summary characteristics of small strongyle egg per gram values in correlation with preservation method and flotation solution

S.C.	Fresh samples			Formalin		SAF			
	NaCl	NaNO$_3$	Sheather's	NaNO$_3$	Sheather's	NaNO$_3$	Sheather's	NaNO$_3$	Sucrose
Average	360.35	506.0	706.00	382.150	304.95	221.30	139.85	54.90	40.20
Median	297.00	525.00	570.00	263.00	239.00	147.00	120.00	35.00	25.00
Min	20.00	112.00	6.00	72.00	61.00	26.00	20.00	0.00	0.00
Max	868.00	994.00	2320.00	1346.00	1088.00	1088.00	442.00	232.00	148.00
SD	253.95	290.13	547.67	336.60	233.76	245.60	121.67	59.74	42. 25

solutions, but only with the assumption that data from one sample had the same EPG value in all three flotation solutions. The presumption is unrealistic because of the relatively uneven distribution of eggs in a sample and therefore the frequency is affected by the location in the faeces. The different input information produces significant errors and makes direct comparison of results impossible without previous modification. We tried to limit this problem by using homogenization.

It is possible to assess if there is any relationship between flotation solutions within one preservation method according to the correlation matrix (Table 2). Correlation coefficients for different preservation methods for the same flotation solution did not indicate any linear relationship. Relative dispersion of EPG in fresh, frozen and preserved samples is described by the coefficient of variation in Figure 1.

solution for faecal suspension and method of faecal preservation which affects the results.

According to our results the most efficient reagent for fresh samples was Sheather's solution with regards to strongyle eggs. Values of EPG for *Parascaris equorum* were comparable in all three reagents. Another publication presented sodium chloride and Rinaldi's solutions as the most efficient for strongyles, sodium nitrate and Rinaldi's solution for *Parascaris equorum* and sucrose solution for *Anoplocephala spp.* (1). Our results were different as we obtained the lowest faecal count for strongyle eggs from sodium chloride solution. Rinaldi's solution is based on the use of mercury iodide which is toxic and dangerous for the environment and therefore a safety cabinet must be used and special waste control is required (1). This was the reason for replacing it with different flotation solutions in our study.

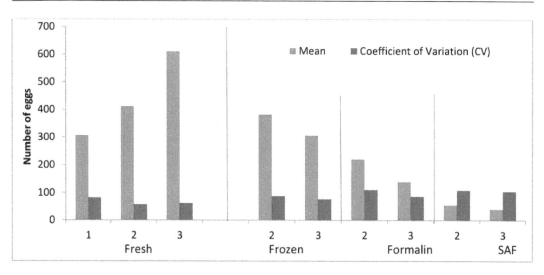

Figure 1. Correlation between value of small strongyle egg per gram and preserved method in different flotation solution. 1 – sodium chloride solution, 2 – sodium nitrate solution, 3 – Sheather's solution

DISCUSSION

The aims of this study were to identify the most efficient flotation solution for quantifying equine parasites using the FLOTAC technique; to identify the most suitable method for preservation of samples and to investigate whether the results obtained from different methods are comparable. We attempted to compare the flotac solutions recommended in the literature (1). Previously we have used a saturated sodium chloride solution and our results for EPG in fresh samples did not indicate any correlation between FLOTAC and McMaster. It is known that there is some interaction between the flotation

It is interesting that Sheather's solution seemed to be most efficient for fresh samples, but with preserved samples it showed a lower EPG than the sodium nitrate solution. The most suitable flotation solution for preserved samples was sodium nitrate with no difference in preservation methods used. Another advantage when examining frozen samples was that most of the strongyle eggs had not been destroyed in contrast to the situation with the preservation methods. This result is in contrast to other studies performed on sheep, where the majority of *Haemonchus contortus* eggs were damaged and EPG decreased after freezing (-10 °C and -170 °C in liquid nitrogen) for seven days (15).

EPG of *Ostertagia circumcincta* decreased after freezing in -10 °C (16).

Our results showed that SAF is not a suitable preservation reagent for equine faecal samples as indicated by the lowest strongyle EPG and *Parascaris equorum* egg values.

We tried to identify the most suitable preservation method for equine faecal samples as we were not aware of any previous publications on this topic. It is known that strongyles eggs are very fragile and should be examined within 48 hours of collection after being stored at fridge temperatures (17). This could be a problem when there are many samples from numerous herds. We tried various conservation methods which are used in human parasitology, such as freezing, preservation in formalin and SAF. Preservation in 5% formalin produced more accurate results than other preservation methods (1). In general, it is advisable not to freeze faecal samples.

The latter paper showed that dog faecal samples preserved in 5% formalin had a higher value of EPG when compared to those preserved in 10% formalin, SAF or frozen (9). A short communication (18) on the diagnosis of lungworm (*Dictyocaulus filaria, Muellerius capillaris, Protostrongylus rufescens*) in sheep using the FLOTAC apparatus reported that the highest faecal count was from samples preserved in 5% formalin when compared with data from fresh samples and those preserved in 10% formalin or frozen. The results from our study indicate that samples preserved in 5% formalin were very variable in both flotation solutions and in only one case EPG was higher than in a fresh sample.

Our results were unexpected because, in our study, freezing seemed to be the best preservation method for equine faecal samples in comparison with preservation in 5% formalin or SAF. We anticipated that conditions of -80°C would destroy most of the strongyle eggs and that the remaining eggs would be damaged. However, in defrosted samples, a minimum number of strongyle eggs were destroyed and a high EPG value was recorded in 10 out of 40 samples, the EPG count being higher than in fresh samples. This appears paradoxical but may be explained by the high aggregation of helminth eggs in faecal samples. To minimize the unequal distribution of eggs in faeces, careful homogenization of the samples is recommended. The finding that strongyle eggs "survive" such low temperatures is of great concern when considering the possibilities for elimination of strongyle eggs on grazing land. Further studies are required to discover if these "surviving" strongyle eggs would in fact be infective. An egg hatch assay would be useful.

CONCLUSION

Our study showed that the most suitable flotation solution for equine faecal samples seems to be Sheather's solution for fresh samples, but NaNO$_3$ for preserved samples. The most efficient preservation method according to our results was freezing.

ACKNOWLEDGEMENTS

The study was supported by grant IGA VFU 41/2013/FVL.

REFERENCES

1. Cringoli, G., Rinaldi, L., Maurelli, M. P., Utzinger, J. (2010). FLOTAC: new multivalent techniques for qualitative and quantitative compromicroscopic diagnosis of parasites in animals and humans. Nat. Protoc. 5, 503-515.
http://dx.doi.org/10.1038/nprot.2009.235
PMid:20203667

2. Cringoli, G. (2006). FLOTAC, a novel apparatus for a multivalent faecal egg count technique. Vet. Parasitol. 48, 381-384.

3. Utzinger, J., Rinaldi, L., Lohouringnon, L. K., Rohner, F., Zimmermann, M. B., Rschannen, A. B., N´Goran, E. K. N., Cringoli, G. (2008). FLOTAC: a new sensitive technique for the diagnosis of hookworm infection in humans. Trans. R. Soc. Trop. Med. Hyg. 102, 84-90.
http://dx.doi.org/10.1016/j.trstmh.2007.09.009
PMid:18028969

4. Jeardon, A., Abdykdaueva, G., Usubalieva, J., Ensink, J. H. J., Cox, J., Matthys, B., Rinaldi, L., Cringoli, G., Utzinger, J.(2010). Accuracy of the Kato-Katz, adhesive tape and FLOTAC techniques for helminth diagnosis among children in Kyrgyzstan. Acta. Trop. 116, 185-192.
http://dx.doi.org/10.1016/j.actatropica.2010.08.010
PMid:20800568

5. Knopp, S., Speich, B., Hattendorf, J., Rinaldi, L., Mohammed, K. A., Khamis, I. S., Mohammed, A. S., Albonico, M., Rollinson, D., Marti, H., Cringoli, G., Utzinger, J. (2011). Diagnostic accuracy of Kato-Katz and FLOTAC for assessing anthelmintic drug efficacy. Plos. Negl. Trop. Dis. 4, e1036.
http://dx.doi.org/10.1371/journal.pntd.0001036
PMid:21532740 PMCid:PMC3075226

6. Rinaldi, L., Veneziano, V., Morgoglione, M. E., Pennacchio, S., Santaniello, M., Schioppi, M., Musella, V., Fedele, V., Crignoli, G. (2009). Is gastrointestinal strongyle faecal egg count influenced by hour of sample collection and worm burden in goats? Vet. Parasitol. 163, 81-86.
http://dx.doi.org/10.1016/j.vetpar.2009.03.043
PMid:19414222

7. Gaglio, G., Rinaldi, L., Brianti, E., Giannetto, S. (2008). Use of the FLOTAC technique for the diagnosis of Aelurostrongylus abstrusus in the cat. Parasitol. Res. 103, 1055-1057.
http://dx.doi.org/10.1007/s00436-008-1091-4
PMid:18618146

8. Rinaldi, L., Calabri, G., Carbone, S., Carrella, A., Cringoli, G. (2007). Crenosoma vulpis in dog: first case report in Italy and use of the FLOTAC technique for copromicroscopic diagnosis. Parasitol. Res. 101, 1681-1684.
http://dx.doi.org/10.1007/s00436-007-0713-6
PMid:17805573

9. Cringoli, G., Rinaldi, L., Maurelli, M. P., Morgoline, M. E., Musella, V., Utzinger, J. (2011). Ancylostoma caninum: Calibration and comparison of diagnostic accuracy of flotation in tube, McMaster and FLOTAC in faecal samples of dogs. Experiment. Parasitol. 128, 32-37.
http://dx.doi.org/10.1016/j.exppara.2011.01.014
PMid:21295030

10. Schnyder, M., Maurelli, M. P., Morgoglione, M. E., Kohler, L., Deplazes, P., Torgerson, P., Cringoli, G., Rinaldi, L. (2011). Comparison of faecal techniques including FLOTAC for copromicroscopic detection of first stage larvae of Angiostrongylus vasorum. Parasitol. Res. 109, 63-69.
http://dx.doi.org/10.1007/s00436-010-2221-3
PMid:21181189

11. Cringoli, G., Rinaldi, L., Veneziano, V., Capelli, G., Scala, A. (2004). The influence of flotation solution, sample dilution and choise of McMaster technique in estimating the faecal egg counts of gastrointestinal strongyles and Dicrocoelium dendriticum in sheep. Vet. Parasitol. 123, 121-131.
http://dx.doi.org/10.1016/j.vetpar.2004.05.021
PMid:15265576

12. Rinaldi, L., Russo, T., Schioppi, M., Pennacchio, S., Cringoli, G. (2007). Passalurus ambiguus: new insights into copromicroscopic diagnosis and circadian rhythm of egg excretion. Parasitol. Res. 101, 557-561.
http://dx.doi.org/10.1007/s00436-007-0513-z
PMid:17372763

13. Levecke, B., De Wilde, N., Vandenhoute, E., Vercruysse, J. (2009). Field validity and feasibility of four techniques for the detection of Trichuris in simians: a model for monitoring drug efficacy in public health? PLos. Negl. Trop. Dis. 3, e366.
http://dx.doi.org/10.1371/journal.pntd.0000366
PMid:19172171 PMCid:PMC2621347

14. Pietrzak-Johnston, S. M., Bishop, H., Walhquist, S., Moura, H., De Oliviera Da Silva, N., Pereira Da Silva, S., Nguyen-Dinh, P. (2000). Evaluation of commercially available preservatives for laboratory detection od Helminths and Protozoa in human fecal specimens. J. Clin. Microbiol. 38, 1959-1964.
PMid:10790128; PMCid:PMC86633

15. Van Wyk, J., Wyk, L. (2002). Freezing of sheep faeces invalidates Haemonchus contortus faecal egg counts by the Mc Master technique. Onderstepoot J. Vet. Res. 69, 299-304.
PMid:12625382

16. Cabaret, J. (1981). Quantitative diagnostics of occurrence of small strongyle eggs and protostrongylides larvae in sheep. Effect of duration and selective method of preservation (in French: Diagnostic quantatif des oeufs de strongles digestifs et des larves de protostrongylides Cheb les ovins. Influence de la duree et du made de conservation des reces). Recueil de Medicine Vétérináre 157, 347-349.

17. Coles, G., Bauer, C., Borqsteede, F. H., Geerts, S., Klei, T. R., Taylor, M. A., Waller, P. J. (1992). World assessment of the advancement of veterinary parasitology (W.A.A.V.P.) methods for the detection of anthelmintic resistance in nematoda of veterinary importance. Vet. Parasitol. 44(1-2), 35-44.
http://dx.doi.org/10.1016/0304-4017(92)90141-U

18. Rinaldi, L., Maurelli, M. P., Musella, V., Santaniello, A., Coles, G. C., Cringoli, G. (2010). FLOTAC: An improved method for diagnosis of lungworm infection in sheep. Vet. Parasitol. 169, 395-398.
http://dx.doi.org/10.1016/j.vetpar.2010.01.008
PMid:20149543

28

PHENOTYPIC AND GENOTYPIC CHARACTERISTICS OF ENTEROCIN PRODUCING ENTEROCOCCI AGAINST PATHOGENIC BACTERIA

Sandra Mojsova[1], Kiril Krstevski[2], Igor Dzadzovski[2],
Zagorka Popova[2], Pavle Sekulovski[1]

*[1]Food Institute, Faculty of Veterinary Medicine-Skopje,
Ss. Cyril and Methodius University in Skopje, Republic of Macedonia
[2]Veterinary Institute, Faculty of Veterinary Medicine-Skopje,
Ss. Cyril and Methodius University in Skopje, Republic of Macedonia*

ABSTRACT

The study investigated the antimicrobial activity of 13 enterococcal strains (*E. faecalis* -8, *E. faecium*-2, *E. hirae*-2, *E. spp.*-1) isolated from our traditional cheeses against pathogen microorganisms. Also, it includes the detection of the following enterocin structural genes: enterocin A, enterocin B, enterocin P, enterocin L50A/B, bacteriocin 31, enterocin AS48, enterocin Q, enterocin EJ97 and cytolysin by using PCR method. All isolates inhibited growth of *L. monocytogenes* and *L.innocua*. One isolate had a broader antimicrobial activity. None of the isolates showed inhibitory activity against *S. enteritidis*, *E. coli and Y. enterocolitica*. The genes enterocin P, cytolysin and enterocin A were the most frequently detected structural genes among the PCR positive strains. No amplification was obtained in two *strains E. faecalis*-25 and *E. faecalis*-86. Three different genes were identified in some strains. With the exclusion of strains possessing a virulence factor, such as cytolysin, producers of more than one enterocins could be of a great technological potential as protective cultures in the cheese industry.

Key words: traditional cheese, enterococci, enterocins, antimicrobial activity

INTRODUCTION

The presence of pathogens in the dairy industry posses a potential risk and a constant concern in the field of food safety for consumers, food business operators and government authorities. A number of food borne disease outbreaks have been associated with these products (1). Although most of these outbreaks were closely related with the consumption of dairy products made from raw milk, post-processing contamination must be taken into account as an important risk factor in the manufacture of such products (2).

Corresponding author: Mojsova Sandra, MSc, DVM
E-mail address: kostova.sandra@fvm.ukim.edu.mk
Present address: Food Institute, Faculty of Veterinary Medicine
Ss. Cyril and Methodius University in Skopje
Lazar Pop-Trajkov 5-7, 1000 Skopje,
Republic of Macedonia

Enterococci as a part of lactic acid bacteria (LAB) present a complex, divergent and significant group of bacteria in terms of their interaction with food and humans. Enterococci are omnipresent bacteria and are dominant residents of the digestive tract of humans and animals but their presence it's not unusual in the surrounding environment like soil, surface waters, plants and vegetables. They can also be found in food, especially in cheese (3). They are found in a high percentage as a part of the dairy microflora. They are especially found in a high percentage in many artisanal made cheeses traditionally produced in the countries from the Mediterranean region, mostly from raw ewe's or goat's milk. There is a widely spread opinion that these types of bacteria initially became contaminants from animal organic waste, water or milking equipment and storage tanks, and consequently became an essential component of artisanal cultures (4). These types of bacteria have a fundamental role in the ripening process of traditionally made cheeses (5). As a contribution to their involvement in the unique and specific peculiar taste and flavor, the enterococci also have the ability to protect from various pathogens (6). Recently, the scientific community has increased its interest in enterocins, encouraged by the fact that they act against food-borne pathogens, mostly against *L. monocytogenes, S.aureus, B. cereus* and vegetative cells and spores of *C. botulinum* (7, 8).

Lactic acid bacteria for centuries have been used in food and feed conservation and their preservative effects are mainly due to the decreasing of pH values and the formation of organic acids, principally lactic acid (9, 10, 11). Bacteriocins are ribosomally synthesized polypeptides that possess antimicrobial activity and are commonly pH and heat tolerant and are rapidly digested by proteases in the human digestive tract due to their proteinaceous nature (12). Bacteriocins can also inhibit adulteration of food by preventing the outgrowth of non-pathogen and pathogen bacteria. The bacteriocin or bacteriocin-producing LAB except cytolysin, can be used as safe alternatives to chemical preservatives in foods (11, 13), because they are harmless to eukaryotic cells.

Beside the clear evidence that bacteriocinogenic enterococci and their bacteriocins are well known in the literature, the exploration in this field is still an actual subject of the research, as the isolation and characterization of the enterocin producing enterococci from different geographical areas, which have tradition for making artisanal dairy products, could perhaps give new data about the diversity and ecology of *Enterococcus* strains and their enterocins.

The objectives of this study were to identify bacteriocinogenic enteroccoci isolated from Macedonian traditional cheeses, as well as to determine the existence of bacteriocin structural genes.

MATERIAL AND METHODS

Bacterial strains

A collection of 13 Enterococcus strains that were previously isolated from traditional white pickled (brined) cheese from different regions of Macedonia were tested for presence of bacteriocin structural genes. The enterococci were isolated on a selective agar (KAA, Oxoid, UK) and identified by polymerase chain reaction (PCR) amplification of a part of 16S rRNA gene (14). Species determination was performed using PCR protocol for species-specific enterococcal targets (14, 15). Additionally, isolates negative on species-specific PCR were further determined by BLAST analysis of the 16S rRNA sequences, using available sequence data from GenBank.

The following cultures were tested for sensitivity to enterocins: *L. monocytogenes* (NCTC 11994), *L. innocua* (cheese isolate), *S. aureus* (cheese isolate), *P. aeruginosa* (NCTC 10662), *B. cereus* (NCTC 7464), *S. enteritidis* (meat isolate), *E. coli* (NCTC 9001) and *Y. enterocolitica* (ATCC 11303).

Bacteriocin production assay

For the detection of antimicrobial activity, 50 µl of an overnight culture of the indicator strain was added to 5ml molten soft semisolid Plate count agar (PCA), mixed and poured onto a solid PCA agar plate. A single colony of each enterococcus to be tested for antimicrobial activity was transferred with a sterile loop. Agar plates were incubated for 24 h at 37°C in aerobic condition. The antimicrobial activity was visually detected by observing clear zones around the tested strain. To test the proteinaceous nature of the inhibitors, 10 µl of trypsin solution was deposited on the side of each spot of bacterial growth. The absence of inhibition in the trypsin-spotted zone indicated protease sensitivity.

Detection by PCR of enterocin structural genes

All isolates have been tested for the presence of the following bacteriocin structural genes: enterocin A (entA), enterocin B (entB), enterocin P (entP), enterocin L50A/B (entL50A-entL50B), bacteriocin 31 (bac31), enterocin AS48 (entAS48), enterocin Q (entQ), enterocin EJ97 (E21) and cytolysin (cyl) using specific enterocin PCR primers (Table 1).

Primers have been used in combinations giving four different duplex and two single-plex PCR reactions, as described in Table 1 and Table 2. All PCR reactions were set in a final volume of 20 µl, consisting of 17 µl PCR mixture and 3 µl DNA template, using Taq PCR Mastermix Kit (Qiagen, USA). Positive controls were included in PCR assays for detection of EntA, EntB, EntP, E21, EntAS48 and cyl genes, whereas positive controls weren't available for EntQ, Ent1071, Bac31, EntL50. Control DNA was obtained from isolates (FIFL-20, FIFL-36, FIFL-29, FIVRE-19) belonging to the culture collection of the Food Institute in which the presence of above mentioned structural genes has been confirmed by PCR.

The thermal profiles used for the amplification were the following: initial denaturation at 94° C for 3 minutes followed by 40 cycles of denaturation at 94 °C for 40 seconds, annealing (50° C for entA and ent Q and 56° C for entP, entB, ent50A/B, bac31, entAS-48, ent1071A/B, E21) for 40 seconds, and elongation at 72° C for 60 seconds. Final extension was at 72° C for 10 minutes.

Table 1. Primers used for PCR detection of bacteriocin genes

Target gene	Primer	Sequence (5'-3')	fragment (bp)	PCR	Reference
Enterocin A	Ent Af Ent Ar	AAA TAT TAT GGA AAT GGA GTG TAT GCA CTT CCC TGG AAT TGC TC	126	1	(16)
Enterocin B	EntBf EntBr	GAA AAT GAT CAC AGA ATG CCT A GTT GCA TTT AGA GTA TAC ATT TG	162	4	(16)
Enterocin Q	EntQf EntQr	ATG AAT TTT CTT CTT AAA AAT GGT ATC GCA TTA ACA AGA AAT TTT TTC CCA TGG CAA	105	1	(17)
Enterocin P	EntPf EntPr	TAT GGT AAT GGT GTT TAT TGT AAT ATG TCC CAT ACC TGC CAA AC	120	2	(16)
Enterocin L50 A/B	EntL50f EntL50r	TGG GAG CAA TCG CAA AAT TAG ATT GCC CAT CCT TCT CCA AT	98	3	(17)
Bacteriocin 31	Bac31f Bac31r	TAT TAC GGA AAT GGT TTA TAT TGT TCT AGG AGC CCA AGG GCC	123	3	(16)
Enterocin AS48	EntAS48f EntAS48r	GAG GAG TTT CAT GAT TTA AAG A CAT ATT GTT AAA TTA CCA AGC AA	340	4	(16)
Enterocin EJ97	E21f E21r	GCA GCT AAG CTA ACG ACT AGGGGAATTTGAACAGA	279	5	(18)
Cytolysin	Cylf Cylr	ACT CGG GGA TTG ATA GGC GCT GCT AAA GCT GCG CTT	688	6	(19)

The thermal profile for cytolysin was the following: initial denaturation at 95° C for 2 minutes followed by 40 cycles of denaturation at 95 °C for 30 seconds, annealing at 56 °C for 90 seconds, elongation 72 °C for 90 seconds and final extension was at 72° C for 10 minutes. The amplification products were analysed by electrophoresis in 2.5% agarose gel at 7 V/cm for 1.5 h in Tris-acetate-EDTA buffer and revealed in ethidium bromide (20 μg/mL). The gel was photographed using UV light.

RESULTS

Bacteriocin-producer isolates were identified as *E. faecalis* (n=8), *E. faecium* (n=2) and *E. hirae* (n=2). Species determination for one of the isolates (*E.spp.-90)* was inconclusive: despite the positive identification using 16S rRNA PCR, BLAST analysis of the amplified part of 16s RNA sequence revealed 100% similarity with *Lactococcus lactis* subsp. *lactis*. This finding imposes the necessity for further and deeper analysis of this isolate.

The 13 isolates were screened for antibacterial activity, since they may produce enterocins that can control the growth of the tested indicator bacteria. All of the isolates showed the activity predominantly against *L. monocytogenes* (Fig. 1), mostly showing larger inhibition zone for *L. monocytogenes* than *L. innocua*.

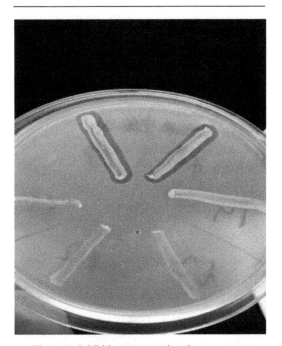

Figure 1. Inhibition areas against *L. monocytogenes* as a result of bacteriocin activity

Three of the isolates (*E. faecalis-31, E.faecalis-32, E. hirae-36*) were found to be inhibitory against *S. aureus* and *P. aeruginosa*,

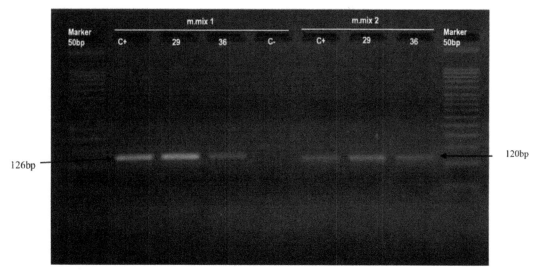

Figure 2. Agar gel visualisation of PCR products obtained with two duplex PCR reactions (PCR1 and PCR2). Lane Marker 50bp is 50 bp ladder, lanes C+ positive controls and lanes C- negative controls. Tested samples (29, 36) are in the lanes between positive and negative controls

but only two of them were found to be inhibitory against *B. cereus (E. faecalis-31 and E. hirae-36).* None of the isolates were found to be inhibitory against *S. enteritidis, Y. enterocolitica* and *E. coli* (Table 2).

enterococci (Table 2). *E. faecalis*-4, *E.faecium*-15, *E. faecium*-29 and *E. hirae*-36 had three different structural enterocin genes. *E. faecalis*-31, *E. faecalis*-32, *E. faecalis*-51, *E. faecalis*-77 and *E. spp.* had only one structural enterocin gene.

Table 2. Enterocin genes and antimicrobial activity towards pathogens and their inhibition

Isolate	Source	Enterocin genes	Inhibition							
			L. monocyt	L. innocua	S. aureus	B.cereus	P. aerugin.	Y. enterocol.	S. enteritidis	E. coli
E. fl-4	**Cheese**	P,B,cyl	+	+	-	-	-	-	-	-
E. fl-8	**Cheese**	P,cyl	+	+	-	-	-	-	-	-
E. fm-15	**Cheese**	A,B,P	++	+	-	-	-	-	-	-
E. fl-25	**Cheese**	/	++	+	-	-	-	-	-	-
E. fm-29	**Cheese**	A, B, P	+++	+	-	-	-	-	-	-
E. fl-31	**Cheese**	Cyl	+	+	+	+	+	-	-	-
E. fl-32	**Cheese**	Cyl	+	+	+	-	+	-	-	-
E. h-36	**Cheese**	A, P, EJ97	+++	++	+	+++	++	-	-	-
E. fl-51	**Cheese**	Cyl	+	+	-	-	-	-	-	-
E. h-52	**Cheese**	P, EJ97	+++	++	-	-	-	-	-	-
E. fl-77	**Cheese**	AS-48	+	+	-	-	-	-	-	-
E. fl-86	**Cheese**	/	+	+	-	-	-	-	-	-
E.spp. 90	**Cheese**	A	++	+	-	-	-	-	-	-

+ weak inhibition (1 - 2 mm), ++ moderate inhibition (3 - 4mm) , +++ strong inhibition (>4 mm)

The most frequent bacteriocin structural genes in this study were enterocin P, enterocin A and cytolysin, followed by enterocin B. Less frequent genes were EJ97 and AS-48. Enterocin Q, bacteriocin 31 and enterocin L50 were not found in the tested

Two of the isolates (*E. faecalis -25* and *E. faecalis-86),* did not harbour any of the tested bacteriocins.

A gene for cytolysin was detected in 5 isolates of *E. faecalis* (*E. faecalis-4, E. faecalis-8, E. faecalis-31, E. faecalis-32, E. faecalis -51).*

DISCUSSION

Results from previous studies report identical findings that most enterocin producing enterococci show antilisterial activity, while a small part of them also show inhibitory activity against *Staphylococcus aureus* and *Bacillus spp.* (7, 20, 21). Gram-negative bacteria are mostly resistant to many enterocins and the absence of inhibitory activity against them is in agreement with the data that most of the bacteriocins produced by *Enterococcus* strains inhibit the growth of closely related bacteria and activity against Gram-negative bacteria is very rare (22, 23). Though, we found inhibitory activity against *Pseudomonas aeruginosa.* There are reports that certain lactic acid bacteria especially the class 2 bacteriocins - pediocins can inhibit a limited number of Gram-negative bacteria including *Pseudomonas, Shigella* sp. *Salmonella* sp. (24, 25).

According to our PCR results, different bacteriocin structural genes are spread among enterococcal strains. Enterocin A, B and P were the most prevalent among enterococci which is in accordance with the results obtained for enterococci isolated from different sources of food and feed, animal isolates, clinical and nonclinical human isolates (26), enterococci isolated from artisan food of animal origin (27) and Spanish goats milk cheeses (28). Earlier study showed that entAS-48 was widely distributed throughout E. faecalis (29), but there are also authors who did not detect the presence of enterocin AS-48 (27, 28). Contrary to our findings, no equivalence in results was found with this authors. Only in two isolates (*E. faecalis-25* and *E. faecalis-86)*, we could not detect presence of any of the tested enterocin genes. Still, these isolates showed inhibitory activity against. *L. monocytogenes* and *L. innocua.* This could be explained with the possible presence of other already known bacteriocins (non-tested in this study) or possible existence of novel bacteriocins. As previously published by Ozdemir et al., (30), bacteriocin production is correlated to the species. However, contrary to their findings we found in our study *E. hirae* and *E. faecalis* as bacteriocin producers.

Enterocin A and P belong to the family of pediocins and they are grouped as Class II 1, which are effective mostly against listeria (31). Over the past ten years, class II bacteriocins produced by LAB have brought a significant attention to their potential application in food industry as natural preservatives and in the medical sector as antibiotic supplements or antiviral agents (7, 32). Enterocin

B belongs to the subgroup II 3, which are part of the non-pediocin type enterocin. Enterocin AS-48 belongs to the class of cyclic antibacterial peptides (33). It should be underlined that only one of our isolates (*E. faecalis-77)* showed exclusively the *entAS-48* gene, which is opposite to the previous findings in the literature that this enterocin is widely distributed among *E. faecalis* and *E. faecium* (29).

The combination of three different enterocin genes was observed in four strains (*E. faecalis-4, E. faecium-15, E. faecium-29, E. hirae-36).* Combination of two enterocin genes was observed in two strains (*E. faecalis-8, E. hirae-52).* According to the reviewed literature enterocin B is found predominantly with enterocin A, considering the fact that transport genes for enterocin B producers are not found (26, 34). In this study enterocin B was found with enterocin A, but it was also found in combination with enterocin P. It is considered by some authors that the reason for the high incidence of enterocin A, B and P genes in enterococcal bacteriocinogenic strains that are isolated from food is not only to antagonize bacteria but also to reinforce the competition of the selected strains against the competitors of the same species (35). Another combination of two genes is enterocin P and EJ97 and enterocin P, enterocin A and enterocin EJ97. These combinations, which were not found in the previous studies, were found in two of our isolates (*E. hirae-36* and *E. hirae-52).*

Enterocin EJ97 belongs to enterocins synthesized without a leader peptide that is active against Gram-positive bacteria as well as enterococci, several species of *Bacillus, Listeria* and strains of *S.aureus* (36). Even though both strains (*E. hirae -36* and *E. hirae-52)* posses the same structural gene EJ97, *E. hirae-36* had a larger zone of inhibition. This could be explained by two possible hypotheses: the antimicrobial activity was reinforced by the presence of enterocin P and enterocin A or eventual presence of "silent" gene(s) in *E. hirae-52.* Various authors report the presence of bacteriocin silent genes in enterococci (26, 37, 38).

Cytolysin was found only in *E. faecalis* isolates, which is the species with the highest occurrence of virulence genes. According to our results, it can be concluded that there is no large zone of inhibition around the strain that harbour a gene for cytolysin. Cytolysin is the only two-peptide lantiobiotic isolated from genus *Enterococcus* with cytolitic activity. Cytolysin is not considered useful due to the fact that it's a virulence factor (39), so these strains are not safe for application.

CONCLUSION

Results of this study showed that further analysis of certain strains as adjunct cultures for the process of fermentation of dairy products is needed. Also further studies should be conducted in order to identify new antimicrobial substances produced by the enterococcal strains.

Due to the fact that cytolysin's virulence factor is not considered useful, so these strains are not safe for application. The usefulness of the strains that are free of cytolysin genes should be investigated, because these strains could be candidates for safe and practical use. Having in mind the potential of the strains, the future challenge will be optimizing the conditions during the fermentation process, as well as the composition of the medium in order to achieve better production of bacteriocin substances.

As a conclusion, our investigation gives a clear evidence of bacteriocin producing enterococci in traditional artisanal-produced cheese. The main bacteriocinogenic species was *E. faecalis*. Enterocin structural genes can be found in many different combinations, some of them reported for the first time in this study.

REFERENCES

1. Mead, P.S., Slutsker, L., Dietz, V., Mccaig, L.F.; Bresee, J.S.; Shapiro, C.; Griffin, P.M.; Tauxe, R.V. (1999). Food-related illness and death in the United States. Emerg. Infect. Dis. 5, 607-625. http://dx.doi.org/10.3201/eid0505.990502 PMid:10511517 PMCid:PMC2627714

2. De Buyser, M.L., Dufour, B., Marie, M., Lafarge, V. (2001). Implication of milk and milk products in foodborne diseases in France and in different industrialized countries. Int. J. Food. Microbiol. 67, 1-17. http://dx.doi.org/10.1016/S0168-1605(01)00443-3

3. Giraffa, G. (2002). Enterococci from foods FEMS Microbiology Reviews 26 pp. 163–171. http://dx.doi.org/10.1111/j.1574-6976.2002.tb00608.x PMid:12069881

4. Folquie-Moreno, M. R., Sarantinoupulos, P., Tsakalidou, E., De Vuyst, L. (2006). The role and application of enterococci in food and health. Int. J. Food. Microbiol. 106, 1-24. http://dx.doi.org/10.1016/j.ijfoodmicro.2005.06.026 PMid:16216368

5. Manolopoulou, E., Sarantinopoulos, P., Zoidou, E., Aktypis, A., Moschopoulou, E., Kandarakis, IG. (2003). Evolution of microbial populations during traditional Feta cheese manufacture and ripening. Int J Food Microbiol. 82(2):153–161. http://dx.doi.org/10.1016/S0168-1605(02)00258-1

6. De Vuyst, L.,. Vandamme E. J. (1994). Antimicrobial potential of lactic acid bacteria, p. 91-142. InL. de Vuyst and E. J. Vandamme (ed.), Bacteriocins of lactic acid bacteria: microbiology, genetics and applications. Blackie Academic & Professional, London, United Kingdom.

7. Cleveland, J., Montville, T.J., Nes, I.F., Chikindas, M.L. (2001). Bacteriocins: safe natural antimicrobials for food preservation. Int. J. Food. Microbiol. 71,1-20. http://dx.doi.org/10.1016/S0168-1605(01)00560-8

8. Deegan, I. H., Cotter, P. D., Hill, C., Ross, P. (2006). Bacteriocins: biological tools for bio-preservation and shelf-life extension. Int Dairy J. 16, 1058-1071. http://dx.doi.org/10.1016/j.idairyj.2005.10.026

9. O'Sullivan, L., Ross, R.P., Hill, C. (2002). Potential of bacteriocin producing lactic acid bacteria for improvements in food safety and quality. Biochimie 84, 593–604. http://dx.doi.org/10.1016/S0300-9084(02)01457-8

10. Klaenhammer, T. R., Barrangou, R., Buck, B. L., Azcarate-Peril, M. A., Altermann, E. (2005). Genomic features of lactic acid bacteria effecting bioprocessing and health. FEMS Microbiol Rev. 29, 393–409. http://dx.doi.org/10.1016/j.fmrre.2005.04.007 PMid:15964092

11. Casaus, P., Nilsen, T., Cintas, LM., Nes, IF., Hernández, PE., Holo, H. (1997). Enterocin B, a new bacteriocin from Enterococcus faecium T136 which can act synergistically with enterocin A. Microbiology 143(Pt 7):2287-2294. http://dx.doi.org/10.1099/00221287-143-7-2287 PMid:9245817

12. Galvez, A., Abriouel, H.; Lopez, R.L.,Ben Omar, N. (2007). Bacteriocin-based strategies for food biopreservation. Int. J. Food. Microbiol. 120, 51–70. http://dx.doi.org/10.1016/j.ijfoodmicro.2007.06.001 PMid:17614151

13. Bennik, M. et al. (1998). A novel bacteriocin with a YGNGV motif from vegetable-associated Enterococcus mundtii: full characterization and interaction with target organisms. Biochim. Biophys. Acta, 1373, 47-58. http://dx.doi.org/10.1016/S0005-2736(98)00086-8

14. Dutka-Malen S, Evers S, Courvalin P. (1995). Detection of glycopeptide resistance genotypes and identification to the species level of clinically relevant enterococci by PCR. J Clin Microbiol., 33(1): 24-27.

15. Jackson, C.R., Fedorka-Cray, P.J., Barrett, J.B. (2004). Use of a genus- and species-specific multiplex PCR for identification of enterococci. J Clin Microbiol. 42, 3558–3565. http://dx.doi.org/10.1128/JCM.42.8.3558-3565.2004 PMid:15297497 PMCid:PMC497640

16. Yousuf NMK, Dawyndt P, Abriouel H (2005). Molecular Characterization, technological properties and safety aspects of enteroccocci from Husuwa, an African fermented sorghum product. J Appl. Microbiol. 98, 216-228.
http://dx.doi.org/10.1111/j.1365-2672.2004.02450.x
PMid:15610435

17. Ben Belgacem Z, Abriouel H, Ben Omar (2010). Antimicrobial activity, safety aspects and some technological properties of bacteriocinogenic Enterococcus faecium from artisanal Tunisian meat. Food Control 21, 462-470.
http://dx.doi.org/10.1016/j.foodcont.2009.07.007

18. Sanchez-Hidalgo, M., Maqueda, M., Galvez, A., Valdivia, E. and Martinez-Bueno, M. (2003). The genes coding for enterocin EJ97 production by Enterococcus faecalis EJ97 are located on a conjugative plasmid. Appl Environ Microbiol. 62, 1633–1641.
http://dx.doi.org/10.1128/AEM.69.3.1633-1641.2003
PMCid:PMC150074

19. Vankerckhoven, V., Van Autgaerden, T., Vael, C., Lammens, C., Chapelle, S., Rossi, R., Jabes, D., Goossens, H. (2004). Development of a multiplex PCR for the detection of asa1, gelE, cylA, esp and hyl genes in enterococci and survey for virulence determinants among European hospital isolates of Enterococcus faecium. J Clin Microbiol. 42, 4473–4479.
http://dx.doi.org/10.1128/JCM.42.10.4473-4479.2004
PMid:15472296 PMCid:PMC522368

20. Franz, C., Van Belkum, MJ., Holzapfel, WH., Abriouel, H., Gálvez, A. (2007). Diversity of enterococcal bacteriocins and their grouping into a new classification scheme. FEMS Microbiol Rev. 31: 293-310.
http://dx.doi.org/10.1111/j.1574-6976.2007.00064.x
PMid:17298586

21. Giraffa, G. (1995). Enterococcal bacteriocins: their potential as anti-Listeria factors in dairy technology. Food Microbiol 12, 291–299.
http://dx.doi.org/10.1016/S0740-0020(95)80109-X

22. Gong H. S., Meng X.C., Wang H. (2010). Plantaricin MG active against Gram negative bacteria produced by Lactobacillus plantarum KLDS1 isolated from "Jiaoke" a traditional fermented cream from China. Food Control, 21, 89-96.
http://dx.doi.org/10.1016/j.foodcont.2009.04.005

23. Todorov., S. D., Dicks, L.M.T, (2005a). Lactobacillus plantarum isolated from molasses produces bacteriocins active against Gram-negative bacteria. Enzyme and Microbial Technology, 36. 318-326.
http://dx.doi.org/10.1016/j.enzmictec.2004.09.009

24. Laukova A., Czikkova S., Vasilkova Z., Juris P., Marekova M (1998). Occurrence of bacteriocin production among environmental enterococci. Letters in Applied microbiology 27, 178-182.
http://dx.doi.org/10.1046/j.1472-765X.1998.00404.x
PMid:9750323

25. Kwon DY, Koo M S, Ryoo CR, Kang CH, Min KH, Kim WJ (2002). Bacteriocin produced by Pediococcus sp. in kimchi and its characteristics. J. Microbiol. Biotechnol. 12, 96-105.

26. De Vuyst L., Foulquie Moreno M.R., Revets H. (2003). Screening for enterocins and detection of hemolysin and vancomycin resistance in enterococci of different originsInt. J. Food Microbiol., 84, 299–318.
http://dx.doi.org/10.1016/S0168-1605(02)00425-7

27. Valenzuela AS, Ben-Omar N, Abriouel H, Lopez RL, Veljovic K, Canamero MM, Topisirovic MKL, Galvez A. (2009). Virulence factors, antibiotic resistance, and bacteriocins in enterococci from artisan foods of animal origin. Food Control. 20, 381-385.
http://dx.doi.org/10.1016/j.foodcont.2008.06.004

28. Martin-Platero, A. M., Valdivia E, Maqueda M, Martinez-Bueno M. (2009) . Characterization and safety evaluation of Enterococci isolated from Spanish goats' milk cheeses. Int J of Food Microbiol, 132: 24-32.
http://dx.doi.org/10.1016/j.ijfoodmicro.2009.03.010
PMid:19375810

29. Joosten H. M., Rodriguez E, Nunez M (1997). PCR detection of sequences similar to the AS-48 structural gene in bacteriocin-producing enterococci. Lett Appl Microbiol. 24, 40–42.
http://dx.doi.org/10.1046/j.1472-765X.1997.00349.x
PMid:9024003

30. Ozdemir, G,B., Oryasin, E., Biyuik, H. H., Ozteber, M., Bozdogan, B. (2011). Phenotypic and genotypic characterisation of bacteriocins in enterococcal isolates of different sources. Indian Journal of Microbiology. 51 (2): pp 182-187.

31. Eijsink VG, Skeie M, Middelhoven PH, Brurberg MB, Nes IF. (1998). Comparative Studies of Class IIa Bacteriocins of Lactic Acid Bacteria. Appl Environ Microbiol.; 64 (9): 3275–3281.
PMid:9726871 PMCid:PMC106721

32. Wachsman, M. B., Castilla, V., de Ruiz Holgado, A. P., de Torres, R. A., Sesma, F., Coto, C. E. (2003). Enterocin CRL35 inhibits late stages of HSV-1 and HSV-2 replication in vitro. Antiviral Res 58, 17–24.
http://dx.doi.org/10.1016/S0166-3542(02)00099-2

33. Nes, I.F., Diep, D.B., Havarstein, L.S., Brurberg, M.B., Eijsink, V., Holo, H., (1996). Biosynthesis of bacteriocins in lactic acid bacteria. Antonie van Leeuwenhoek 70, 113-128.
http://dx.doi.org/10.1007/BF00395929
PMid:8879403

34. Franz, C.M.A.P., Holzaphel, W.H. Stiles, M.E. (1999). Enterococci at the crossroads of food safety? Int. J. Food. Microbiol. 47, 1–24. http://dx.doi.org/10.1016/S0168-1605(99)00007-0

35. Ben Omar, N., Castro, A., Lucas, R., Abriouel, H., Yousif, N.M.K., Franz, C.M.A.P., Holzapfel, W.H., Pérez-Pulido, R. et al. (2004). Functional and safety aspects of Enterococci isolated from different Spanish foods. Syst Appl Microbiol 27, 118-130. http://dx.doi.org/10.1078/0723-2020-00248 PMid:15053328

36. Gálvez, A., Valdivia Hikmate Abriouel, E., Mendez, E.C., Martínez-Bueno, M, Maqueda, M. (1998). Isolation and characterization of enterocin EJ97, a bacteriocin produced by Enterococcus faecalis EJ97Archives of Microbiology ; 171(1): 59-65.

37. Eaton, T.J, Gasson, M.J. (2001). Molecular screening of Enterococcus virulence determinants and potential for genetic exchange between food and medical isolates Appl. Environ. Microbiol., 67, 1628–1635. http://dx.doi.org/10.1128/AEM.67.4.1628-1635.2001 PMid:11282615 PMCid:PMC92779

38. Semedo T. S, Martins M. A., Lopes M. F. S., Figueiredo Marques J. J., Tenreiro R., Barreto Crespo M. T (2003). Comparative study using type strains and clinical and food isolates to examine hemolytic activity and occurrence of the cyl operon in enterococci J. Clin. Microbiol., 41, 2569–2576. http://dx.doi.org/10.1128/jcm.41.6.2569-2576.2003

39. Pangallo, D, Harichova, J, Karelova, E, Drahovska, H, Chovanova, K, Feriane, P, Turna, J, Timko, J. (2004). Molecular investigation of enterococci isolated from different environmental sources. Biologia 59, 829-837.

Permissions

All chapters in this book were first published in MVR, by De Gruyter Open; hereby published with permission under the Creative Commons Attribution License or equivalent. Every chapter published in this book has been scrutinized by our experts. Their significance has been extensively debated. The topics covered herein carry significant findings which will fuel the growth of the discipline. They may even be implemented as practical applications or may be referred to as a beginning point for another development.

The contributors of this book come from diverse backgrounds, making this book a truly international effort. This book will bring forth new frontiers with its revolutionizing research information and detailed analysis of the nascent developments around the world.

We would like to thank all the contributing authors for lending their expertise to make the book truly unique. They have played a crucial role in the development of this book. Without their invaluable contributions this book wouldn't have been possible. They have made vital efforts to compile up to date information on the varied aspects of this subject to make this book a valuable addition to the collection of many professionals and students.

This book was conceptualized with the vision of imparting up-to-date information and advanced data in this field. To ensure the same, a matchless editorial board was set up. Every individual on the board went through rigorous rounds of assessment to prove their worth. After which they invested a large part of their time researching and compiling the most relevant data for our readers.

The editorial board has been involved in producing this book since its inception. They have spent rigorous hours researching and exploring the diverse topics which have resulted in the successful publishing of this book. They have passed on their knowledge of decades through this book. To expedite this challenging task, the publisher supported the team at every step. A small team of assistant editors was also appointed to further simplify the editing procedure and attain best results for the readers.

Apart from the editorial board, the designing team has also invested a significant amount of their time in understanding the subject and creating the most relevant covers. They scrutinized every image to scout for the most suitable representation of the subject and create an appropriate cover for the book.

The publishing team has been an ardent support to the editorial, designing and production team. Their endless efforts to recruit the best for this project, has resulted in the accomplishment of this book. They are a veteran in the field of academics and their pool of knowledge is as vast as their experience in printing. Their expertise and guidance has proved useful at every step. Their uncompromising quality standards have made this book an exceptional effort. Their encouragement from time to time has been an inspiration for everyone.

The publisher and the editorial board hope that this book will prove to be a valuable piece of knowledge for researchers, students, practitioners and scholars across the globe.

List of Contributors

Uzunov Risto, Hajrulai-Musliu Zehra, Stojanovska-Dimzoska Biljana,
Dimitrieska-Stojkovic Elizabeta and Todorovic Aleksandra
Food Institute, Faculty of Veterinary Medicine, Skopje, Republic of Macedonia

Stojkovski Velimir
Institute for Reproduction and Biomedicine, Faculty of Veterinary Medicine-Skopje,Republic of Macedonia

Mujeebur Rehman Fazili
Veterinary Clinical Complex, Faculty of Veterinary Sciences & Animal Husbandry, Shere Kashmir Universityof Agricultural Sciences & Technology of Kashmir, Shuhama, Srinagar, Kashmir, India

Nida Handoo, Mohd Younus Mir and Beenish Qureshi
Division of Veterinary Surgery & Radiology, Faculty of Veterinary Sciences & Animal Husbandry, Shere Kashmir University of Agricultural Sciences & Technology of Kashmir, Shuhama, Srinagar, Kashmir, India

Marjan Piponski, Tanja Bakovska, Marina Naumoska, Tatjana Rusevska,
Gordana Trendovska Serafimovska and Hristina Andonoska
Pharmaceutical Company Replek Farm Ltd., Quality Control Department
st. Kozle 188, 1000 Skopje

Rabecca Tono
Zonal Veterinary Clinic, Zuru Kebbi State, Nigeria

Olufemi Oladayo Faleke and Abdullahi Alhaji Magaji
Department of Veterinary Public Health and Preventive Medicine,
Faculty of Veterinary Medicine, Usmanu Danfodiyo University Sokoto, Nigeria

Musbaudeen Olayinka Alayande
Department of Veterinary Entomology and Parasitology, Faculty of Veterinary Medicine, Usmanu Danfodiyo University Sokoto, Nigeria

Akinyemi Olaposi Fajinmi
Nigeria Institute of Trypanosomosis and Onchocerciasis Research, Kaduna, Nigeria

Emmanuel Busayo Ibitoye
Department of Theriogenology and Animal Production, Faculty of Veterinary Medicine, Usmanu Danfodiyo University Sokoto, Nigeria

Opsomer Geert
Department of Reproduction, Obstetrics and Herd Health, Faculty of Veterinary Medicine, Ghent University, Belgium

Fatih Alkan and Arzu Kotan
Pendik Veterinary Control Institute, Department of Pharmacology, Laboratory of Residue. 34890 Pendik, Istanbul, Turkey

Nurullah Ozdemir
Namik Kemal University, Veterinary Faculty, Department of Pharmacology and Toxicology, Degirmenalti Mevkii, 59030 Tekirdag, Turkey

Aliye Sağkan Öztürk and Serkan İrfan Köse
Department of Internal Medicine, Faculty of Veterinary Medicine, Mustafa Kemal University, 31040, Hatay, Turkey

Nuri Altuğ
Department of Internal Medicine, Faculty of Veterinary Medicine, Namık Kemal University, 59030, Tekirdağ, Turkey

Oktay Hasan Öztürk
Department of Biochemistry, Faculty of Medicine, Akdeniz University, 07985, Antalya, Turkey

Velev Romel
Department of Pharmacology and Toxicology, Faculty of Veterinary Medicine, University "Ss. Cyril and Methodius", Skopje, R. Macedonia

Krleska-Veleva Natasa
Replek Farm, Kozle 188, 1000 Skopje, R. Macedonia

Salah H. Afifi and Diefy A. Salem
Department of Pathology, Faculty of Veterinary Medicine, Assiut University, Assiut, Egypt

Reham El-Kashef and A. Sh. Seddek
Department of Forensic Medicine and Toxicology, Faculty of Veterinary Medicine, South Valley University, Kena, Egypt

Aleksandra Domanjko Petrič
Clinic for Surgery and Small Animal Medicine, Veterinary Faculty, University of Ljubljana, Cesta v Mestni log 47, 1000 Ljubljana, Slovenia

Genova Krasimira, Stancheva Nevyana, Angelov Geno and Mehmedov Tandju
Faculty of Veterinary Medicine, University of Forestry, Sofia, Bulgaria

Dimitrova Ivona
Agronomy Faculty, University of Forestry, Sofi a, Bulgaria

Nakev Jivko
Agricultural Institute, Shumen, Bulgaria

Georgieva Svetlana
Faculty of Agriculture, Trakia University, Stara Zagora, Bulgaria

Goran Stojković and Marija Soklevska,
University "Ss. Cyril and Methodius", Faculty of Natural Sciences and Mathematics, Institute of Chemistry, Skopje, Republic of Macedonia

Elizabeta Dimitrieska-Stojković and Romel Velev
University "Ss. Cyril and Methodius", Faculty of Veterinary Medicine – Skopje, Institute for Food, Skopje, Republic of Macedonia

Aleksandar Cvetkovikj and Miroslav Radeski
Veterinary Institute, Faculty of Veterinary Medicine, Ss. Cyril and Methodius University in Skopje, Lazar Pop-Trajkov 5-7, 1000 Skopje, Republic of Macedonia

Vangjel Stevanovski and Dijana Blazhekovikj-Dimovska
2Fishery Department, Faculty of Biotechnical Sciences, St. Kliment Ohridski University in Bitola, Partizanska bb, 7000 Bitola, Republic of Macedonia

Vasil Kostov
Fishery Department, Institute of Animal Science, Ss. Cyril and Methodius University in Skopje, Bul. Ilinden 92-a, 1000 Skopje, Republic of Macedonia

Judita Zymantiene, Rasa Zelvyte, Vaidas Oberauskas and Ugne Spancerniene
Department of Anatomy and Physiology, Veterinary Faculty of Lithuanian University of Health Sciences, Tilzes st. 18, LT 47181 Kaunas, Lithuania

Mojsova Sandra, Jankuloski Dean, Sekulovski Pavle, Angelovski Ljupco,
Ratkova Marija and Prodanov Mirko
Food institute, Faculty of veterinary medicine University of "Ss. Cyril and Methodius" in Skopje

Valentina Urumova, Mihni Lyutzkano and Vladimir Petrov
Department of Veterinary Microbiology, Infectious and Parasitic Diseases Faculty of Veterinary Medicine, Trakia University, 6000 Stara Zagora, Bulgaria

Romel Velev
Department of Pharmacology and Toxicology, Faculty of Veterinary Medicine - Skopje, "Ss. Cyril and Methodius" University in Skopje, R. Macedonia

Toni Tankoski and Maja Tankoska
Veterinary Practice Toni, Makedonski Prosvetiteli b.b., T.C. Ohrigjanka lok. 1, 6000 Ohrid, R. Macedonia

Irena Celeska and Igor Ulchar
Department of Pathophisiology, Faculty of Veterinary Medicine-Skopje, Ss. Cyril and Methodius University in Skopje

Aleksandar Janevski and Igor Dzadzovski
Department of Farm Animal Health, Faculty of Veterinary Medicine-Skopje, University Ss. Cyril and Methodius University in Skopje

Danijela Kirovski
Department of Physiology and Biochemistry, Faculty of Veterinary Medicine, University of Belgrade

Sohee Bae, Jina Kim, Li Li, Aeri Lee, Hyunjoo Lim, Junemoe Jeong,
Seung Hoon Lee, Oh-kyeong Kweon and Wan Hee Kim
Department of Veterinary Clinical Sciences, College of Veterinary Medicine and Research Institute for Veterinary Science, Seoul National University, 1 Gwanak-ro, Gwanak-gu, Seoul 151-742, Republic of Korea

Ivan Pavlović and Snežana Ivanović
Scientific Veterinary Institute of Serbia, V. Toze 14, 11000 Belgrade, Serbia

Aleksandar Dimitrić
Agrimatco DOO, Narodnog Fronta 73/I, 21000 Novi Sad, Serbia

Mensur Vegara
Department of International Environment and Development Studies Norwegian University of Life Science (NMBU) Campus As, Postboks 5003, No-1432 Aas, Norway

Ana Vasić
Faculty of Veterinary Medicine, Belgrade University, Bul.Oslobođenja 18, 11000 Belgrade, Serbia

Slavica Živković and Bojana Mijatović
Agricultural School PKB, Pančevački Put 39, 11000 Krnjača-Belgrade, Serbia

Ljupche Kochoski
Faculty of Biotechnical Sciences Bitola, University "St. Kliment Ohridski" – Bitola, Partizanska bb, 7000 Bitola, Macedonia

Zoran Filipov, Ilcho Joshevski, Stevche Ilievski and Filip Davkov
ZK Pelagonija Bitola, Boris Kidrik 3, 7000 Bitola, Macedonia

Shanis Barnard, Matteo Chincarini, Stefano Messori and Nicola Ferri
Istituto Zooprofilattico Sperimentale dell'Abruzzo e del Molise 'G. Caporale', Campo Boario, 64100 Teramo, Italy

Lucio Di Tommaso and Fabrizio Di Giulio
Servizio Sanità Animale Dipartimento di Prevenzione della ASL di Pescara, Via Paolini 47 65100 Pescara, Italy

Roman Pepovich
Department of Infectious Pathology & Hygiene, Technology and Control of Food of Animal Origin, Faculty of Veterinary Medicine, University of Forestry, Sofia, Bulgaria

Branimir Nikolov and Kalin Hristov
Department of Obstetrics, Gynecology, Biotechnology of Reproduction & Pathological Anatomy and Biochemistry, Faculty of Veterinary Medicine, University of Forestry, Sofia, Bulgaria

Ivo Sirakov and Elena Nikolova
Department of Virology and Viral Diseases, National Diagnostic and Research Veterinary Institute, Sofia, Bulgaria

Krasimira Genova
Department of Animal Breeding Science, Faculty of Veterinary Medicine, University of Forestry, Sofia, Bulgaria

Radka Hajiolova and Boika Beltova
Department of Pathophysiology, Faculty of Medicine, Medical University, Sofia, Bulgaria

Oliver Stevanović
PI Veterinary Institute of Republic Srpska „Dr. Vaso Butozan" Branka Radičevića 18, 78000 Banja Luka, Bosnia and Herzegovina

Maciej Janeczek and Aleksander Chrószcz
Department of Biostructure and Animal Physiology, Department of Veterinary Medicine Wroclaw University of Environmental and Life Sciences, Kożuchowska 1/3 51-531, Poland

Nemanja Marković
Institute of Archaeology, Kneza Mihaila 35/IV, 11000, Belgrade, Serbia

Oluyinka O. Okubanjo and Ologunja J. Ajanusi
Department of Veterinary Parasitology and Entomology, Faculty of Veterinary Medicine, Ahmadu Bello University, Zaria-Nigeria

Victor O. Sekoni
Department of Veterinary Public Health and Reproduction, College of Veterinary Medicine, Federal University of Agriculture, Abeokuta-Nigeria

Adewale A. Adeyeye
Department of Theriogenology and Animal Production, Faculty of Veterinary Medicine, Usmanu Danfodiyo University, Sokoto-Nigeria

Ahmed Tunio, Shamasuddin Bughio, Jam Kashif Sahito and Muhammad Ghiasuddin Shah
Faculty of Animal Husbandry and Veterinary Sciences, Sindh Agriculture University, Tandojam 70060, Pakistan

Mahdi Ebrahimi
Faculty of Veterinary Medicine, Universiti Putra Malaysia

Shazia Parveen Tunio
Social Science Research Institute, Tandojam, Pakistan

Eva Vavrouchova, Stepan Bodecek and Olga Dobesova
University of Veterinary and Pharmaceutical Sciences, Faculty of Veterinary Medicine, Equine Clinic, Brno, Czech Republic

Sandra Mojsova and Pavle Sekulovski
1Food Institute, Faculty of Veterinary Medicine-Skopje, Ss. Cyril and Methodius University in Skopje, Republic of Macedonia

Kiril Krstevski, Igor Dzadzovski and Zagorka Popova
2Veterinary Institute, Faculty of Veterinary Medicine-Skopje, Ss. Cyril and Methodius University in Skopje, Republic of Macedonia

Index

Printed in the USA
CPSIA information can be obtained
at www.ICGtesting.com
JSHW051326221024
72173JS00006B/1296